SECOND EDITION

HAND
REHABILITATION

A PRACTICAL GUIDE

Library of Congress Cataloging-in-Publication Data

A catalog record for this book is available from the Library of Congress

ISBN 0-443-07642-1

Distributed in the United Kingdom by Churchill Livingstone, Robert Stevenson House, 1–3 Baxter's Place, Leith Walk, Edinburgh EH1 3AF, and by associated companies, branches, and representatives throughout the world.

Medical knowledge is constantly changing. As new information becomes available, changes in treatment, procedures, equipment and the use of drugs become necessary. The editors/authors/contributors and the publishers have, as far as it is possible, taken care to ensure that the information given in this text is accurate and up to date. However, readers are strongly advised to confirm that the information, especially with regard to drug usage, complies with the latest legislation and standards of practice.

The Publishers have made every effort to trace the copyright holders for borrowed material. If they have inadvertently overlooked any, they will be pleased to make the necessary arrangements at the first opportunity.

Acquisitions Editor: *Carol Bader*
Production Supervisor: *Laura Mosberg Cohen*
Desktop Coorinator: *Kathy Jo Dunayer*
Cover Design: *Jeannette Jacobs*

Printed in the United States of America

Last digit is the print number: 9   8   7   6   5   4

We dedicate this book
to the founders of
The Union Memorial Hospital's
Raymond M. Curtis Hand Center:
Raymond M. Curtis, M.D.
E.F. Shaw Wilgis, M.D.
Gaylord L. Clark, M.D.
Frederik C. Hansen, Jr., M.D.
Rodney W. Schlegel, P.T., E.C.S.,
and
Janice Maynard, O.T.R.,
and to all of the hand
and upper extremity patients
past, present, and future.

Contributors

Bonnie Aiello, B.S., P.T., C.H.T.
Clinical Specialist, Raymond M. Curtis Hand Center, The Union Memorial Hospital, Baltimore, Maryland

Mallory S. Anthony, R.P.T., M.M.Sc., C.H.T.
Senior Hand Therapist, Raymond M. Curtis Hand Center, The Union Memorial Hospital, Baltimore, Maryland

Arlynne Pack Brown, P.T., C.H.T.
Formerly Raymond M. Curtis Hand Center, The Union Memorial Hospital, Baltimore, Maryland

Gaylord L. Clark, M.D.
Assistant Professor, Department of Orthopedic Surgery, Johns Hopkins University School of Medicine; Attending Hand Surgeon, Raymond M. Curtis Hand Center, The Union Memorial Hospital, Baltimore, Maryland

Frank DiGiovannantonio, O.T.R./L.
Formerly Raymond M. Curtis Hand Center, The Union Memorial Hospital, Baltimore, Maryland

Dale Eckhaus, O.T.R./L., C.H.T.
Senior Hand Therapist, Raymond M. Curtis Hand Center, The Union Memorial Hospital, Baltimore, Maryland

Lauren Valdata Eddington, R.P.T., C.H.T.
Senior Hand Therapist, Raymond M. Curtis Hand Center, The Union Memorial Hospital, Baltimore, Maryland

Anne Edmonds, P.T., C.H.T.
Senior Hand Therapist, Raymond M. Curtis Hand Center, The Union Memorial Hospital, Baltimore, Maryland

Gregory Hritcko, M.S., O.T.R./L., C.H.T.
Southern Tier Hand Therapy, Vestal, New York; Formerly Raymond M.Curtis Hand Center, The Union Memorial Hospital, Baltimore, Maryland

Donna M. Keegan, M.Ed., C.V.E., C.R.C.
Program Coordinator, Raymond M. Curtis Hand Center, The Union Memorial Hospital, Baltimore, Maryland

Beth Farrell Kozera, O.T.R./L., C.H.T.
Formerly Raymond M. Curtis Hand Center, The Union Memorial Hospital, Baltimore, Maryland

Paige E. Kurtz, M.S., O.T.R./L.
Senior Hand Therapist, Raymond M. Curtis Hand Center, The Union Memorial Hospital, Baltimore, Maryland

Sharon Leilich, M.P.T.

Formerly Raymond M. Curtis Hand Center, The Union Memorial Hospital, Baltimore, Maryland

Ann Leman-Domenici, M.S.W., L.C.S.W.-C.

Senior Social Worker, Department of Social Work, Raymond M. Curtis Hand Center, The Union Memorial Hospital, Baltimore, Maryland

Lynne F. Murphy, M.S., O.T.R./L.

Formerly Raymond M. Curtis Hand Center, The Union Memorial Hospital, Baltimore, Maryland

Mary Schuler Murphy, O.T.R./L., C.H.T.

Clinical Specialist, Raymond M. Curtis Hand Center, The Union Memorial Hospital, Baltimore, Maryland

Rebecca J. Saunders, P.T., C.H.T.

Senior Hand Therapist, Raymond M. Curtis Hand Center, The Union Memorial Hospital, Baltimore, Maryland

Jane Imle Schmidt, P.T., C.H.T.

Clinical Coordinator, Central Maryland Rehabilitation Center, Columbia, Maryland; Formerly Raymond M. Curtis Hand Center, The Union Memorial Hospital, Baltimore, Maryland

Barbara Steinberg, O.T.R./L., C.H.T.

Senior Hand Therapist, Raymond M. Curtis Hand Center, The Union Memorial Hospital, Baltimore, Maryland

Jennifer Stephens, M.S., P.T.

Hand Therapy of Oakland, Oakland, California; Formerly Raymond M. Curtis Hand Center, The Union Memorial Hospital, Baltimore, Maryland

Lorie Theisen, O.T.R./L., C.H.T.

Clinical Specialist, Raymond M. Curtis Hand Center, The Union Memorial Hospital, Baltimore, Maryland

Linda Coll Ware, O.T.R./L., C.H.T.

Clinical Specialist, Raymond M. Curtis Hand Center, The Union Memorial Hospital, Baltimore, Maryland

E.F. Shaw Wilgis, M.D.

Associate Professor, Departments of Orthopedic Surgery and Plastic Surgery, Johns Hopkins University School of Medicine; Chief, Division of Hand Surgery, and Director, Raymond M. Curtis Hand Center, The Union Memorial Hospital, Baltimore, Maryland

Neal B. Zimmerman, M.D.

Instructor, Department of Orthopedic Surgery, Johns Hopkins University School of Medicine, Attending Hand Surgeon, Raymond M. Curtis Hand Center, The Union Memorial Hospital, Baltimore, Maryland

Foreword to the Second Edition

As many of us began in hand therapy some twenty years ago we were idealistic, eager to learn, honored to work beside skilled hand surgeons, and fortunate to develop professional friendships with colleagues across the United States and throughout the world. At that time, our common thread was an unquenchable thirst for knowledge. Very little was published on hand rehabilitation, and the hand surgery literature was limited. Our common goal was to ensure the highest quality of care and functional outcome for each and every patient. This standard of care and demand for excellence was exemplified by hand surgeons and hand therapists alike. Both professionals recognized they would be successful in their quest for knowledge if they worked closely together and shared their experiences. Twenty years later, as the professions have worked closely together, there are a large number of publications that now serve as valuable references, adding greatly to our knowledge base of the upper extremity.

The second edition of *Hand Rehabilitation: A Practical Guide* exemplifies one of the outstanding works in the literature contributing to our depth and breadth of knowledge in this area of medicine. The senior editors, Gaylord Clark, M.D., E.F. Shaw Wilgis, M.D., Bonnie Aiello, P.T., C.H.T., Dale Eckhaus, O.T.R./L., C.H.T., and Lauren Valdata Eddington, R.P.T., C.H.T., have selected complex areas of the upper extremity and have shared with us their seasoned clinical expertise, which has been acquired through many years of direct patient care. Rarely do you find a written work reflective of such clinical expertise, but these authors have done so in a precise and succinct manner.

The written work itself is a blending of occupational therapy, physical therapy, and hand surgery technical and clinical skills and knowledge. Medical conditions and surgical procedures are explained, along with the purpose and rationale for the surgeries. Both conservative management and postsurgical rehabilitation are reviewed and potential postoperative complications are addressed. Throughout the book, numerous pictures of custom-made splints are shown as well as many excellent illustrations.

References and/or suggested readings serve to complete each chapter. In the second edition, six additional chapters have been added to expand the scope of upper extremity medical conditions and procedures.

Two of the editors of this publication, Drs. Clark and Wilgis, along with Raymond Curtis, MD, established the Raymond Curtis Hand Center, Union Memorial Hospital in Baltimore, Maryland, in 1975. The center is considered one of the most well-known and highly regarded in the country with a leading industrial rehabilitation program. The philosophy of the center is to provide a team approach to medical care for upper extremity medical conditions. *Hand Rehabilitation: A Practical Guide* is reflective of their philosophy and the authors' ongoing commitment to the highest quality of care. Interestingly, and refreshingly evident, I might add, is that the authors have carefully crafted their standards for patient care and team approach in this written work.

In today's health care world it has become increasingly difficult to maintain continuity of care for patients due to managed health care plans restricting providers and/or denying the physician's referral to therapy. We can all be indebted to the authors for creating a written work that reflects the tremendous value the surgeon-therapist relationship and team approach to patient care add to positively impacting the patient's final outcome. Hand rehabilitation and hand surgery are both fortunate to have this immensely valuable contribution in the literature.

Nancy M. Cannon, O.T.R., C.H.T.
Director
The Hand Rehabilitation Center of Indiana
Indianapolis, Indiana

Foreword to the First Edition

The impetus for my becoming a hand surgeon started with Raymond M. Curtis twenty years ago during my residency at Johns Hopkins Hospital. Dr. Curtis, one of the pioneers in hand surgery, emphasized meticulous preoperative planning, precise surgical technique, and the importance of hand rehabilitation. Before the advent of hand therapy as a specific discipline, he spent many hours performing therapy on his own patients, both preoperatively and postoperatively. Through his vision, The Union Memorial Hospital created the Hand Center, one of the first hand rehabilitation centers in the world, with a staff of outstanding surgeons dedicated to surgery of the hand.

After Dr. Curtis retired, the Hand Center continued to grow and develop under the direction of Drs. Shaw Wilgis and Gaylord Clark. Today, the Raymond M. Curtis Hand Center is recognized worldwide as a center of innovation and excellence in the rehabilitation of hand disorders. Among its accomplishments are the work evaluation protocols and the BTE work simulator that were developed there.

It is an honor for me to write the foreword for this text, *Hand Rehabilitation: A Practical Guide,* for it is Drs. Curtis, Wilgis, and Clark who were my mentors. Learning the indications for and how to perform hand surgery is, however, only one-half of the equation. Hand therapy preoperatively and postoperatively is the most critical factor in achieving the best possible results for our patients. It is through Bonnie Aiello, Dale Eckhaus, and Lauren Valdata Eddington that I learned these principles.

Based on over twenty years of experience, the authors have written a practical guide to hand rehabilitation to commonly seen disorders. The 43 individual chapters start with basic principles of wound management, sensory evaluation, desensitization, and sensory re-education. Each chapter is organized alike, with an introduction, treatment purposes, goals, and indications and techniques for nonoperative and postoperative therapy. Each chapter provides for each topic a list of possible complications to alert the therapist, followed by an evaluation timetable to measure the patient's progress. Each chapter concludes with a current bibliography and suggested readings. The staff at The Union Memorial Hospital has performed a great service to the field of hand surgery by providing therapists, surgeons, and hand fellows with practical and useful guidelines we can all use in pursuing our goal of achieving the best possible functional results for our patients with disorders of the hand and upper extremity.

Andrew J. Weiland, M.D.
Surgeon in Chief
The Hospital for Special Surgery
Professor
Divisions of Orthopaedics and Plastic Surgery
Department of Surgery
Cornell University Medical College
New York, New York

Preface

Hand Rehabilitation: A Practical Guide began as a small-scale project and grew into a department-wide endeavor involving the hand therapists and hand surgeons at the Raymond M. Curtis Hand Center. It originated from our own need to organize the vast amount of valuable information we have gathered from being part of such a unique setting. Our purpose was to create a valuable teaching tool for new graduates, hand fellows, hand therapists, and surgeons that would relate therapeutic approaches to various diagnoses.

The book is designed to provide guidelines and a stimulus for therapists to analyze diagnoses of hand and upper extremity patients. We do not want this book to be viewed as a "protocol" to treat, or a "cookbook" for the non-professional to "follow directions." It is to be an adjunct of one's knowledge, a guideline for different treatment methods, and a resource for information. The information provided and the format it is presented in can be used in a number of treatment settings. The book is an educational tool to be used in combination with the knowledge and training of the professional.

Our first edition has been available since 1993, and we now present our second edition. Our revised publication is more comprehensive than our original. We hope our goal of providing a resource for quality care of hand and upper extremity patients is achieved.

The Editors and Authors

Acknowledgments

The editors and contributors thank Nancy Frisk Millner for her tireless patience and expert help in preparing our manuscript from our initial drafts to the completed project. Without her assistance, the preparation of this book would have been nearly impossible.

Peter Andrews is thanked for his photographic expertise and his flexibility in working with us.

Dr. Peter Innis, Dr. Michael A. McClinton, Dr. J. Russell Moore, Dr. John O'Donnell, Dr. Anne B. Redfern, and Dr. Neal B. Zimmerman are thanked for their reviews and critiques of the manuscript drafts.

The therapists would like to thank Dr. Gaylord L. Clark for his contribution of surgical procedures to the chapters of this book.

Contents

Wounds 1

Mallory S. Anthony

Those of us involved with the treatment of hand injuries know how detrimental even a small wound can be to hand function. Almost all hand structures are made up of dense connective tissue, and essential to normal hand function is the ability of these strong connective tissue structures to glide in relation to one another. The formation of scar tissue after wounding can significantly impede gliding and thus decrease function. A thorough understanding of wound management throughout all phases of wound healing (i.e., inflammation, fibroplasia, epithelialization, contraction, and scar maturation) is important in developing a comprehensive treatment program.

During the initial phases of wound healing, we must concentrate on the preservation of function by preventing edema and subsequent fibrosis, as well as maintaining gliding surfaces. We must facilitate wound closure based on our knowledge of wound healing and effective dressing techniques.

During the final phases of wound healing, the scar maturation phase, our role is to apply controlled stress to the scar, thereby increasing gliding potential and allowing the most functional outcome.

The following guideline suggests evaluation and wound care techniques that should help the clinician expedite wound closure, minimize scar formation, and achieve optimum functional results.

DEFINITION

A disruption of the anatomic or functional continuity of tissue

I. Wound classification[1]
  A. Tidy wound: clean laceration, minimal tissue damage, minimal contamination (Fig. 1-1A).

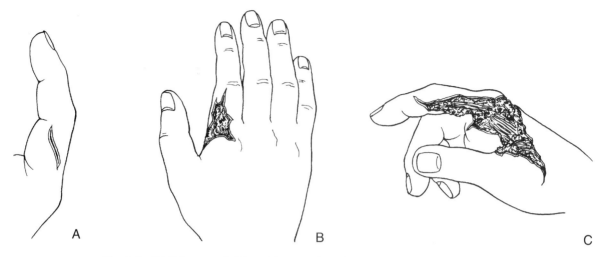

Fig. 1-1. **(A)** Tidy wound, **(B)** untidy wound, and **(C)** wound with tissue loss.

B. Untidy wound: significant amount of tissue damage (e.g., crush injury), uncertainty regarding viability of deeper structures, may have higher degree of contamination (Fig. 1-1B).

C. Wound with tissue loss: deeper vital structures may be involved (vessels, tendon, nerve, bone); may require soft tissue coverage (Fig. 1-1C).

   1. Split-thickness skin grafts (STSG) (epidermis and part of dermis) or full-thickness (FTSG) (epidermis and entire underlying dermis): replace skin in areas where adequate subcutaneous tissues remain to protect underlying parts and vascularize the graft.

   2. Flap coverage is necessary when the wound bed has exposed vital structures or when the bed has either a poor chance or no chance of providing vascularization for a graft.

D. Infected wound: presently or potentially infected.

SURGICAL PURPOSE

To achieve complete healing of soft tissue, to minimize scar formation, and to allow for the maximum function of the underlying anatomic components (e.g., tendon, nerve, blood vessels, bone, etc.).

TREATMENT GOAL

   I. Promote wound closure as quickly as possible with minimal scar formation.

  II. Restore active range of motion (AROM) and passive range of motion (PROM) in involved area, through scar management, splinting, stretching, and range of motion (ROM) exercises.

III. Maintain full ROM of all uninvolved joints of the upper extremity.
IV. Increase strength and promote return of upper extremity function to optimum level.

INDICATIONS/PRECAUTIONS FOR THERAPY

I. Indications
   A. Primary closure: immediate wound closure, for example, tidy wound (sutures, grafts).
   B. Delayed primary closure: wound left open following injury because the degree of bacterial contamination or the extent of vascular impairment is in doubt (usually left open 4 to 5 days, then closed with minimal risk of infection); for example, untidy wounds.
   C. Secondary intention: wound closes through natural biologic processes of epithelialization, inflammation, fibroplasia, scar maturation, and contraction. Commonly used for heavily contaminated wounds and for extensive superficial wounds with tissue loss.
II. Precautions
   A. Infection
   B. Damage to deep vital structures
   C. Extreme pain
   D. Severe edema

THERAPY

I. Pretreatment evaluation
   A. Wound history
      1. Mechanism, force, duration of injury
      2. Time interval between injury and onset of treatment: acute versus chronic
   B. Patient history
      1. Age
      2. Occupation and avocational interests
      3. Alcohol, tobacco, or caffeine use
      4. Metabolic status: underlying disease affecting circulation (e.g., diabetes, vascular disorders)
      5. Nutritional status
      6. Medications (i.e., steroids, anticoagulants)
   C. Subjective evaluation
      1. Pain (location, description, frequency, what relieves pain, etc.); pain scale rating
      2. Presence of paresthesias
      3. Sensory loss (i.e., threshold and discrimination testing) (see Ch. 7, Sensory Evaluation)
   D. Objective wound evaluation
      1. General inspection of upper extremity

    a. Edema
       i. Description: pitting, brawny, hard, or mobile
      ii. Objective measurement: circumferential measurements or volumetrics
    b. Color
    c. Temperature
2. Location of wound
    a. Anatomic landmarks
3. Wound type
    a. Tidy
    b. Untidy
    c. Wound with tissue loss
    d. Wound with exposed vital structures
    e. Infected wound
4. Type of closure
    a. Primary closure
    b. Delayed primary closure
    c. Secondary intention
    d. Closure: sutures, staples, Steri-strips, graft, or flap
    e. Fixation: K-wire, pull-out wire, external fixator
5. Configuration
    a. Size
    b. Shape
    c. Depth (can use sterile cotton-tipped applicator)
6. Inflammatory response
    a. Normal (5 to 7 days, up to 2 weeks)
    b. Prolonged or abnormal (2 to 4 weeks or longer)
       i. Infection (edema, redness, warmth, pain)
      ii. Cellulitis (redness and edema extending well beyond wound boundaries)
     iii. Lymphangitis (streaking redness)
     iv. Venous obstruction (cyanotic blue appearance of surrounding skin)
      v. Arterial insufficiency (pallor of surrounding skin)
7. Integrity of tissue[2]
    a. Viability or nonviability of wound edges; note signs of dehiscence
    b. Maceration: moist and white appearance of skin
    c. Hematoma/seroma: collection of blood and/or serum, usually clotted
    d. Bleb: a blood- or serum-filled blister
8. Exudate
    a. Color/consistency: bloody, serous, serosanguinous, pus, purulent, or dark red
    b. Amount: slight, minimal, moderate, severe
    c. Odor: presence or absence of foul odor
9. Wound bed
    a. Color and extent of granulation tissue (red wound[3])
    b. Presence of epithelial budding (small pink islets forming within the wound)

      c. Presence of adherent fibrinous exudate and debris (yellow wound[3])

      d. Presence of dark, thick eschar (black wound[3])

  10. Other measurements/observations

      a. Active and passive ROM measurements (if indicated)

      b. Activities of daily living (ADL)

      c. Psychosocial skills

II. Wound management

  A. Debridement and cleansing to assist in removal of exudate and necrotic tissue, decrease surface contamination, and control wound pathogens.[4]

    1. Whirlpool

      a. Debrides superficial necrotic material.

      b. Recommended temperature is 94°F (34.4°C) to 98°F (36.6°C) (higher temperatures may increase edema).[5]

      c. Degree of agitation and duration depends on viability of tissues and patient comfort.

      d. Also creates sedation and analgesic effect (may aid in decreasing pain).

      e. Additives: at present no meaningful data exist to substantiate the therapeutic benefit of additives. Also, povidone–iodine and sodium hypochlorite, common additives, can be cytotoxic if not diluted properly.[4]

    2. Irrigation

      a. Debrides superficial necrotic material.

      b. Uses sterile water or antiseptic solution in water pik or syringe to flush out wound.

      c. Not a commonly used method.

    3. Debridement

      a. Selective (removes only necrotic material).

         i. Topical application of enzymes (Travase, Elase, Collagenase).

        ii. Manual debridement with surgical instruments. Care must be taken not to disturb delicate granulation tissue and migrating epithelium at wound margins. Debridement should be relatively painless since only nonviable tissue is removed. (Assess patient's sensibility.)

       iii. Autolytic debridement (self-digestion of necrotic tissue by enzymes naturally present in wound fluids); facilitated by synthetic occlusive dressings.[4]

      b. Nonselective debridement (removes both nonviable and viable tissue from the wound; chosen for wounds containing excessive necrotic tissue).

         i. Wet to dry dressings. Be careful not to remove new epithelium and granulation tissue when removing these dressings.

        ii. Whirlpool or irrigation.

       iii. Hydrogen peroxide. Use with care: foaming effervescence may wash away healthy tissue. May be more cytotoxic than bactericidal.[4] Mainly used to help loosen dried exudate or debris. (Should not be used on closed wounds.[4])

  c. Debridement of blisters
   i. Controversial: consult with treating physician.
   ii. Debride blisters if plasma fluid begins to leak or becomes cloudy; or if the blister covers a joint.[6]

B. Dressings
 1. Purpose
  a. Provide physiologic environment for wound
  b. Protect from further trauma and bacterial contamination
  c. Antisepsis
  d. Pressure to help decrease edema
  e. Immobilization
  f. Debridement if needed
 2. Components
  a. Contact layer: dry, adherent, or nonadherent
  b. Intermediate layer: absorptive, protective, and supportive
  c. Outer layer: holds dressing in place
 3. Types
  a. Adherent dressing used when amount of necrotic tissue is greater than viable tissue and debridement is necessary. Necrotic tissue is debrided when the dressings *are removed.*
   i. Wet to dry dressing: saline-soaked sterile gauze placed directly on wound, then covered with dry gauze pads and outer wrap (Fig. 1-2).
   ii. Wet to wet dressing: same as wet to dry, except the dressing is periodically soaked with more saline to keep it moist (Fig. 1-3).
  b. Nonadherent dressing used on tidy wounds (i.e., surgical incision, donor site) and open wounds composed primarily of viable granulation tissue, to minimize tissue disruption (Fig. 1-4).
   i. Vaseline gauze
   ii. Adaptic
   iii. Xeroform
  c. Permeable dressing used for draining wounds: dry dressing with secondary absorbent layer to draw wound secretions away by capillary action (Fig. 1-5).
  d. Occlusive dressing
   i. Provides moist environment and expedites rate of epithelialization, but may create an environment more conducive to maceration and increased bacterial proliferation. Use primarily on clean, noninfected wounds.
   ii. Many types of occlusive, microenvironmental dressings are available, which vary in their degree of permeability. They are categorized as films, foams, hydrocolloids, and hydrogels[7] (Fig. 1-6). They are

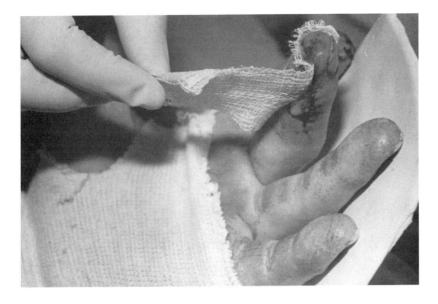

Fig. 1-2. Wet to dry dressing.

especially beneficial for treatment of chronic wounds, when healing is depressed and prolonged, and in treatment of wounds with exposed vital structures, where a moist environment is essential for tissue survival. See references 4 and 7 for more specific information on microenvironmental dressings.

e. Wound packing
   i. Used with large deep wounds with dead space, to keep superficial portions of wound open while deeper layers contract.[7] A fine mesh strip gauze, such as Nu Gauze, is commonly used.
   ii. Avoid tight packing, as it may cause tissue ischemia.

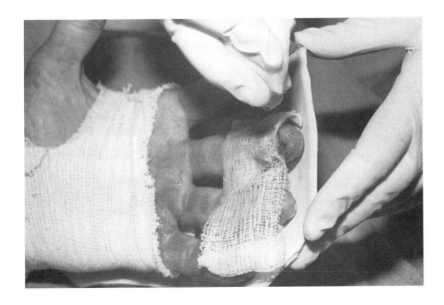

Fig. 1-3. Wet to wet dressing.

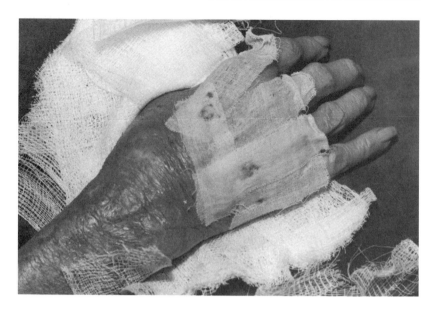

Fig. 1-4. Nonadherent dressing.

C. Topical agents
  1. Mercurochrome (5 percent solution): liquid antibacterial
     agent applied to small open areas to promote drying; usu-
     ally left open.
  2. Silver nitrate (AgNO$_3$): applied with a stick and rolled across
     hypertrophic granulation tissue to cauterize and flatten this
     raised tissue. (Please note this form of AgNO$_3$ should be dis-
     tinguished from the 0.5 antimicrobial solution, frequently
     used for burn wound care.) Table salt may also be used to
     flatten hypertrophic granulation tissue.
  3. Silvadene: antimicrobial agent; bacteriostatic; keeps eschar
     soft and wound from drying.[4,7] Frequently used on burn
     wounds.

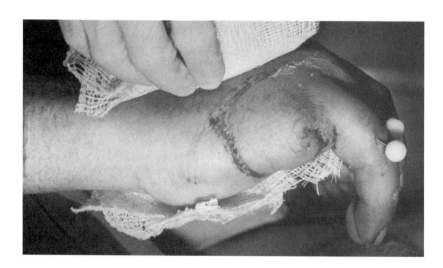

Fig. 1-5. Dry dressing.

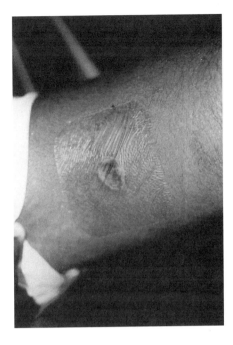

Fig. 1-6. Semipermeable dressing.

    4. Bacitracin and Neosporin: antimicrobial agents; provide moist environment for dry wounds.

    5. Povidone–iodine (Betadine): studies have shown that povidone–iodine is cytotoxic if not diluted properly and offers no advantage over cleansing with saline.[4]

D. Choice of dressing changes as wound status changes

E. If wound is clean and healing well, topical antimicrobial agents are not needed. However, if wound is heavily contaminated and needs to be disinfected, use topical antibiotics (e.g., Silvadene [silver sulfadiazine], Neosporin, bacitracin) as opposed to antiseptics (e.g., povodine–iodine, hydrogen peroxide, boric acid, alcohols, chlorohexidene, merthiolate), which may be cytotoxic.[8]

F. Patients may do daily dressing changes at home, depending on their reliability and the severity of their wound.

III. Early therapeutic intervention

A. Edema control

    1. Effects of edema on wound healing[9]

        a. Decreases arterial, venous, and lymphatic flow.

        b. Increases risk of infection.

        c. Decreases motion, which could lead to permanent tissue shortening and fibrosis.

    2. Therapeutic management of edema

        a. Elevation

        b. ROM exercise (combined with elevation)

        c. Intermittent compression

           i. Fluid flushing massage

          ii. Vasopneumatic devices (e.g., Jobst)

         iii. String wrapping

           d. Continuous compression (consult physician for use over recent arterial repairs)
-       i. Coban wraps
-       ii. Ace wraps
-       iii. Compressive garments (Jobst, tubigrip, Isotoner gloves)
-       iv. Air splints

           e. Thermal agents
-       i. Moist heat in elevated position (after inflammatory phase)
-       ii. Cryotherapy for acute edema (contraindicated over recent arterial repairs)

           f. Microdyne

B. ROM
1. Maintain ROM in uninvolved joints
2. Prevent remodeling of scar in shortened position

C. Splinting
1. Early protective splinting
   - a. Avoid undue stress to wound and healing structures.
   - b. Decrease development of shortened remodeled scar.

D. Pain management

IV. Late therapeutic intervention

A. Scar assessment[2]
1. Location—note involvement of joints or tendons.
2. Type—note hypertrophic, keloid, or widespread scars.
3. Texture—note if scars are immature (thick, rigid, and raised), mature (flattened and softened), or if fibrous bands (frequently seen in burn wounds) are present.
4. Size: length and height can be measured with a ruler.
5. Vascularity: immature scars are red-purplish, raised, and blanch to touch. Mature scars are more skin tone and no longer blanch.
6. Sensibility: some scars are hypersensitive, while others totally lack sensation.
7. Pigmentation: hyperpigmentation or loss of pigmentation should be noted.

B. Scar management
1. Pharmacologic
   - a. Colchicine, β-aminoproprionitrile (BAPN); clinical application limited at present.
2. Mechanical
   - a. Surgical excision
   - b. Skin grafting
   - c. Therapeutic application of stress (to realign collagen fibers in a more orderly and parallel configuration; application of pressure to theoretically decrease vascularity and oxygen, thereby retarding collagen synthesis).[10]
     - i. Compressive techniques
       - A. Pressure garments (Fig. 1-7)
       - B. Silastic molds and gel sheets (Fig. 1-8)

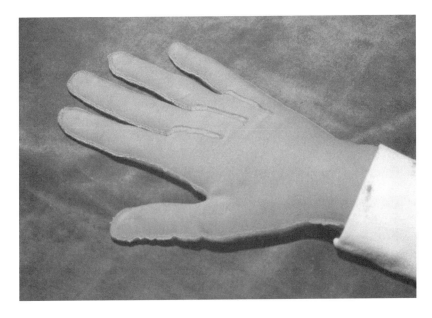

Fig. 1-7. Compressive garment.

      ii. Splinting. (Requires low-load, long duration application of stress for permanent elongation of scar.)
     iii. AROM and PROM exercise
     iv. Deep friction massage
      v. Mechanical vibration
   d. Thermal agents to increase tissue extensibility before stretching and ROM exercise.
      i. Superficial heat (paraffin, hot packs, fluidotherapy)
     ii. Deep heat (ultrasound)
3. Functional
   a. Exercises and activities to increase strength, endurance, and function in the injured extremity

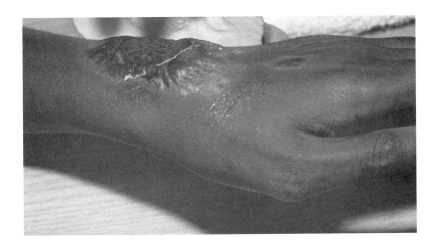

Fig. 1-8. Elastomer mold.

COMPLICATIONS

    I. Infections
   II. Wound dehiscence
  III. Abnormal scar formation
      A. Hypertrophic
      B. Keloid

EVALUATION TIMELINE

Wound status and type of dressing should be assessed at every treatment, during initial and discharge evaluations, and each time a progress evaluation is indicated for that patient, up until the wound is healed. After wound closure, description of scar and resulting limitations of motion, strength, and function should be noted.

REFERENCES

1. Noe JM: Wound Care. 2nd Ed. Chesebrough-Pond's Inc., Greenwich, 1985
2. Baldwin JE, Weber LJ, Simon CLS: Clinical Assessment Recommendations. p. 21. 2nd Ed. American Society of Hand Therapists, Chicago, IL, 1992
3. Cozzell J: The new red, yellow, black color code. Am J Nurs 10:1014, 1989
4. Feedar JA, Kloth LC: Conservative management of chronic wounds, p. 135. In Kloth LC, McCulloch JM, Feedar JA (eds): Wound Healing: Alternative in Management. FA Davis, Philadelphia, 1990
5. Mullins PT: Use of therapeutic modalities in upper extremity rehabilitation. p. 1495. In Hunter JM, Mackin EJ, Callahan AD (eds): Rehabilitation of the Hand: Surgery and Therapy. 4th Ed. Mosby, St Louis, 1995
6. Howell JW: Management of the acutely burned hand for the non-specialized clinician. J Phys Ther 69:1077, 1989
7. Evans RB, McAuliffe JA: Wound classification and management. p. 217. In Hunter JM, Mackin EJ, Callahan AD (eds): Rehabilitation of the Hand: Surgery and Therapy. 4th Ed. Mosby, St Louis, 1995
8. Evans RB: An update on wound management. Hand Clin 7:409, 1991
9. Walsh M, Muntzer E: Wound management. p. 153. In Stanley BG, Tribuzi SM (eds): Concepts in Hand Rehabilitation. FA Davis, Philadelphia, 1992
10. Hardy MA: The biology of scar formation. Phys Ther 69:1014, 1989

SUGGESTED READINGS

Alvarez O, Rozint J, Wiseman D: Moist environment for healing: matching the dressing to the wound. Wounds 1:35, 1989
Arem AJ, Madden JW: Effects of stress on healing wounds: I. intermittent non-cyclical tension. J Surg Res 20:93, 1976
Ahn ST, Monafo WW, Mustoe TA: Topical silicone gel: a new treatment for hypertrophic scars. Surgery 106:781, 1989
Brennan SS, Foster ME, Leaper DJ: Antiseptic toxicity in wounds healing by secondary intention. J Hosp Infect 8:263, 1986

Bruster J, Pullium G: Gradient pressure. Am J Occup Ther 37:485, 1983

Bryant W: Clinical Symposia: Wound healing. CIBA Pharmaceutical Co, Summit, 1977

Burkhalter WE: Wound classification and management. p. 167. In Hunter JM, Schneider LH, Mackin EJ, Callahan AD (eds): Rehabilitation of the Hand: Surgery and Therapy. 3rd Ed. Mosby, St. Louis, 1990

Carrico T, Merhof A, Cohen I: Biology of wound healing. Surg Clin North Am 64:721, 1984

Clark JA, Cheng JC, Leung KS, Leung PC: Mechanical characterization of human postburn hypertrophic skin during pressure therapy. J Biomech 20:397, 1987

Cohen K: Can collagen metabolism be controlled: theoretical considerations. J Trauma 25:410, 1985

Cohn GH: Hyperbaric oxygen therapy: promoting healing in difficult cases. Postgrad Med Oxygen Ther 79:89, 1986

Davies D: Scars, hypertrophic scars, and keloids. Br Med J Clin Res 290:1056, 1985

Donnell M: Pros and cons of wound care techniques for the upper extremity. Practice forum. J Hand Ther 3:128, 1991

Dow Corning Wright Monograph: Silastic gel sheeting. Arlington, TN, 1989

Groves AR: The problem with scars. Burns 13:S15, 1987

Henning JP, Roskam Y, Van Gemert MJ: Treatment of keloids and hypertrophic scars with an argon laser. Lasers Surg Med 6:72, 1986

Hunt TK (ed): Wound Healing and Wound Infection: Theory and Surgical Practice. Appleton-Century-Crofts, East Norwalk, CT, 1980

Hunt TK, Dunphy J: Fundamentals of Wound Management. Appleton-Century-Crofts, East Norwalk, CT, 1979

Hunt TK, Hussain Z: Wound microenvironment. p. 274. In Cohen IK, Diegelman RF, Lindblad WJ (eds): Wound Healing: Biochemical and Clinical Aspects. WB Saunders, Philadelphia, 1992

Hunt TK, Lavan FB: Enhancement of wound healing by growth factors. N Engl J Med 321:111, 1989

Jensen LL, Parshley PF: Postburn scar contractures: histology and effects of pressure treatment. J Burn Care Rehabil 5:119, 1984

Johnson CL: Physical therapists as scar modifiers. Phys Ther 64:1381, 1984

Johnson CL: Wound healing and scar formation. Top Acute Care Trauma Rehabil 1:1, 1987

Kanzler MH, Gorsulowsky DC, Swanson NA: Basic mechanisms in the healing cutaneous wound. J Dermatol Surg Oncol 12:1156, 1986

Katz BE: Silastic gel sheeting is found to be effective in scar therapy. Cosmetic Dermatol 1992

Kloth LC, Feedar JA: Acceleration of wound healing with high voltage, monophasic, pulsed current. Phys Ther 68:503, 1988

Kloth LC, McCulloch JM, Feedar JA: Wound Healing: Alternatives in Management. FA Davis, Philadelphia, 1990

Lawrence JC: The aetiology of scars. Burns 13:S3, 1987

Linares HA, Kischer CA, Dobrkovsky M, Larson DL: On the origin of the hypertrophic scar. J Trauma 13:70, 1973

Madden JW: Wound healing: the biological basis of hand surgery. p. 181. In Hunter JM, Schneider LH, Mackin EJ, Callahan AD (eds): Rehabilitation of the Hand: Surgery and Therapy. 3rd Ed. Mosby, St. Louis, 1990

Malick MH, Carr JA: Flexible elastomer molds in burn scar control. Am J Occup Ther 34:603, 1980

Martin GR, Peacock EE: Current perspectives in wound healing. In Cohen IK, Diegleman RF, Lindblad WJ (eds): Wound Healing: Biochemical and Clinical Aspects. WB Saunders, Philadelphia, 1992

McAuliffe JA, Seltzer DG: HIV disease: basic science and treatment implications. p. 261. In Hunter JM, Mackin EJ, Callahan AD (eds): Rehabilitation of the Hand: Surgery and Therapy. 4th Ed. Mosby, St. Louis, 1995

Michlovitz SL: Thermal Agents in Rehabilitation. 2nd Ed. FA Davis, Philadelphia, 1990

Nathan R, Taras JS: Common infections in the hand. p. 251. In Hunter JM, Mackin EJ, Callahan AD (eds): Rehabilitation of the Hand: Surgery and Therapy. 4th Ed. Mosby, St. Louis, 1995

Nicolai JP, Bronkhorst FB, Smale CE: A protocol for the treatment of hypertrophic scars and keloids. Aesthetic Plast Surg 11:29, 1987

Noe JM: Dressing the acutely injured hand. p. 241. In Wolfort FG (ed): Acute Hand Injuries: A Multispecialty Approach. Little, Brown, Boston, 1980

Noe JM, Keller M: Can stitches get wet? Plast Reconstr Surg 81:82, 1988

Peacock EE: Wound Repair. 3rd Ed. WB Saunders, Philadelphia, 1984

Peacock EE, Madden JW, Trier WC: Biologic basis for the treatment of keloids and hypertrophic scars. South Med J 63:755, 1970

Perkins K, Davey RB, Wallis K: Current materials and techniques used in a burn scar management programme. Burns 13:406, 1987

Pollack SV: Wound healing: a review. J Dermatol Surg Oncol 5:389, 1979

Quinn KJ: Silicone gel in scar treatment. Burns 13:S33, 1987

Quinn KJ, Evans JH, Courtney JM et al: Non-pressure treatment of hypertrophic scars. Burns 12:102, 1985

Reid W: Hypertrophic scarring and pressure therapy. Burns 13:S29, 1987

Rodeheaver G, Bellamy W, Kody M et al: Bactericidal activity and toxicity of iodine-containing solutions in wounds. Arch Surg 117:181, 1982

Rose MP, Deitch EA: The clinical use of a tubular compression bandage, Tubigrip, for burn-scar therapy: a critical analysis. Burns 12:58, 1985

Ross R: Wound healing. Sci Am 220:40, 1969

Rudolph R: Wide spread scars, hypertrophic scars, and keloids. Clin Plast Surg 14:253, 1987

Smith KL: Wound care for the hand patient. p. 172. In Hunter JM, Schneider LH, Mackin EJ, Callahan AD (eds): Rehabilitation of the Hand: Surgery and Therapy. 3rd Ed. Mosby, St Louis, 1990

Smith KL: Wound care for the hand patient. p. 232. In Hunter JM, Mackin EJ, Callahan AD (eds): Rehabilitation of the Hand: Surgery and Therapy. 4th Ed. Mosby, St. Louis, 1995

Surveyer JA, Cloughtery DM: Burn scars: fighting the effects. Am J Nurs 83:746, 1983

Ware LC, Anthony MS: Burns and open wounds of the hand. pp. 1–18. In: Home Study Course 95-2. Topic: The Wrist and Hand. Orthopaedic Section, APTA, Inc, 1995

Weeks P, Wray C: Hand Management: A Biological Approach. Mosby, St. Louis, 1973

Wessling N, Ehleben CM, Chapman V et al: Evidence that use of a silicone gel sheet increases range of motion over burn wound contractures. J Burn Care Rehabil 6:503, 1985

Westaby S (ed): Wound Care. Mosby, St Louis, 1986

Wheeland RG: The newer surgical dressings and wound healing, Dermatol Clin 5:393, 1987

Wiseman DM et al: Wound dressings: design and use. p. 562. In Cohen IK, Diegelman RF, Lindblad WJ (eds): Wound Healing: Biochemical and Clinical Aspects. WB Saunders, Philadelphia, 1992

Appendix 1-1

Wound Healing Phase Timetable

I. Epithelialization (begins within a few hours after wounding)
   A. Regeneration of epithelial layer through four stages: mobilization, migration, proliferation, and differentiation of epithelial cells.
   B. Covers exposed dermis.
   C. May be complete in 6 to 48 hours after suturing (longer in wound healing by secondary intention).

II. Inflammatory (substrate or lag phase: from wounding to 3 to 5 days)
   A. Vascular response (5 to 10 minutes of vasoconstriction followed by vasodilation)
   B. Phagocytosis (neutrophils and macrophages rid wound of bacteria and foreign debris)

III. Fibroplasia (latent phase: days 4 to 5 to days 14 to 28)
   A. Fibroblasts enter wound and begin synthesizing collagen (scar tissue).
   B. Tensile strength increases with deposition of collagen.
   C. Angiogenesis (neovascularization): capillary budding begins, to form new blood vessels.
   D. Formation of granulation tissue (new collagen and new capillaries, red in appearance).

IV. Scar maturation or remodeling (days 14 to 28 up to several years)
   A. Strength increases through gradual intramolecular and intermolecular cross linking of collagen molecules.
   B. Changes occur in form, bulk, and architecture of collagen (i.e., ongoing collagen synthesis versus lysis cycle; more organized orientation of collagen fibers with applied stress).
   C. Appearance of scar will change from red and raised to a more pale and flat as maturation occurs.

V. Contraction (days 4 to 5 up to day 21)
   A. Movement of wound margins toward center of wound defect.
   B. Myofibroblasts (a modified fibroblast) thought to be responsible for wound contraction.

Appendix 1-2

Wound Healing Process

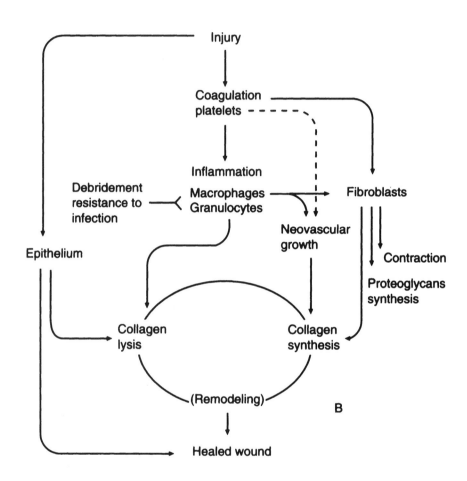

(From Levenson S, Seifter E, Van Winkle W: Nutrition. p. 286. In Hunt TK, Dunphy J (eds): Fundamentals of Wound Management. Appleton-Century-Crofts, East Norwalk, CT, 1979, with permission.)

Skin Grafts and Flaps

2

Mallory S. Anthony

Wounds with significant tissue loss often require skin grafts or flaps for adequate wound closure. In the hand, replacement of soft tissue warrants special attention since maximum functional outcome is imperative. Dorsal skin must be thinner, more elastic, and loose enough not to restrict flexion; it must provide a barrier to cover tendons and joints.[1] Volar skin must be thicker and tougher (to withstand pressure and friction caused by grasp and pinch), be loose and elastic enough to allow motion, and retain its function of sensibility.[1]

The immediate short-term goals for soft tissue replacement are (1) to encourage primary healing, (2) to prevent infection, and (3) to preserve the viability of exposed underlying structures.[2] The long-term benefits of adequate skin replacement are to (1) provide a durable skin cover to withstand everyday use, (2) provide sensation at key points in the hand, (3) permit mobility of underlying structures, especially tendons, (4) permit later reconstruction procedures on the deep structures, if necessary, and (5) prevent the development of contractures.[2]

Skin grafts are used to replace skin in areas where adequate circulation is available, and underlying structures are protected by adequate subcutaneous tissue.[2] A split-thickness skin graft (STSG) is generally obtained from the thigh, buttock, or abdomen. These skin grafts (1) are more suitable on large and contaminated wounds, (2) take more readily, (3) are less prone to infection, and (4) offer a large supply of donor sites. One major disadvantage is its increased tendency to contract during healing. Meshing of an STSG is occasionally indicated on suboptimal wound beds, where the risk of infection and/or hematoma is great, and meshing is necessary to allow drainage of exudate and/or blood.[2] Meshing may also be used in cases of donor site shortage, such as extensive burns, to allow expansion of graft.[2]

A full-thickness skin graft (FTSG) is generally obtained from the hypothenar eminence, medial aspect of the arm, or groin. These skin

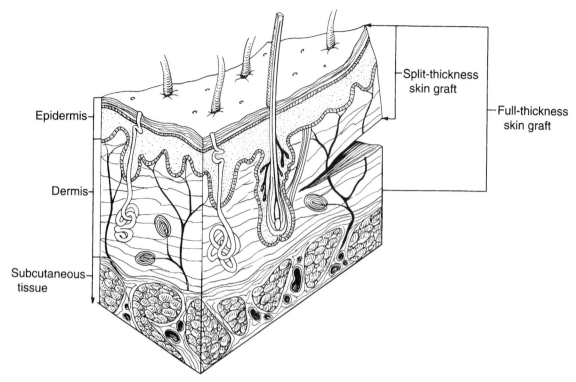

Fig. 2-1. Split- and full-thickness skin grafts.

grafts (1) provide increased durability, (2) afford better protection, (3) establish better sensibility, (4) contain more epidermal appendages, (5) contract less than STSGs, (6) provide increased cosmesis and color match, and (7) are more suitable for small, clean wounds (Fig. 2-1).

Firm "take" of a skin graft requires good recipient bed vascularity, free from increased levels of bacteria and devitalized tissue. After application of a skin graft, the graft first survives by transudate from the wound (plasmatic circulation).[1] Later, the ingrowth of capillary buds into the skin graft from the wound bed provides the necessary vascularity. Optimal beds for skin grafts include muscle and fascia. Suboptimal beds include denuded bone or tendon.

Skin flaps are needed for soft tissue coverage when the recipient bed provides poor vascularity and when vital structures are exposed.[3] A skin flap consists of dermis and subcutaneous tissue elevated from its underlying bed. It maintains vascularity through its base (pedicle). A flap can be classified as pedicle or free. A pedicle flap remains attached to the recipient site and requires later detachment. A free flap is transferred by dividing its vascular pedicle and resuturing the pedicle to recipient vessels in the recipient site.

A pedicle flap may be classified according to its vascular supply from the skin, which is present in four vascular layers. These layers are the subdermal, subcutaneous, fascial, and muscular layers shown in Figure 2-2.

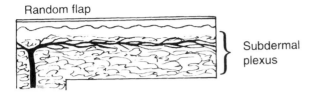

Random flap

Subdermal
plexus

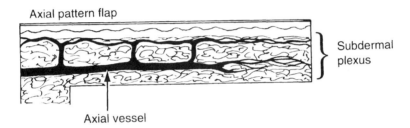

Axial pattern flap

Subdermal
plexus

Axial vessel

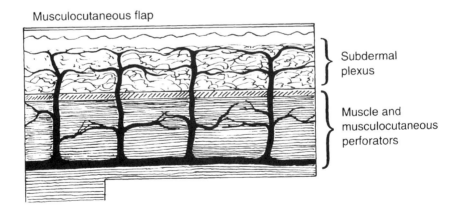

Musculocutaneous flap

Subdermal
plexus

Muscle and
musculocutaneous
perforators

Fig. 2-2. Types of pedicle flaps.

A flap that receives its blood supply from the subdermal layer is called a random flap[3] (Fig. 2-2). The vascular supply of an axial flap comes from the subcutaneous, fascial, or muscular layer[3] (Fig. 2-2).

Pedicle flaps can provide sufficient tissue coverage in all but the most massive defects.[3] However, the hand must be dependent during attachment, resulting in prolonged immobilization; these flaps require a minimum of two operative procedures; the blood supply upon which the pedicle flap is initially dependent is cut at the time of detachment, making the flap dependent on peripheral vascularity (less dependable and robust); and the flap may be avulsed by a very young or incompetent patient (Fig. 2-3).

The edges of all these skin flaps initially depend on nutrition by perfusion through microcirculation, before neovascularization (capillary budding) occurs and sufficient blood supply has grown across into the flap from the surrounding tissues. Approximately 3 weeks is required before healing is sufficient to allow pedicle division.

A free flap provides immediate vascularity. Vein grafts are sometimes necessary if the vascular pedicle is stretched at the repair site. Free flaps offer many advantages over the pedicle flap: (1) The recipient limb is mobile and free of prolonged attachment to the donor, permitting elevation and early mobilization; (2) free flaps frequently require only one operative procedure; (3) they bring their own blood supply, increasing the potential for healing, especially in a poorly vascularized and scarred bed; and (4) they can be cut to fit the defect with incomparable precision (almost limitless choice of size and thickness).[4]

Independent of the type of soft tissue coverage chosen for the patient, our role is to promote wound healing, decrease edema, provide effective scar management, and help restore optimal range of motion (ROM) and function for these patients.

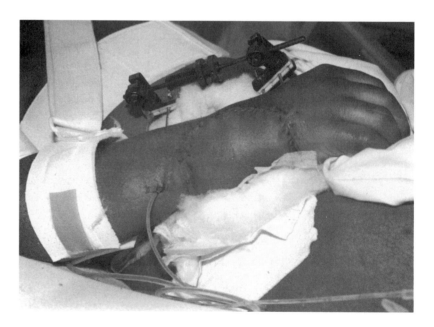

Fig. 2-3. Pedicle flap from groin for soft tissue defect. External fixator for treatment of distal forearm fracture.

DEFINITIONS

 I. Graft: a portion of tissue, such as skin, periosteum bone, or fascia that is severed free and transferred to correct a defect in the body. A graft may consist of skin only (skin graft), or it may be a composite of tissues such as skin, muscle, or bone (composite graft).[5]

 II. Flap: a portion of tissue *partly* severed from its place of origin to correct a defect in the body, as in pedicle flaps or completely severed from its origin as in free flaps. A flap may also consist of skin only (including its subdermal plexus of vessels), or it may be a composite of tissues such as skin, muscle, or bone (composite flap).[5] A flap contains its own vascular supply (Fig. 2-4).

 III. Types of tissue transfers
   A. Free tissue transfers
     1. STSG: a free graft of skin that includes the epidermis and part of the dermis. (May be meshed where moderate serous drainage is expected or when recipient bed is suboptimal for vascularity.)
     2. FTSG: a free graft of skin that includes the whole thickness of epidermis and dermis. Contains dermal appendages and nerve endings, with the exception of subcutaneous sweat glands and some pacinian corpuscles.

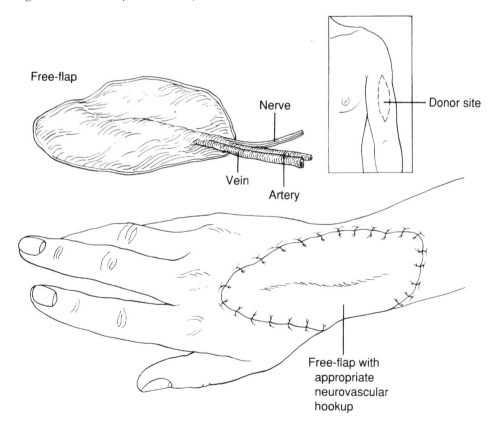

Fig. 2-4. Various flaps may be considered for coverage.

3. Free vascularized tissue transfer: a composite flap with its vascular pedicle completely cut and transferred to the recipient site for immediate microvascular anastomoses (e.g., free groin flap, free latissimus flap).

B. Pedicled flaps (require later detachment)
   1. Random: designed to fit the recipient defect without attention to specific nutrient vessels in the pedicle.[5] There is no anatomically recognized arterial or venous system, and it receives its blood supply from the dermal-subdermal plexus (e.g., Z-plasty, V–Y advancement, rotation flap, transposition flap).
   2. Axial: designed so that the pedicle has within it identifiable, direct, cutaneous vascular elements.[5]
      a. Cutaneous: axial flaps whose vessels supply skin alone and proceed directly to it (e.g., groin flap).
      b. Fasciocutaneous: axial flaps whose vessels first supply fascia (e.g., lateral arm flap).
      c. Myocutaneous or musculocutaneous: axial flaps whose vessels first supply muscle (e.g., latissimus dorsi flap).
      d. Island flap: axial flap whose pedicle has been reduced to the point that it consists only of nutrient blood vessels with or without nerves (e.g., neurovascular digital island flap).

IV. Location of grafts/flaps
   A. Local (from skin adjacent to the defect); for example, transposition (Z-plasty), advancement (V–Y advancement), or rotation (Fillet flap).
   B. Regional (from elsewhere on the limb); for example, lateral arm flap, cross-finger flap, or thenar flap.
   C. Distant (from other parts of the body); for example, abdominal or groin flap.

SURGICAL PURPOSE

To provide wound coverage of open areas to protect underlying structures. Each graft type has a very specific reason for being used, and each has well-defined risk/benefit ratios.

TREATMENT GOALS

I. Provide adequate wound care and promote wound healing of graft, flap, and/or donor site.
II. Restore active ROM (AROM) and passive ROM (PROM) in affected areas underlying flaps/grafts.
III. Maintain full ROM of all uninvolved joints.
IV. Return to optimum level of function.

INDICATIONS FOR TISSUE COVERAGE

I. Split-thickness and full-thickness grafts are used to replace skin in areas where adequate subcutaneous tissues remain to protect underlying structures, and where adequate circulation is available.

II. Flaps are indicated in wounds where there is bone devoid of periosteum, tendon devoid of paratenon, cartilage devoid of perichondrium, or exposed vital structures.

PRECAUTIONS FOR THERAPY

I. Decreased graft/flap viability
   A. Infection (cardinal signs: warmth, redness, pain, and edema)
   B. Mechanical problems: establishment of barrier between bed and graft (e.g., hematoma)
   C. Inadequate preparation of recipient bed
   D. Inadequate surgical technique

II. Damage and repair to deep vital structures

III. Extreme pain

IV. Severe edema

THERAPY

I. Preoperative management
   A. Provide sterile whirlpool, dressing changes, and debridement of recipient wound area, if indicated, in preparation for tissue coverage.
   B. Patient education to prepare patient for pedicle or free flap. This may include instruction in one-handed techniques and information regarding the type of clothing that will best accommodate the arm while it is attached, as in the case of a groin flap.
   C. Maximize ROM and increase strength in muscle to be transferred for planned functional muscle flap (nonemergency basis).

II. Postoperative evaluation
   A. Please refer to wound management evaluation, Chapter 1.
   B. Graft/flap viability assessment (general guidelines).[3]
      1. Observe color
         a. Random pattern flap
            i. *Pink*: healthy.
            ii. *Pale* with faint *blue/gray tinge*: inadequate arterial supply.
            iii. *Angry red* first, then progressively *purple red* and *purple blue*: inadequate venous supply.
         b. Axial pattern flap
            i. *Very pale pink*: healthy.
            ii. *Waxy pallor* (white tinged with yellow or brown): vascular compromise.

      c. Free flaps
         i. *Pink*: healthy.
        ii. *White* or *mottled appearance*: arterial problems.
      iii. *Dusky blue*: venous problems.
  2. Observe refill after blanching by fingertip pressure or by running a blunt point across flap.
    a. Slow refill (> than 2 seconds) with pale flap: arterial insufficiency.
    b. Rapid refill with bluish flap: venous insufficiency (e.g, kinking of pedicle).
  3. Temperature of flap
    a. Marked decrease in temperature between flap and tissue adjacent to flap may indicate impaired blood flow.
  4. Monitor pulsatile flow within the flap.

III. Postoperative management (skin grafts)[1,6]

  A. Grafts immobilized and protected 4 to 5 days for STSG and 5 to 7 days for FTSG.

  B. 5 to 7 days postoperatively may begin daily dressing changes with nonadherent gauze.

    Please note: Loss of a graft is usually the result of shear forces, fluid accumulation under graft, tension, or purulence. Care must be taken during dressing changes not to rub the healing graft.

  C. Seventh postoperative day, begin *gentle* ROM exercises (under supervision of therapist only). May want to exercise without dressing in place to avoid a shearing force on the wound.

  D. Elevation to decrease edema (no compressive wraps until at least 2 weeks postoperatively, and only after consulting the treating physician).

  E. 1 week postoperatively, sterile whirlpool and wound care to clean wound and stimulate local circulation.

  F. 10 to 14 days: gentle application of topical lubricant to healed areas, as graft sites are dry due to lack of secondary protective skin structures.

  G. 2 weeks postoperatively, pressure garments and compressive wraps may be used over a well-vascularized graft to decrease edema, if shearing forces are avoided, and after consulting treating physician.

  H. 3 to 4 weeks postoperatively: gentle massage and scar-softening modalities.

  I. Splinting
    1. Early/protective: to immobilize joints in functional position, eliminate tension on repaired structures, and protect the healing graft.
    2. Late (6 weeks): to apply stress to scar and increase ROM.

  J. Continue ROM exercises and add activities to increase strength, endurance, and function.

  K. Monitor return of sensation.

  L. Caution patients against exposure of either graft donor or recipient sites to the sun for at least 6 months.

IV. Postoperative management (flaps)[6]
   A. Pedicle (axial)
      1. Left attached 2 to 4 weeks (to allow new vascular ingrowth to the flap from the recipient bed).
      2. Use gauze pads in areas where maceration is a problem.
      3. String wrapping or coban to free digits and retrograde massage to decrease edema if no stress is placed on attachment.
      4. Maintain ROM in uninvolved joints.
      5. After flap detachment
         a. Promote wound healing.
         b. Decrease edema.
         c. Regain active and passive motion in uninvolved joints.
         d. Re-establish active and passive ROM in affected area.
         e. Scar management.
   B. Free tissue transfer[3,6]
      1. Vascular status is critical in the first few days postoperatively. (Patient is kept warm and should abstain from caffeine and nicotine.)
      2. Elevation to heart level only to decrease edema. Extensive elevation may impair arterial inflow.
      3. 8 to 10 days: flap should be stable.
         a. Wound care for donor and recipient sites. (If wounds are dry and healing well, minimal dressing is required. If not, whirlpool may be initiated once the flap is thought to be stable by treating physician.)
         b. Monitor vascularity: observe color, temperature, and capillary refill time.
         c. Continue elevation for edema control (no compressive wraps until at least third postoperative week, and only with physician approval).
         d. AROM to uninvolved joints.
      4. 2 weeks: AROM of involved joints if vascular status is stable.
      5. 3 to 4 weeks: gentle massage, scar-softening modalities, and compressive wraps if vascular status is stable.
      6. 6 to 8 weeks: splinting and passive ROM exercise as healing permits.
      7. 8 weeks: patient can resume normal daily activities using the hand.
      8. Continue ROM exercises and add activities to increase strength, endurance, and function.
      9. Heavy and stressful activities allowed at 3 months.
      10. Monitor return of sensation.
   C. Functional muscle flap (free tissue transfer)[6]
      1. Immobilized for 3 weeks in relaxed position. During this immobilization phase, once vascular stability is achieved (usually by 1 to 2 weeks), and with physician approval, PROM of uninvolved joints may be initiated.
      2. Continue gentle PROM exercise until preoperative ROM is achieved.

3. As clinical signs of reinnervation are noted (4 to 7 months postoperatively), active-assistive ROM exercises may be initiated.
4. Muscle stimulation, active exercise, and resistive exercise may be added as muscle strengthens.

V. Donor sites
   A. Monitor donor site for development of hypertrophic scar.
   B. Massage with topical lubricant and application of pressure may be initiated for scar management, as wound healing permits.
   C. Be aware of loss of sensibility in donor site and educate patient, if a nerve has been taken for a transfer.

POSTOPERATIVE COMPLICATIONS

I. Loss of graft/flap
   A. Hematoma or seroma
   B. Infection
   C. Vascular compromise
      1. Kinking of pedicle attachment.
      2. Compression of arterial supply for free flap.
      3. Inadequate preparation of recipient bed.
II. Extreme pain
III. Severe edema
IV. Excess scarring due to a long interval between injury and time of coverage

EVALUATION TIMELINE

Graft/flap viability status should be assessed at initial evaluation, and during every treatment session until the graft or flap is well taken. Joint motion affected by graft/flap should be assessed when changes occur or at least once a month. Mobility and description of scar should be assessed, as well as sensory status, strength, and function during these follow-up evaluations.

REFERENCES

1. Browne EZ: Skin grafts. p. 1711. In Green DP (ed): Operative Hand Surgery. 3rd Ed. Churchill Livingstone, New York, 1993
2. Smith PF: Skin loss and scar contractures. p. 31. In Burke FD, McGrouther DA, Smith PJ (eds): Principles of Hand Surgery. Churchill Livingstone, New York, 1990
3. Lister G: Skin flaps. p. 1741. In Green DP (ed): Operative Hand Surgery. 3rd Ed. Churchill Livingstone, New York, 1993
4. Lister G: Emergency free flaps. p. 1127. In Green DP (ed): Operative Hand Surgery. 2nd Ed. Churchill Livingstone, New York, 1988

5. Chase RA: Skin and soft tissue. p. 1. In: Atlas of Hand Surgery. Vol. 2. WB Saunders, Philadelphia, 1984

6. Singer DI, Moore JH, Bryon PM: Management of skin grafts and flaps. p. 277. In Hunter JM, Mackin EJ, Callahan AD (eds): Rehabilitation of the Hand: Surgery and Therapy. 4th Ed. Mosby, St. Louis, 1995

SUGGESTED READINGS

(Please also refer to wound management suggested readings.)

Beasley RW: Hand Injuries. WB Saunders, Philadelphia, 1981

Brown PW: Open injuries of the hand. p. 1533. In Green DP (ed): Operative Hand Surgery. 3rd Ed. Churchill Livingstone, New York, 1993

Browne EZ: Complications of skin grafts and pedicle flaps. Hand Clin 2:353, 1986

Jabaley ME: Recovery of sensation in flaps and skin grafts. p. 583. In Tubiana R (ed): The Hand. Vol. 1. WB Saunders, Philadelphia, 1981

Ketchum L: Skin and soft tissue coverage of the upper extremity. Hand Clin 4(1), 1985

Lister G: The theory of the transposition flap and its practical application in the hand. Clin Plast Surg 8:115, 1981

Lister G: Injury. p. 1. In: The Hand: Diagnosis and Indications. 2nd Ed. Churchill Livingstone, New York, 1984

Lister GD: Free skin and composite flaps. p. 1103. In Green DP (ed): Operative Hand Surgery. 3rd Ed. Churchill Livingstone, New York, 1993

Michon J: Complex hand injuries: surgical planning. p. 196. In Tubiana R (ed): The Hand. Vol. 2. WB Saunders, Philadelphia, 1985

Morrison WA, Gilbert A: Complications in microsurgery. p. 145. In Tubiana R (ed): The Hand. Vol. 2. WB Saunders, Philadelphia, 1985

Tsuge K, Kanaujia RR, Steichen JB: Comprehensive Atlas of Hand Surgery. Year Book Medical Publishers, Chicago, 1989

Ware LC, Anthony MS: Burns and open wounds of the hand. Chp. 2. In Home Study Course 95-2. Topic: The Wrist and Hand. Orthopedic Section, APTA, Inc., 1995

Weeks P, Wray C: Wound healing and tissue coverage. p. 3. In: Hand Management: A Biological Approach. Mosby, St. Louis, 1973

Wolfort FG: Acute Hand Injuries: A Multispeciality Approach. Little, Brown, Boston, 1980

Appendix 2-1

Type of Soft Tissue Coverage	Vascularity/Take	Donor Site Closure
STSG	3 days	Secondary intention
FTSG	5–7 days	Primary intention
Pedicled flaps	Approximately 3 weeks	Primary closure or skin graft
Free tissue transfer	Immediate	Primary closure or skin graft

STSG, split-thickness skin graft; FTSC, full-thickness skin graft.

Burns

3

Beth Farrell Kozera

Hand burns are the most common of all thermal injuries.[1–3] In terms of long-term functional well-being, severe hand burns can result in the most crippling deformities.

Normal skin serves several functions essential for life:

1. Guards against invasion of bacteria.
2. Regulates body temperature.
3. Prevents excess loss of body fluids.
4. Protects deeper structures from injury.
5. Protects against ultraviolet rays of the sun.
6. Protects nerve endings responsible for sensation.

When a burn injury has occurred and skin is lost, the body is vulnerable to infection, fluid loss, and injury to deeper structures.[4]

Functional and cosmetic results following burn injuries are directly related to the severity of the burn and the body's biologic response in terms of infection and scar formation.[5] The severity of thermal injuries depends on the level of underlying destruction. Superficial partial-thickness burns involve destruction of the epidermis and possible portions of the dermis whereas in deep partial-thickness burns, most of the dermal layers are destroyed. There is complete destruction of the epidermal and dermal layers in full-thickness burns.

Wound severity is sometimes unclear and not always determined until several days following burn injury because a burn "evolves" over several days. It is possible for a deep partial-thickness burn to convert into a full-thickness burn if left untreated. It is not surprising, therefore, that several treatment approaches have arisen in recent years: conservative treatment with topical antibiotics to permit spontaneous healing, early total excision and immediate grafting, delayed excision and grafting (later than 14 days), and sequential tangential excision and grafting.[5]

Therapeutic intervention of the burned upper extremity requires a therapist trained specifically in wound/graft care, splinting to prevent deformities/contractures, edema control, scar management, and pain control. Close monitoring of the patient's response to treatment (wound status, range of motion [ROM], skin integrity) is necessary to determine whether treatment methods are effective. As well, close communication with the surgeon is vital initially postoperatively, and throughout the course of treatment. The following protocol serves as a guideline for treatment of thermal injuries to the hand/upper extremity.

DEFINITION

Injuries to soft tissues caused by contact with dry heat (e.g., fire), moist heat (e.g., steam or hot liquid), chemicals, electricity, friction, or radiant energy.[6] The following is a discussion of thermal injuries according to the level of injury (Fig. 3-1).

    I. Partial-thickness burns[7]
        A. Superficial partial-thickness: first or second degree burn (i.e., destruction of epidermis and possibly portions of upper dermal layers). Appears red, bright pink, blistered, wet, and soft. Painful. No grafting necessary for healing.
        B. Deep partial-thickness[2]: deep second degree burn. Destruction of epidermis and greater portion of dermal layer (hair follicles, sweat glands). Appears red or white, wet, soft, elastic. Sensation may be diminished. Potential conversion to full-thickness burn.

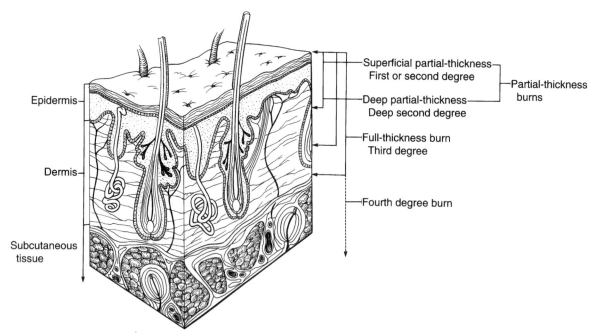

Fig. 3-1. Categorization of thermal injuries according to level of injury.

II. Full-thickness burn[2,7]

Third degree burn. Destruction of entire epidermis and dermal layers (hair follicles, nerve endings, sweat glands). Requires skin grafting. Appears white or tan, waxy, dry, leathery, nonelastic.

III. Fourth degree burn

Deep soft tissue damage to fat, muscle, and bone.

IV. Electrical burn[7]

Thrombosed blood vessels, destruction of nerves along pathway, possible fractures, dislocations. Requires surgical excision of necrotic tissue. Possible amputation.

TREATMENT AND SURGICAL PURPOSE

To prevent deformity where burns have occurred and to restore parts where damaged or lost. Of greatest concern is the loss of skin and joint mobility in critical areas such as with the wrist and digits. Proper splinting to prevent deformity and maintain function is essential. Skin resurfacing is frequently required to achieve joint motion and underlying tendon gliding. Resurfacing where scar contractures exist that cause deformity will also necessitate skin grafting.

TREATMENT GOALS

I. Maximize functional recovery through prevention of the following:
   A. Contractures
   B. Infection
   C. Edema
   D. Muscle disuse atrophy
   E. Tendon adherence
   F. Capsular shortening
II. Control pain.
III. Achieve wound closure by protecting regenerating epithelial cells.[1]
IV. Maintaining or regaining full ROM.
V. Stretching of healing skin.
VI. Promote functional independence.
VII. Control/remodel scar.

INDICATIONS FOR SURGERY

I. Tangential excision/grafting: indicated for deep partial-thickness burns.
II. Full-thickness excision: indicated for full-thickness burns.
III. Thermal burn: may require an escharotomy.
IV. Electrical burn: may require fasciotomy.[3]

POSTOPERATIVE INDICATIONS/ PRECAUTIONS FOR THERAPY

I. Contraindications for open wounds
   A. Excessive heat on burn wound (will cause sloughing).
   B. Serial casting.
   C. Overstretching and vigorous exercise.[2,7–9]
   D. Occlusive dressing (interferes with evaluation of perfusion).[3]
   E. Splinting straps may interfere with circulation. Gauze wraps may be an alternative.
   F. Pressure areas caused by splinting may increase severity of burn.[8]
   G. Discontinue ROM to exposed joints or tendons.[7]
   H. Discontinue ROM if patient complains of deep joint pain.[7]
   I. Cellulitis[7]
II. Contraindications during entire rehabilitation program
   A. Patient should avoid the following:
      1. Strong sunlight
      2. Rubbing skin
      3. Contact with heat, radiators
      4. Cold weather: patient should wear gloves.
      5. Vascular insufficiency may lead to compartment syndrome if not treated.[1]
      6. Ice packs

POSTOPERATIVE THERAPY

I. See graft care guidelines for specific management.
II. See wound care guidelines for specifics on management of wounds.
III. Superficial partial-thickness burns
   A. First 48 hours: keep hand elevated.[3,8] Sterile whirlpool. See physician regarding debridement approach. Dress with nonadherent dressing. Begin gentle active range of motion (AROM) and passive range of motion (PROM) to pain tolerance. High voltage pulsed galvanic stimulation (HVPC) may be indicated to control edema and pain.[1] Splinting as indicated.
   B. Two days to healing of wounds: encourage independence in activities of daily living (ADL); full mobility.[2,7,9]
IV. Deep partial-thickness burns if *not grafted*
   A. Up to 72 postoperative hours: keep hand elevated.[3,8] Irrigate wound with saline. Remove debris. Dress with nonadherent dressing. Edema control as indicated. Pain control as indicated. Begin gentle AROM. AROM exercise should be performed every hour.[1]
      1. Lumbrical plus position
      2. Abduction/adduction of fingers

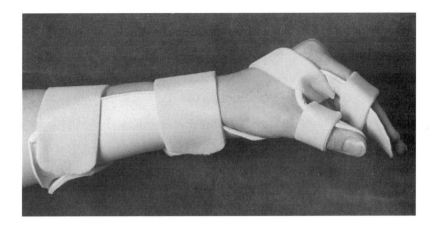

Fig. 3-2. Splint design to be used with dorsal hand burns.

For dorsal hand burn, hook and fist exercises may be initiated as soon as viability of the extensor tendons is known.[1] Splint in intrinsic-plus position; that is, wrist 20 degrees to 30 degrees extension; metacarpophalangeal (MCP) joints: 70 degrees flexion; interphalangeal (IP) joints full extension; thumb abducted and extended[1,7] (Fig. 3-2).

  B. Once edema has decreased: splint only at night and during rest periods. Begin PROM to tolerance. Provide patient with sponge to encourage increased ROM. Encourage use of hand for light activities.

  C. Once wound has healed: begin gradual strengthening as tolerated.

V. Full-thickness burn: excision/grafting or deep partial-thickness burn

  A. Immediately postoperative: Hand is elevated.[3,8] Splint in intrinsic plus position unless the dorsal surface of the hand and fingers are grafted; then splint with fingers in abduction, and consider use of fingernail hooks for proper positioning and tension (Fig. 3-3).

  B. 72 hours postoperative: First dressing change.[7] Consult with patient's physician about appropriate type of dressing. Splint at all times. Continue to keep hand elevated. Pain control as indicated.

  C. 5 to 7 days: Daily dressing changes. Take off splint to exercise. Begin gentle AROM exercises as described in Section IV A.[7,8] Encourage light ADL.[7] Begin sterile whirlpool as soon as edema has minimized. Discontinue whirlpool if edema increases with its use.

  D. Over 7 days: Decrease splinting time unless patient begins to develop deformities. Begin PROM to tolerance (stretching of thumb and web space).[7] Encourage use of hand for all self-care activities.

  E. Once tissue is healed: Begin friction massage. Begin retrograde massage if needed. Apply elastomer molds or gel sheets to

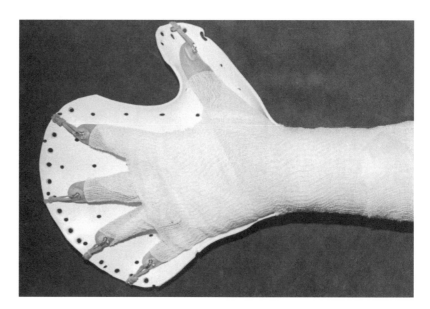

Fig. 3-3. Splint for dorsal hand and finger grafts.

patient's scars (Fig. 3-4). Assess the maturity and stability of new skin before proceeding with pressure therapy. Tubigrip gloves are applied first after wound closure. Custom burn garments can be ordered and then applied when higher shear forces can be tolerated.[10] (Fig. 3-5) Elastomer inserts may be worn under compressive garments.[2] Begin occupational training as soon as edema is minimal and patient presents with a good grip. Keep in mind that contractures sometimes do not

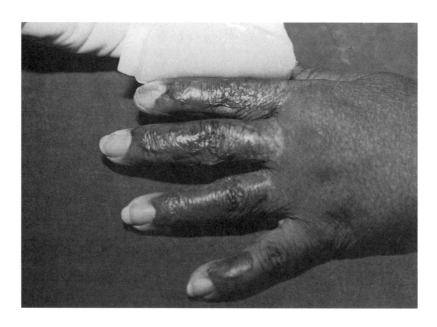

Fig. 3-4. Gel sheet application for scar management.

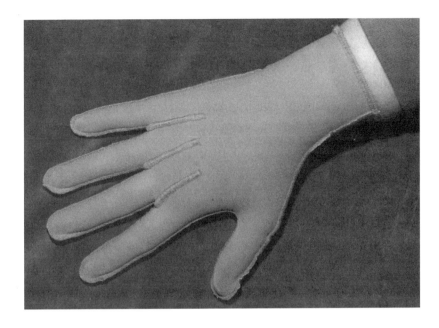

Fig. 3-5. Compressive garments are used to minimize hypertrophic scarring.

develop until 2 to 3 weeks postoperatively. Patient should continue to see his/her therapist for splinting and elastomer adjustments as needed.

POSTOPERATIVE COMPLICATIONS

   I. Infection
  II. Contractures
 III. Associated joint disorders (stiff elbow, shoulder)
 IV. Fractures under the burn wound
  V. Osteomyelitis
 VI. Electrically induced heart arrhythmias (electrical burns only)
 VII. Pain
VIII. Vascular insufficiency (primarily during the first 72 hours)
 IX. Skin maceration (especially when wearing compressive garments)
  X. Poor hygiene (especially when wearing compressive garments, elastomer molds, etc.)

EVALUATION TIMELINE

  I. ROM
    A. Superficial partial-thickness burns: up to 72 hours postoperatively
    B. Deep partial-thickness burns *not grafted*: up to 72 hours postoperatively
 II. Sensory
    For all burns: evaluate as soon as wounds have healed.
 III. Strengthening: For all burns: evaluate as soon as all wounds have healed, edema is minimized, and patient presents with a good grip.

REFERENCES

1. Howell JW: Management of the acutely burned hand for the non-specialized clinician. J Phys Ther 69:1077, 1989
2. Hopkins HL, Smith HD: Willard and Spackman's Occupational Therapy. 6th Ed. Lippincott-Raven, Philadelphia, 1983
3. Salisbury RE, Dingeldein GP: The burned hand and upper extremity. p. 1523. In Green DP (ed): Operative Hand Surgery. 2nd Ed. Vol. 2. Churchill Livingstone, New York, 1988
4. Ware LC, Anthony MS: Orthopaedic Physical Therapy: Burns and Open Wounds of the Hand. Home Study Course 95-2. Orthopaedic Section APTA (American Physical Therapy Association) LaCrosse, 1995
5. Frist W, Ackroyd F, Burke J et al: Long-term functional results of selective treatment of hand burns. Am J Surg 149: 516, 1985
6. Dorland's Illustrated Medical Dictionary. 27th Ed. WB Saunders, Philadelphia, 1988
7. Malick M, Carr J: Manual on Management of the Burned Patient. Harmanville Rehabilitation Center, Pittsburgh, 1982
8. Ostergren G: Burn care. p. 103. In Ziegler EM (ed): Current Concepts in Orthotics: A Diagnosis and Related Approach to Splinting. Roylan Medical Products, Chicago, 1984
9. Puddicombe BE, Nardone MA: Rehabilitation of the burned hand. p. 281. In Grossman JA (ed): Hand Clinics: Burns of the Upper Extremity. Vol. 6. No. 2. WB Saunders, Philadelphia, 1990
10. Kealy GP, Jensen KT: Aggressive approach to physical therapy management of the burned hand. Phys Ther 68: 683, 1988

SUGGESTED READINGS

Belliappa PP, McCabe SJ: The burned hand. In Kasdan ML (ed): Hand Clinics. Vol. 9. WB Saunders, Philadelphia, 1993

Clarke HM, Wittpenn GP, McLeod AM et al: Acute management of pediatric hand burns. In Grossman JAI (ed): Hand Clinics. Vol. 6. WB Saunders, Philadelphia, 1990

Fisher SV, Helm PA: Comprehensive Rehabilitation of Burns. Williams & Wilkins, Baltimore, 1982

Groencvett F, Kreis W: Burns of the hand. Neth J Surg 6:167, 1985

Habal MB: The burned hand: a planned treatment program. J Trauma 18:587, 1978

Harrison DH, Parkhouse N: Experience with upper extremity burns: the Mount Vernon experience. In Grossman JAI (ed): Hand Clinics. Vol. 9, WB Saunders, Philadelphia, 1990

Levine NS, Buchanan T: The care of burned upper extremities. p. 107. In Ruberg RL (ed): Clinics in Plastic Surgery: Advances in Burn Care. Vol. 13. No. 1. WB Saunders, Philadelphia, 1988

Robson MC, Smith DJ, Vanderzee AJ: Making the burned hand functional. In Salisbury RE (ed): Clinics in Plastic Surgery. Vol. 19. WB Saunders, Philadelphia, 1992

Sykes PJ: (Review Article) Severe burns of the hand: a practical guide to their management. J Hand Surg (Br) 16:6, 1991

Dupuytren's Disease 4

Dale Eckhaus

Dupuytren's disease is often cited as being of genetic origin.[1,2] The disease primarily affects individuals of Northern European descent.[1-3] It is often associated with other conditions such as chronic alcoholism, epilepsy, diabetes mellitus, and chronic pulmonary disease.[1-4] Disease onset is usually in the fifth to seventh decade of life.[3] Men are more often affected than women.[1,2] In most instances the ulnar side of the hand is affected.[2,5] The disease can have a slow or rapid progression.[2]

Individuals may sometimes exhibit a Dupuytren's diathesis. In those instances, there is a strong family history, the disease begins at an early age, and there is evidence of fibromatosis in areas other than the volar surface of the hand.[3]

The disease is an active cellular process in the fascia of the hand.[1,3,6] It often presents initially as a nodule in the pretendinous bands of the ring and little fingers.[2,3,5] This is followed by the appearance of tendon-like cords, which are due to the pathologic change in normal fascia.[3,6] The thickening and shortening of the fascia causes contracture.[2]

Nonoperative treatment has been ineffective. Attempts to use splints, steroid injections, and vitamin E have not been helpful.[3,7]

Surgery is indicated when the metacarpophalangeal (MCP) joint contracts to 30 degrees, as this deformity becomes a functional problem. Some surgeons feel that any amount of proximal interphalangeal (PIP) joint contracture warrants surgery. Others feel that 15 degrees or greater is an indication for surgery.[1,3,6] A contracture of a PIP joint is more of a concern than an MCP joint contracture because of their differences in capsular ligament structure.[5]

Many methods of surgical treatment have been reported. No one method has been established.[3] Postoperative management also varies. A common goal of the various methods is to promote wound healing, which minimizes scar and maximizes scar mobility.

DEFINITION

Disease of fascia of palm and digits (Figs. 4-1 and 4-2).

SURGICAL PURPOSE

Dupuytren's contractures frequently interfere with normal hand function. The deformities are caused by abnormal thickening and contracture of the palmar fascia and its extensions. Surgery is the only method of correcting the problem. The surgical release of the contracture can be made through varied skin incisions. Neurovascular and tendon elements are frequently in close proximity with the diseased tissues and, therefore, are vulnerable to injury. Recurrences of the contractures can occur. Some surgeons use skin grafts to reduce the chances of recurrence. Postoperative hand therapy is an important adjunct in the care of this disease.

TREATMENT GOALS

I. Maintain range of motion (ROM) of uninvolved joints and digits.
II. Control postoperative edema.
III. Promote wound healing, especially in open palm techniques.
IV. Improve active ROM (AROM) and passive ROM (PROM) for both extension and flexion.
V. Control and guide scar formation.

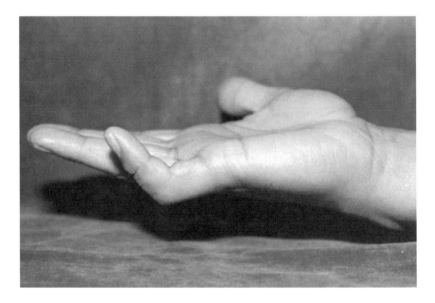

Fig. 4-1. Preoperative positioning of a hand with Dupuytren's disease.

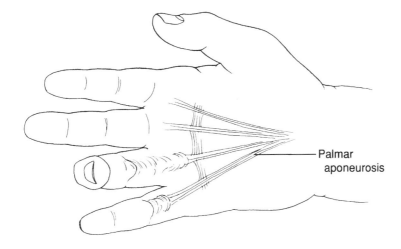

Palmar
aponeurosis

Fig. 4-2. Dupuytren's disease
affects the fascia of the hand.

NONOPERATIVE INDICATIONS/
PRECAUTIONS FOR THERAPY

Nonoperative treatment, including splinting, has not been effective.

POSTOPERATIVE INDICATIONS/
PRECAUTIONS FOR THERAPY

    I. Indications: following surgery of the diseased fascia
   II. Precautions
      A. Intraoperative complications involving the neurovascular bundles
      B. Concomitant surgical procedures such as capsulectomy
      C. Skin grafts

POSTOPERATIVE THERAPY

    I. During first week, postoperative dressing and splint are replaced
      with a thin, nonadhesive dressing and either a volar or dorsal
      removable thermoplastic extension splint. Splints are used periodi-
      cally during the day and worn throughout the night while sleeping
      (Fig. 4-3).
   II. Whirlpool with extremity positioned horizontally is used early in
      treatment with an open palm technique or open wounds that result
      from complications of surgical incisions or grafts.
  III. Wound care treatment is used with appropriate wounds, especially
      the open techniques.
  IV. Edema control methods are instituted.

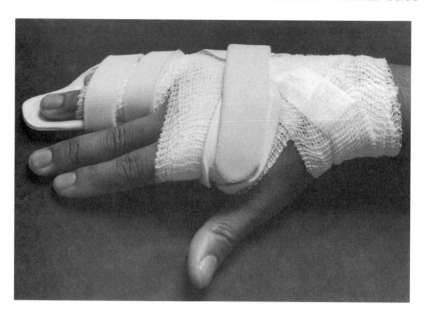

Fig. 4-3. Postoperative thermoplastic extension splint.

V. Active, active assisted, and passive range of motion exercises are initiated with first treatment session. Delay or special care in motion may be necessitated by grafts.

VI. Scar management techniques, including molded materials, are used when wounds are closed and sometimes over nonadherent dressings (Fig. 4-4).

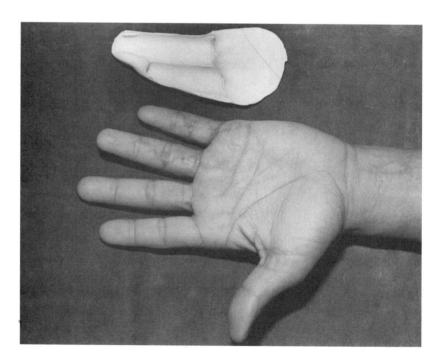

Fig. 4-4. Molded materials are used for scar management.

VII. Light activities of daily living (ADL) are permitted in early postoperative phase.

VIII. Light strengthening exercises, progressing to heavier resistance, is introduced once wounds are healed, edema is controlled, and pressure to area is well tolerated.

IX. Splints are adjusted and various types are used to achieve full extension and flexion.

X. Splints with scar molds are used for up to 6 months or more.

POSTOPERATIVE COMPLICATIONS

I. Hematoma
II. Edema
III. Skin necrosis
IV. Infection
V. Stiffness
VI. Pain
VII. Reflex sympathetic dystrophy (RSD)
VIII. Recurrence of disease

EVALUATION TIMELINE

I. Initial evaluation of first postoperative visit
   A. Assess the following
      1. Wound and skin condition
      2. Edema
      3. Pain
      4. Sensibility
      5. AROM and PROM
      6. Management of ADL

II. Re-evaluation at 4-week intervals
   Assess strength when wounds are closed and palmar surface can tolerate pressure.

REFERENCES

1. McFarlane RM, Albion U: Dupuytren's disease. p. 867. In Hunter JM, Schneider LH, Mackin EJ, Callahan AD (eds): Rehabilitation of the Hand. 3rd Ed. Mosby, St. Louis, 1990

2. Dupuytren's contracture. p. 269. In Schumacher HR, Klippel JF, Robinson DR (eds): Primer on Rheumatic Diseases. 9th Ed. Arthritis Foundation, Atlanta, 1988

3. Hill NA, Hurst LC: Dupuytren's contracture. p. 349. In Doyle JR: Landmark Advances in Hand Surgery. In Peterson BL (ed): Hand Clinics. Vol. 5. WB Saunders, Philadelphia, 1989

4. Hueston JT: Dupuytren's contracture. p. 797. In Flynn JE (ed): Hand Surgery. 3rd Ed. Williams & Wilkins, Baltimore, 1982

5. Lamb DW, Kuczynski K: Dupuytren's disease. p. 635. In Lamb DW, Hooper G, Kuczynski K (eds): The Practice of Hand Surgery. 2nd Ed. Blackwell Scientific Publications, Oxford, 1989

6. McFarlane RM: Dupuytren's contracture. p. 553. In Green DP (ed): Operative Hand Surgery. 2nd Ed. Churchill Livingstone, New York, 1988

7. Abbott K, Denny J, Burke FD, McGauther DA: A review to attitudes to splintage in Dupuytren's contracture. J Hand Surg (Br) 12:326, 1987

SUGGESTED READINGS

Colville J: Dupuytren's contracture—the role of fasciotomy. Hand 15:162, 1983

Fietti VG, Mackin EJ: Open palm technique in Dupuytren's disease. p. 995. In Hunter JM, Mackin EJ, Callahan AD (eds): Rehabilitation of the Hand: Surgery and Therapy. 4th Ed. Mosby, St Louis, 1995

Hueston JT: Dupuytren's contracture. p. 864. In Jupiter JB (ed): Flynn's Hand Surgery. 4th Ed. Williams & Wilkins, Baltimore, 1991

Jain AS, Mitchell C, Carus DA: A simple, inexpensive, post-operative management regime following surgery for Dupuytren's contracture. J Hand Surg (Br) 13:259, 1988

McCash CR: The open palm technique in Dupuytren's contracture. Br J Plast Surg 17:271, 1964

McFarlane RM: Dupuytren's contracture. p. 563. In Green DP (ed): Operative Hand Surgery. 3rd Ed. Churchill Livingstone, New York, 1993

McFarlane RM, McGauther DA, Flint M: Dupuytren's disease. In: The Hand and Upper Limb. Vol. 5. Churchill Livingstone, New York, 1990

Sampson SP, Badalamente MA, Hurst LC et al: The use of a passive motion machine in the postoperative rehabilitation of Dupuytren's disease. J Hand Surg 17A:333, 1992

Seyfer AE, Hueston JT: Dupuytren's contracture. In Mitchell MM (ed): Hand Clinics. Vol. 7. WB Saunders, Philadelphia, 1991

Upper Extremity Vessel Repair

5

Lorie Theisen

Injuries to blood vessels rarely occur independent of injuries to other structures of the hand (e.g., bone, tendon, nerve, and blood vessels). It is worthwhile, however, to singularly examine the operative and postoperative management of repaired blood vessels. Keep in mind these other repaired structures and incorporate the appropriate postoperative management guidelines. It is important for the treating therapist to receive information from the surgeon regarding tension and patency of the anastomosed vessel, as well as the integrity of other repaired structures. The postoperative course must then be modified for the individual case.[1]

Generally, the greatest amount of healing in the vascular system occurs within the first 4 weeks postoperatively.[2] More specifically, healing of the endothelial lining, a single cell layer of the vessel wall serving as a permeable barrier between the blood and other cells of the vessel, occurs in the first 2 weeks. Simultaneously, proliferation of the intimal smooth muscle cells occurs, adding structural integrity. Remobilization is initiated after endothelial healing has occurred and, therefore, should not interfere with or cause excessive intimal thickening.[3]

DEFINITION

Surgical procedure for restoration of blood supply.

SURGICAL PURPOSE

Vessel repair is a common procedure used to restore circulation to a part deprived of its blood supply (Fig. 5-1). This includes both veins and arteries. Often magnification or the operating microscope is used to per-

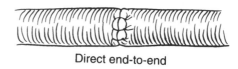

Direct end-to-end

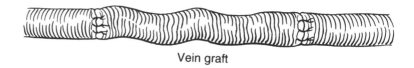

Vein graft

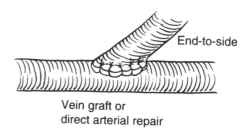

End-to-side

Vein graft or
direct arterial repair

Fig. 5-1. Vessel repair restores circulation to a part deprived of its blood supply.

form these repairs. If direct artery to artery or vein to vein repair cannot be accomplished, vein grafts are used to bridge the gap. Frequently, other adjacent structures such as nerve, bone, muscle, or skin may be damaged. Treatment of these injuries will also be required.

TREATMENT GOALS

Maintain integrity of vessel repair while addressing other specific problems of the injured hand, such as joint stiffness or tendon/soft tissue tightness.

POSTOPERATIVE INDICATIONS/ PRECAUTIONS FOR THERAPY

I. Indications
   Rehabilitation may be indicated following the surgical repair of the vessel for protective splinting, remobilization, and education.
II. Precautions
   A. Follow precautions identified from the surgeon regarding specifics of the vessel repair.
   B. Avoid extremes in temperature to avoid triggering vascular spasm. Arterial spasm can lead to ischemia.[4]
   C. Avoid excessive external compression or pressure via dressing, splints, etc.

   D. Therapy is not indicated where thrombosis or the integrity of the vessel is in question.

   E. Avoid trauma to the soft tissues, particularly when removing any dressing. Dressing changes can trigger vascular spasm.

   F. Vigorous exercise that causes pain may precipitate vasospasm.

   G. Exercise or splints should not decrease digital temperatures. It is recommended that these temperatures be monitored closely.[5]

POSTOPERATIVE THERAPY

   I. Elevation of the injured part above the heart, but the elbow should not be flexed more than 30 degrees. Excessive elevation should be avoided if there is arterial congestion.[6]

  II. Application of protective splinting to preserve the arches of the hand and to preserve maximum ligament length of any immobilized joint, with consideration given to other injuries such as tendon laceration, nerve laceration, fractures, etc.

 III. Observe carefully for signs of vascular compromise, which may include an increase in edema, a decrease in temperature, or an increase in pain. A dusky bluish appearance suggests venous congestion; a pale or white appearance suggests arterial compromise.[7]

 IV. Therapy is initiated between 2 and 4 weeks after surgical repair. Treatment should address problems identified at the initial evaluation such as joint tightness, soft tissue tightness, adhesions preventing tendon gliding, sensory dysfunction, edema, etc.

  V. Continue to instruct the patient in restrictions identified by the surgeon, such as no smoking or caffeine intake.

 VI. Light compressive wrapping may be initiated at 4 to 5 weeks postoperatively after vascularity is stabilized.[8]

POSTOPERATIVE COMPLICATIONS

   I. Arterial occlusion

  II. Venous congestion

 III. Severe edema

 IV. Infection

  V. Cold intolerance

EVALUATION TIMELINE

   I. Initial evaluation at 2 to 4 weeks postoperatively should include assessment of range of motion, edema, sensibility, and temperature.

  II. Progress evaluation every 2 weeks thereafter.

 III. Gross grasp and prehension strength evaluation may be performed at 10 weeks postoperatively, providing guidelines/precautions of other repaired structures are met.

REFERENCES

1. Goldner R: Post-operative management. p. 205. In Urbaniak J (ed): Hand Clinics Microvascular Surgery. Vol. 1. No. 2. WB Saunders, Philadelphia, 1985
2. Kader P: Therapists management of the replanted hand. p. 821. In Hunter J (ed): Rehabilitation of the Hand: Surgery and Therapy. 3rd Ed. Mosby, St. Louis, 1990
3. Wilgis EFS: Ischemic conditions of the upper extremity. p. 4991. In McCarthy J (ed): Plastic Surgery: The Hand. Vol. 8. WB Saunders, Philadelphia, 1990
4. Chase R: Microsurgery. p. 360. In: Atlas of Hand Surgery. Vol. 2. WB Saunders, Philadelphia, 1984
5. Steichen J, Idler R: Surgical aspect of replantation and revascularization. p. 801. In Hunter J (ed): Rehabilitation of the Hand: Surgery and Therapy. 3rd Ed. Mosby, St. Louis, 1990
6. Koman LA: Diagnostic study of vascular lesions. p. 219. In Urbaniak J (ed): Hand Clinics. Vol. 1. No. 2. WB Saunders, Philadelphia, 1985
7. Buncke HJ, Jackson RL, Buncke GM, Chan SW: The surgical and rehabilitative aspects of replantation and revascularization of the hand. p. 1089. In Hunter JM, Mackin EJ, Callahan AD (eds): Rehabilitation of the Hand: Surgery and Therapy. 4th Ed. Mosby, St. Louis, 1995
8. Buncke HJ, Jackson RL, Buncke GM, Chan SW: The surgical and rehabilitative aspects of replantation and revascularization of the hand. p. 1092. In Hunter JM, Mackin EJ, Callahan AD (eds): Rehabilitation of the Hand: Surgery and Therapy. 4th Ed. Mosby, St. Louis, 1995

SUGGESTED READING

Brand P: External stress: effect at the surface. p. 88. In: Clinical Mechanics of the Hand. Mosby, St. Louis, 1985
Brand P: External stress: effect at the surface. p. 129. In: Clinical Mechanics of the Hand. Mosby, St. Louis, 1985
Buncke HJ, Jackson RL, Buncke GM, Chan SW: The surgical and rehabilitative aspects of replantation and revascularization of the hand. p. 1084. In Hunter JM, Mackin EJ, Callahan AD (eds): Rehabilitation of the Hand: Surgery and Therapy. 4th Ed. Mosby, St. Louis, 1995
Kaden PB: Therapists' management of the replanted hand. Hand Clin 2: 179, 1986
MacNeil S, Willette-Green V, Petrilli J: Early protective motion in digital revascularization and replantation. J Hand Ther April-June: 84, 1989

Nerve Repair

6

Beth Farrell Kozera

Peripheral nerves activate the intricately balanced muscles in the upper extremity that enable hand function. With nerve loss, this balance is lost and permanent hand deformities can occur. Understanding the anatomy of the peripheral nervous system, nerve regeneration, and surgical techniques to repair lacerated nerves is vital when rehabilitating patients following nerve repair.

Peripheral nerves are made up of groups of fascicles that contain numerous axons and the enveloping myelin sheath. Fascicles are surrounded with a dense outer coating called the *epineurium*. The epineurium is the site of suture placement in epineural repairs, which is the most commonly used repair for nerve reconstruction. Group fascicular repair is the second most common technique and involves tedious coaptation of individual groups of fascicles.[1] Recovery following nerve repair is least successful when a nerve is repaired under tension. Therefore, if a gap is present following nerve injury, nerve grafting may be necessary.

Therapy following any type of nerve repair is critical for restoring hand function. Care should be taken to avoid stretching of the repaired nerve ends because tension will lead to scarring and may constrict the regenerating axons from achieving functional reinnervation.[1] As the nerve is regenerating, the focus of therapy should be to maintain or promote full mobility of all joints and soft tissue and to prevent hand deformities from occurring. As sensory reinnervation is evident, a sensory re-education program should be initiated.

The following protocol is a guideline for treating patients suffering from peripheral nerve interruption. The addendum section describes the effects of nerve lesions on motor function.

DEFINITION

Approximation of the ends of a lacerated nerve (Fig. 6-1).

TREATMENT AND SURGICAL PURPOSE

To protect against damage and deformity within the defined territory of the injured nerve before its maximum recovery. The goal of surgery is to restore nerve continuity by direct repair or nerve grafting so that an optimum number of nerve fibers will reach their appropriate sensory and/or motor end organs. During the preoperative and postoperative periods, appropriate monitoring and therapy is required to optimize the final result. Patience on the part of those treating or being treated is necessary because of the slow rate of nerve healing.

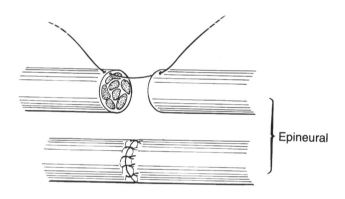

Epineural

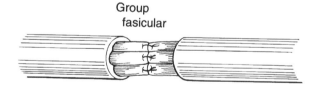

Group
fasicular

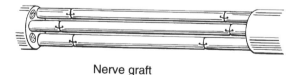

Fig. 6-1. Approximated ends of a lacerated nerve.

Nerve graft

TREATMENT GOALS

I. Restore motor function.
II. Restore sensibility.
III. Minimize recovery time.
IV. Maximize functional recovery. Expected rate of recovery time for nerve repairs is 1 inch per month.[2]
V. Maintain ROM of all upper extremity joints during nerve recovery period.
VI. Provide appropriate preoperative care for delayed repairs or grafts. See section on Postoperative Care with Flexor Tendon Involvement.

POSTOPERATIVE INDICATIONS AND PRECAUTIONS

I. Indications
   A. Primary nerve repair: indicated for a clean, sharply cut nerve in which the damaged ends can be seen and approximated. This type of nerve repair is performed immediately following an injury or within 1 to 3 weeks.[3]
   B. Secondary nerve repair: usually indicated in the presence of a severely crushed or avulsed nerve. This surgery involves recutting the nerve and removal of the neuroma 3 to 6 weeks following injury.[3]
   C. Nerve grafts: usually performed when a direct repair cannot be done without tension or nerve condition is poor. It is often done as a secondary procedure.
II. Precautions
   A. Fractures/dislocations
   B. Stretching of the nerve beyond its elastic limit
   C. Loss of sensation, which could cause secondary injury

POSTOPERATIVE THERAPY FOR PRIMARY OR SECONDARY REPAIR

I. Ulnar and median nerve repairs at the wrist level
   A. 0 to 6 days: rest in dressing with wrist flexed at 30 degrees.
   B. 7 days: position hand in dorsal protection splint with wrist flexed at 30 degrees (Fig. 6-2). For lacerations within the proximal half of the forearm, the elbow is splinted in flexion also. Include a C-bar on the protection splint for median nerve injuries to prevent thumb adduction contracture, active interphalangeal (IP) motion.
   C. 2 weeks: remove sutures. Begin active and passive flexion and extension of IP joints with wrist in flexed position. Begin scar management if wound is healed.

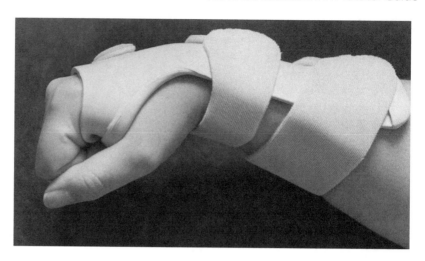

Fig. 6-2. Splinting for wrist level lacerations of median or ulnar nerve.

D. 3 weeks: position wrist in neutral. The test to determine rate of extension splinting is to check for complaints of burning and tingling when gently extending the wrist. Once this has been determined, shape the splint prior to that point of extension.

E. 4 weeks: begin range of motion (ROM) of wrist. Avoid symptoms of irritability. For more proximal lesions in which the elbow was immobilized, begin ROM of elbow when the symptoms are not elicited upon mobilization.

F. 5 weeks: splint only at night and in crowds. Children need to be protected for about 1 week longer than adults. For ulnar nerve lesions, position the hand in a lumbrical block splint to wear during the day and evening.[3] For median nerve repair, if needed, the patient should wear a separate C-bar splint when not wearing a protective splint.[3]

G. 6 weeks: begin wrist extension with fingers extended. Evaluate sensibility. Begin sensory re-education and desensitization program when appropriate. (Refer to sensory evaluation guideline, Ch. 7.)

H. 7 weeks: dynamic splint, if necessary, for joint tightness.

I. 9 to 12 weeks: begin strengthening/work rehabilitation.

II. Radial nerve repair for forearm and above

A. 0 to 6 days: rest in dressing with wrist extended.

B. 7 to 14 days: position hand in forearm based static wrist extension splint with dynamic extension outriggers for fingers and thumb.[3] If lesion more proximal, the elbow should be immobilized.

C. 2 weeks: remove sutures. Begin active and passive flexion and extension of IP joints with metacarpophalangeal (MCP) joints and wrist in extension. Begin friction massage on scar and encourage patient to perform this several times daily, gradually increasing intensity as tolerated. Apply a gel sheet or an elastomer mold to scar once wound is healed.

D. 4 weeks: begin ROM of wrist with fingers extended.

E. 7 weeks: dynamic splint, if necessary, for joint tightness.

F. 9 to 12 weeks: begin strengthening/occupational training.

PREOPERATIVE CARE FOR DELAYED PRIMARY REPAIR OR NERVE GRAFT

I. Goals of therapy

   A. Full passive range of motion (PROM): provide patient with home exercise program to be performed several times a day.

   B. Minimal tendon adherence in the scar: achieved through active movement and scar management techniques.

   C. Promote good skin condition: massage with cream several times a day.

   D. Patient education to avoid injury from sharp objects, heat, pressure areas.

      1. Teach patient to compensate visually for loss of protective sensation.

      2. Have patient wear warm gloves in winter.

      3. Use long-handled cooking utensils.

POSTOPERATIVE CARE WITH FLEXOR TENDON INVOLVEMENT

This is essentially the same as for nerve repair without tendon involvement, except that active flexion of the fingers is postponed until the third or fourth week. Active flexion is performed with the MCP joints in flexion. The major postoperative complication in nerve repair with tendon involvement is flexor tightness of the wrist due to tendon adherence. To help overcome this, scar management techniques are emphasized. Also, finger flexion exercises should be stabilized and performed individually.

POSTOPERATIVE THERAPY FOR NERVE GRAFTS

I. Treatment

   A. 0 to 9 days: wrist is held in neutral, elbow in slight flexion.

   B. 10 days: dressing removed, sutures removed, if needed. Begin very gentle active range of motion (AROM) and PROM.[3,4]

   C. 4 weeks: should expect an advancing Tinel's sign. Begin more progressive AROM and PROM.

   D. 5 weeks: treated like a nerve repair. Refer to the appropriate nerve repair treatment sections.

POSTOPERATIVE COMPLICATIONS

    I. Severe edema
   II. Infection
  III. Neuromas
  IV. Secondary deformity
   V. Severe pain (if noted during ROM exercises, may indicate over-stretching of the nerve)
  VI. Intraneural fibrosis
 VII. Hand burns and/or cuts due to loss of protective sensation

EVALUATION TIME LINE

Evaluations	Time Line
Wound condition	7 days
Edema	7 days
Range of motion	10–14 days
Sensory	6–8 weeks
Manual muscle test	3 months

For sensory and manual muscle testing, re-evaluate once every 6 to 8 weeks thereafter.

ADDENDUM

    I. Effects of nerve lesion on motor function[5,6]
       A. High radial nerve lesion
          1. Wrist drop due to paralysis of wrist extensors.
          2. Diminished abduction and extension of thumb due to paralysis of abductor pollicis longus (APL) and extensor pollicis brevis (EPB).
          3. Inability to extend MCP joints due to paralysis of the long extensors.
          4. Weak grasp and pinch due to the inefficiency of the unopposed long flexors (shortened).
          5. Loss of sensation of the lateral two-thirds of the dorsum of the hand and a portion of the thenar eminence area, as well as the dorsum of the proximal phalanges of the lateral three and one-half fingers.
          6. Weakened supination due to paralysis of the supinator muscle.
       B. Posterior interosseus nerve: presents with the same effects as above, except that sensation is not lost and wrist extension is present, but weakened.

C. Ulnar nerve lesion at the wrist.
  1. Loss of adduction and abduction of the fingers due to paralysis of interossei.
  2. Hyperextension of fourth and fifth MCP joints with flexion of the IP joints due to unopposed action of the extensor digitorum communis (EDC).
  3. Weak thumb adduction due to paralysis of adductor pollicis (AdP).
  4. Loss of opposition of the fifth finger due to paralysis of the opponens digiti quinti.
  5. Weak thumb opposition due to paralysis of the AdP.
  6. Weak MCP flexion due to paralysis of the third and fourth lumbricales.
  7. Weak pinch due to paralysis of the AdP, deep head of the flexor pollicis brevis (FPB), and the first dorsal interosseous.
  8. Weak grasp due to paralysis of the interossei, third and fourth lumbricales, and the flexor digitorum profundus (FDP) of the fourth and fifth fingers.
  9. Sensory nerve loss of volar and dorsal aspects of the medial third of the hand, little finger, and ulnar half of the ring finger.
D. Ulnar nerve lesion in the proximal forearm presents with these additional problems.
  1. Weak IP flexion of IP joints of fourth and fifth fingers due to paralysis of the ulnar half of the FDP.
  2. Weak wrist flexion due to paralysis of the flexor carpi ulnaris (FCU).
E. Median nerve lesion in the proximal forearm
  1. Weak forearm pronation due to paralysis of pronator teres
  2. Weak wrist flexion due to paralysis of flexor carpi radialis (FCR)
  3. Weak finger flexion due to paralysis of flexor digitorum superficialis (FDS)
F. Anterior interosseous nerve (proximal one-third of forearm)
  1. Loss of distal interphalangeal (DIP) joint flexion of the index and middle fingers due to paralysis of FDP to each of these digits
  2. Loss of thumb IP joint flexion due to paralysis of flexor pollicis longus (FPL)
  3. Weak forearm pronation due to paralysis of pronator quadratus
G. Palmar branch of the median nerve (wrist level)
  1. Sensory loss of the central palm area and the palmar surfaces of the lateral three and one-half digits
  2. Weak MCP joint flexion of index and middle fingers due to paralysis of the first two lumbricals
  3. Weak pinch due to paralysis of opponens pollicis (OP), abductor pollicis brevis (APB), and the superficial head of the FPB
  4. Loss of thumb palmar abduction due to paralysis of the APB

REFERENCES

1. Smith KL: Nerve response to injury and repair. p. 609. In Hunter JM (ed): Rehabilitation of the Hand: Surgery and Therapy. 4th Ed. Mosby, St. Louis, 1995
2. Hopkins HL, Smith HD: Willard and Spackman's Occupational Therapy, 6th Ed. p. 468. Lippincott-Raven, Philadelphia, 1983
3. Wilgis EF: Nerve repair and grafting. p. 915. In Green DP (ed): Operative Hand Surgery. 2nd Ed. Vol. 2. Churchill Livingstone, New York, 1988
4. Omer GE, Spinner M: Management of Peripheral Nerve Problems. WB Saunders, Philadelphia, 1980
5. Lampe EW: Clinical Symposium: Surgical Anatomy of the Hand. p. 10. New Jersey Pharmaceutical Division, CIBA-GEIGY Corporation, 1988
6. Tam AM: Nerves. p. 12–1. In Kasch MC, Taylor-Mullins PA, Fullenwider L (eds): Hand Therapy Review Course Study Guide. Hand Therapy Certification Commission, Garner, NC, 1990

SUGGESTED READINGS

Arsham NZ: Nerve injury. p. IV. In Ziegler EM (ed): Current Concepts in Orthotics: A Diagnosis-Related Approach to Splinting. Rolyan Medical Products, Chicago, 1984

Boscheinen MJ, Davey V, Conolly WB: The Hand: Fundamentals of Therapy. p. 60. Butterworth Publishers, Cambridge, 1985

MacKinnon SE, Dellon AL: Surgery of the Peripheral Nerve. Thieme Medical Publishers, New York, 1988

Sunderland S: Nerves and Nerve Injuries. 2nd Ed. Churchill Livingstone, New York, 1978

Trombly CA: Occupational Therapy for Physical Dysfunction. 2nd Ed. p. 357. Williams & Wilkins, Baltimore, 1983

Sensory Evaluation

7

Mallory S. Anthony

The ability of the hand to function and to interact and explore the environment depends on good sensibility. The complexity of the sensory system makes the comprehensive sensory evaluation a challenge to the clinician and creates the need for a battery of tests to provide more accurately a true sensory picture.

The peripheral nerve is composed of motor, sensory, and sympathetic nerve fibers. The sensory evaluation is aimed at examining the sympathetic and sensory nerve fiber integrity. The cell body of the presynaptic sympathetic nerve fibers lies in the anterior horn of the spinal cord, and the postsynaptic sympathetic nerve fibers originate in the neurons of the ganglion located from T_1 to T_7. These unmyelinated fibers will innervate the skin, blood vessels, and hair follicles. The cell body of the sensory nerve fibers lies in the dorsal root ganglia. These sensory nerve fibers terminate in the skin as free nerve endings or end in a number of specialized receptors.

Much controversy exists concerning the neurophysiologic basis of sensory testing. Dellon has done considerable research in this area and outlines end-organ specific tests based on type of stimulus and slowly or rapidly adapting properties of receptors. For example, static two-point is used to test Merkle cell-neurite complex (slowly adapting), and moving two-point is used to test rapidly adapting pacinian and Meissner corpuscles. Others believe that many of these end organs may respond to both high- and low-frequency stimuli, thereby making specific end-organ testing difficult.[1] To further compound this issue, the lack of control of certain variables in our testing compromises accuracy. For example, the difficulty in controlling the velocity and application of force in two-point discrimination and vibration testing (tuning forks) make the results less reliable.[1] The advent of computerized test instruments is making sensory testing more accurate and reliable by controlling many of these variables. For example, the Pressure–Specified Sensory Device (PSSD), introduced by Dellon, gives an actual quantitative measurement of cutaneous pressure threshold from 0.1 to 100 g/mm[2] for one- and two-point discrimination testing.[2] The hand-held device has a dampening mechanism on the surface to reduce oscillations of the examiner's hand. The Automated Tactile Tester (ATT) is another computer-controlled device, which measures the cutaneous perception of touch, vibration, temperature, and pain.[3] This device controls amplitude, rate of application, and duration of stimuli. One disadvantage of computerized test instruments is their high cost. Despite their expense, however, they are invaluable tools that can provide a more accurate assessment of peripheral nerve status, as well as quantitative measures that can be used for research.

Our goals and selection of evaluation tools vary, depending on whether we are examining a nerve compression lesion or a nerve repair. In the case of nerve compression, the larger myelinated fibers, which transmit perception of touch, are most sensitive to ischemia and are affected first. Hence, the first symptoms to develop are related to changes in touch perception, rather than pain or temperature.[2] Nerve compression causes changes in threshold (i.e., the stimulus intensity required to elicit the normal response is altered). In mild compression, the patient may experience a hypersensitive response to stimuli, and symptoms may be elicited only with provocative tests (Table 7-1). Later in the course of nerve compression, the threshold appears to be raised, so that a greater stimulus intensity is required to elicit the same response as before the injury.[4] Threshold tests such as vibration, Semmes–Weinstein monofilaments (touch/pressure), and the PSSD are used to assess this sensory change.

With further compression, and loss of nerve fibers caused by wallerian degeneration, the sensory system will have a diminished number of nerve fibers innervating an area. This decrease in innervation density can be measured by two-point discrimination testing, both moving and static.[5]

In patients following nerve repair, our goals and sensory assessment are directed toward monitoring axonal regeneration and reinnervation

Table 7-1. Nerve Compression Symptoms

Degree of Severity	Pathophysiology	Clinical
Mild	Blood–nerve barrier breakdown	Intermittent paresthesias
Moderate	Demyelination	Mild to moderate abnormal sensory threshold
		Persistent paresthesias
		Abnormal motor threshold
Severe	Axonal loss	Mild to severe abnormal two-point discrimination
		Mild to severe atrophy
		Anesthesia

(Adapted from Dellon,[4] with permission.)

into distal tissue. This will help us evaluate sensory function and indicate the need to begin re-education when necessary.

Factors that affect recovery following nerve repair are (1) time interval between injury and repair, (2) state of stumps at suture line, (3) postoperative stretching and suture line tension, and (4) patient's potential for healing (age, metabolic and nutritional status).[6] The normal rate of axonal regeneration is 1 to 5 mm/day or 1 inch/month if conditions are optimal.

The following protocol is designed to present the components of a comprehensive sensibility evaluation and offer guidelines for the selection of appropriate tests.

DEFINITION

I. Sensation: the conscious perception of basic sensory input. This is what we re-educate.[7]

II. Sensibility: neural events occurring at the periphery, nerve fibers, nerve receptors. This is what we evaluate.[7]

   A. Protective sensibility: return of sensibility as evidenced by the ability to perceive pinprick, touch, and temperature.

   B. Functional sensibility: return of sensibility to a level that enables the hand to engage in full activities of daily living, including those in which vision is occluded while the hand manipulates an object.[8]

   C. Hierarchy of sensibility capacity.[9]

      1. Detection: most simple level of function. Requires that the patient be able to distinguish a single point stimulus from normally occurring atmospheric background stimulation (threshold tests).

      2. Discrimination: the ability to perceive that stimulus A differs from stimulus B. Involves the capacity to detect each stimulus as a separate entity and to distinguish between them (two-point discrimination tests).

      3. Quantification: involves organizing tactile stimuli according to degree. For example: the patient selects which texture is roughest, most irregular, or smooth. (Some sensory re-education techniques incorporate this concept.)

      4. Recognition: most complicated level of function. The ability to identify objects, vision occluded. (Some sensory re-education techniques incorporate this concept as well as the Dellon modification of Moberg pick-up test.)

III. Tactile gnosis: object identification as related to the peripheral nervous system.

IV. Stereognosis: refers to central nervous system (CNS) recognition of objects (cortical).

V. Sensory evaluation: the testing of hand sensibility.

TREATMENT PURPOSE

Nerve injuries or conditions that involve the sensory fibers going to the hand will leave a region of altered sensibility. This sensory deficit may fit a specific pattern. In some cases it is important to document such deficiencies. Documentation of these sensory losses may be important in determining an accurate diagnosis or monitoring the progression of healing in an impaired nerve.

TREATMENT GOALS

   I. Determine the presence of changes in sensibility for nerve compression.
   II. Determine if axonal regeneration is occurring after nerve repair.
   III. Determine the sequence of recovery of sensory submodalities as a guide to instituting sensory re-education after nerve repair.
   IV. Determine the status of sensibility in a way that reflects hand function.

INDICATIONS/PRECAUTIONS FOR EVALUATION

   I. Indications
      A. Peripheral nerve repair, digital nerve repair.
      B. Nerve compressions, contusions.
      C. Replants.
      D. Resurfaced flaps, grafts, and cross-finger flaps.
      E. Brachial plexus injuries.
      F. Crush injuries.
   II. Precautions
      A. Underlying vascular or neuropathic disease, which could lead to nerve ischemia and dysfunction.
      B. Fatigue.
      C. Negative attitude and decreased motivation.
      D. Pain/hypersensitivity.
      E. Excessive callous formation on area being tested.
      F. A distracting or cold testing environment.

THERAPY (EVALUATION)

   I. Patient history
      A. Name, age, sex, dominance, occupation.
      B. Date, nature, and level of injury.
      C. Subjective report of symptoms and what aggravates or relieves these symptoms.

D. Brief assessment of motor function (include grip and pinch), because motor function may affect performance on certain sensibility tests.

E. Patient's medical status.

II. Examination of sympathetic function.[8]

A. Vasomotor changes

1. Temperature, color, and edema (initial warm phase: cold intolerance).

B. Sudomotor change

1. Lack of sweating in autonomous area of sympathetic fibers after denervation.

2. May have increased sweating with nerve irritation.

C. Pilomotor changes

1. Absence of gooseflesh response with complete interruption of sympathetic supply.

D. Trophic changes

1. Skin texture: thin and smooth.

2. Atrophy of finger pulps with long-term denervation.

3. Nail changes: striations, ridges, increased hardness.

4. Hair growth: may fall out in region of denervation or may become longer, finer. May demonstrate increased hair growth (hypertrichosis).[8]

5. Increased susceptibility to injury with slowed healing due to atrophy of epidermis and decreased nutrition and vascularity.[8]

III. Classification of sensibility tests

A. Objective tests: require only passive cooperation of the patient, not subjective interpretation of a stimulus.[8]

1. Ninhydrin test

2. O'Riain wrinkle test

3. Electrodiagnostic tests

B. Threshold tests: determine minimum stimulus that can be perceived by patient.

1. Pain and temperature (heat/cold).

2. Touch/pressure (Semmes–Weinstein monofilaments) (Fig. 7-1) (PSSD).

3. Vibration (Fig. 7-2).

C. Functional tests: assess the quality of sensibility.

1. Moving two-point discrimination (Fig. 7-3).

2. Static two-point discrimination.

3. Localization

4. Dellon modification of Moberg pick-up test.

5. Moberg pick-up test.

IV. Testing variables

A. Testing environment: *quiet,* free from distraction.

B. Patient: *relaxed* and able to concentrate.

C. Be aware of differences between *testing instruments.*

D. Use *standardized method* of testing.

E. *Same examiner* should perform successive tests on a given patient.

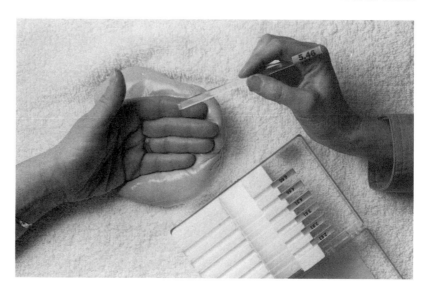

Fig. 7-1. Semmes–Weinstein monofilaments.

      F. Patient's hand should be *fully supported* in examiner's hand or in putty (or similar medium).
  V. Testing techniques
    A. Standard tests
      1. Tinel's sign
        a. Present at site of nerve compression lesion.
        b. Used to monitor level of regenerating sensory axons.
        c. Difficult to test if too much muscle lies over the nerve.
      2. Provocative tests
        a. Direct pressure over suspected compression site.
        b. Manipulation of the extremity to render the nerve locally ischemic, for example, wrist flexion (Phalen's

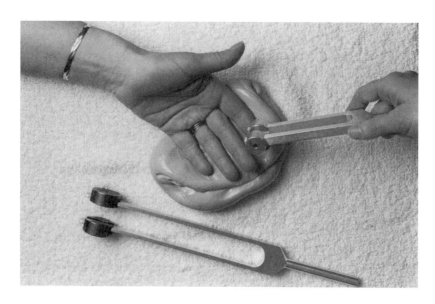

Fig. 7-2. Tuning forks may be used for vibratory testing.

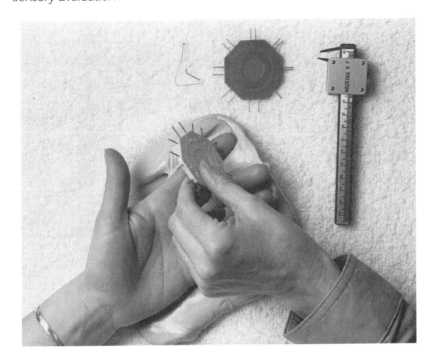

Fig. 7-3. Devices that may be used to assess two-point discrimination.

test) (Fig. 7-4) for median nerve compression at wrist [carpal tunnel syndrome (CTS)], elbow flexion for ulnar nerve compression at elbow (cubital tunnel) (Fig. 7-5), forearm pronation with wrist flexion and ulnar deviation for radial sensory nerve compression[5] (Fig. 7-6).

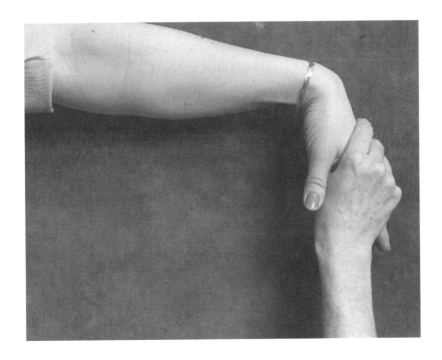

Fig. 7-4. Phalen's test.

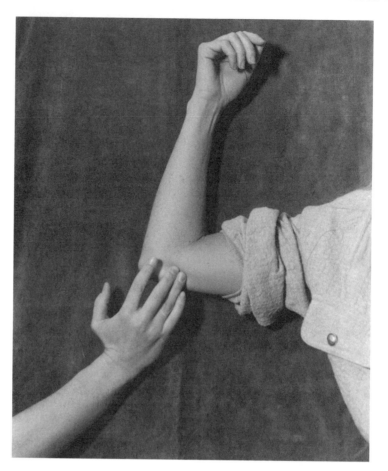

Fig. 7-5. Provocative test for ulnar nerve at elbow (cubital tunnel).

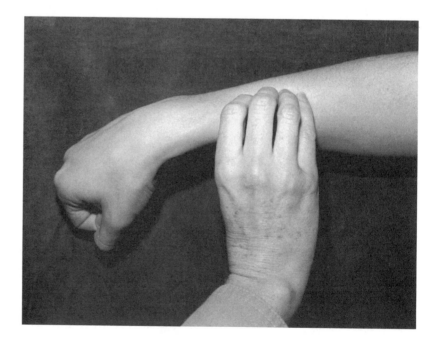

Fig. 7-6. Provocative test for radial sensory nerve compression.

3. Pain assessment
   a. Intensity (rating scale from "no pain" to "unbearable pain").
   b. Location (map out or describe painful area).
   c. Frequency
   d. Type (burning, throbbing, aching, stabbing, tingling, cramping, etc.).
   e. Factors that increase or decrease pain.
   f. Other factors (e.g., patient taking pain medication).
   g. Other tests (McGill Pain Questionnaire, modified Hendler's pain scale, the ATT).
4. Touch/pressure
   a. Semmes–Weinstein monofilaments
      i. Used as a stimulus to establish the threshold of touch ranging from light touch (a necessary component of fine discrimination) to deep pressure (a form of protective sensation).
      ii. Helpful in monitoring return of sensibility in the early months after nerve repair and helpful in assessing early changes in sensibility caused by nerve compression.
      iii. The technique and procedure for administering the Semmes–Weinstein monofilaments test is described in detail in References 1 and 10.
      iv. The minikit can be used and consists of five filaments representing the cut-off forces for each functional level of sensibility (i.e., normal, diminished light touch, diminished protective sensation, and loss of protective sensation). The Weinstein Enhanced Sensory Test also consists of 5 filaments and was designed to increase the ease of portability, speed of testing, and resistance to damage, as well as reduce tip slippage on skin and provide consistent pressures on skin.[8]
      v. Interpretation of test results can be found in Appendices 7-1 and 7-2.
   b. Pressure–specified sensory device
      i. Computer-assisted sensory testing device
      ii. Provides quantitative measurements for the pressure at which two-point discrimination is possible, and for one-point static touch threshold (the threshold estimated by Semmes–Weinstein monofilaments).
      iii. Very sensitive for determining early signs of nerve compression, as it measures the pressure at which two points can be distinguished from one; this threshold becomes abnormal before one-point static.[2]
      iv. May be more sensitive in diagnosing early nerve entrapment syndromes than electrodiagnostic testing.[11]
      v. Can be used as screening tool on job sites to detect early signs of cumulative trauma to peripheral nerves.

           vi. Can be used to monitor progress of neural regeneration.
       vii. An example of PSSD computer printout can be found in Appendix 7-2.
    5. Vibration 30 cps
      a. Tuning fork (30 cps and 256 cps)
        i. Useful in diagnosing digital nerve injuries, in which a perceived difference in vibration exists between the two tested autonomous zones of the digit.
       ii. Useful in detecting earliest sensory changes in nerve compression, since the large group A beta fibers, which carry the perceptions of light touch and vibration, are affected first by the ischemia.
          A. The fingertips of the thumb and index are test sites in median nerve compression.
          B. The tip of the small finger is the test site for ulnar nerve compression.
      iii. Useful following nerve repair to document return of vibration to the affected area. When 30 cps reaches palm, may begin early phase sensory re-education.
      iv. Patient should localize the stimulus because perception of the stimuli may occur through an adjacent peripheral field of a noninjured nerve, for example, radial nerve with a median nerve injury.[6]
       v. The technique and procedure for administering vibration testing are described in Reference 6. The pronged end of the tuning fork is applied to the test site, as suggested by Dellon, because the fingertips have a significant amount of subcutaneous tissue and a more intense stimulus is needed, especially when the threshold level is raised. Also, tuning fork should be warmed before testing, as patient may react to the coldness rather than vibration.
      b. Vibrometer[8]
        i. Many different types available (Bio-Thesiometer, Optacon, Neurometer)
       ii. Has wide range of varying amplitudes
      iii. Has same limitations as other hand-held testing instruments
      iv. Does provide a more quantitative assessment of vibration than the tuning fork.
      c. Automated Tactile Tester
        i. Computer-controlled device that varies the intensity of the stimulus at low and high frequencies of vibration.
       ii. Controls rate and duration of stimulus
      iii. More reliable and sensitive than hand-held instruments.
    6. Moving touch (as described by Dellon)
      a. Used to test return of light and heavy movement following nerve repair.

    b. Helps determine when to begin early phase sensory re-education.[6]

    c. Technique (unpublished protocol and Reference 12): Both light and heavy movement is tested using middle finger to stroke small areas of the extremity, above and below nerve repair site, moving proximal to distal along dysfunctioning nerve distribution. Light versus heavy refers to intensity of the stimulus.

    d. Procedure (unpublished protocol and Reference 12): Patient is instructed to close eyes and then respond to the moving stimulus by indicating whether the stimulus was felt and if so, where. Responses for both light and heavy movement are documented on the sensory evaluation form with appropriate symbols, and a description of "feeling" is recorded.

7. Constant touch (as described by Dellon)

    a. Used to test return of light and heavy touch following nerve repair.

    b. Helps to determine when to begin late phase sensory re-education.

    c. Technique (unpublished protocol and Reference 12). Both light and heavy touch is tested using middle finger to touch different areas on the extremity above and below the nerve repair site, moving proximal to distal along dysfunctioning nerve distribution. Each stimulus should be maintained for no longer than one-half second. Light versus heavy refers to the intensity of the pressure applied.

    d. Procedure: Same as described under moving touch.

8. Moving two-point discrimination

    a. A measure of innervation density (number of functioning nerve fiber-receptors for a given area), and a measure of hand function requiring moving touch,[13,14] for example, object identification (tactile gnosis) and fine manipulative tasks (such as buttoning a button).

    b. Tested when moving touch is perceived at the fingertip, following nerve repair.[6]

    c. Normal values are elevated in later stages of nerve compression (due to decrease in innervation density).

    d. According to methods described by Dellon:[6,14]

       i. Testing is begun with instrument set 6 to 8 mm between the two points.

      ii. The instrument is moved proximally to distally on the fingertip perpendicular to the long axis of the finger with the testing ends side by side.

     iii. The pressure used is just light enough so that the patient can perceive the stimulus without discomfort (skin blanching itself is not a guide to stimulus intensity).

     iv. The patient is required to respond accurately to two out of three stimuli before the distance is narrowed.[10]

    e. The same two-point device should be used for all testing, as the terminal probes can produce significant variations in response.[15,16] Ends should be blunt to ensure testing of touch not pain.

    f. Moving two-point discrimination returns earlier than static two-point (following nerve repair), approaching normal 2 to 6 months before static two-point.[6]

    g. Values for normal and abnormal moving two-point discrimination can be found in Appendix 7-3 (key section of sensory evaluation form).

9. Static two-point discrimination

    a. A measure of innervation density; assesses patient's ability to perform tasks requiring precision grip[14] (i.e., holding a pencil to write or a needle to sew).

    b. Tested when constant touch is perceived at the fingertip, following nerve repair.[6]

    c. Normal values are elevated in later stages of nerve compression (due to decrease in innervation density).

    d. According to methods described by Dellon:[6,14]

      i. Testing is begun with instrument set 6 to 8 mm between the two points.

      ii. The instrument is placed on the fingertip parallel to the long axis of the finger (testing ends lie proximal/distal).

      iii. The pressure used is the same as for moving two-point discrimination.

      iv. The patient is required to respond accurately to two out of three stimuli before the distance is narrowed.[10]

    e. The same two-point device should be used for all testing, as the terminal probes can produce significant variations in response.[15,16] Ends should be blunt to ensure testing of touch not pain.

    f. Static two-point discrimination recovers 2 to 6 months slower than moving two-point and, therefore, is a later assessment of discrimination.

    g. Values for normal and abnormal static two-point discrimination can be found in Appendix 7-3 (key section of sensory evaluation form).

    h. Recommended test instruments for two-point discrimination testing include Disk-Criminator and Boley Gauge.

10. Localization of touch

    a. A more integrated level of perception than simple recognition of stimulus.

    b. May be tested while assessing recovery of vibration, touch/pressure, and two-point discrimination.

    c. May be tested and recorded as a separate function, that is, recording both the site of stimulation and the patient's perceived site of referral on a drawing of the hand (e.g., a touch stimulus to the index may be perceived in the thumb tip).

       d. The patient's record of localization is useful in planning a sensory re-education program.
- B. Additional functional and objective tests
  - 1. Moberg pick-up test

    The patient is asked to pick up a number of everyday objects and put them into a small box, first with involved hand, then with uninvolved, both with eyes open, then eyes closed. Time required and manner of prehension are noted.[6,8,17]
  - 2. Dellon modification of Moberg pick-up test
    - a. Dellon has modified Moberg's test by standardizing the items used and requiring identification of them.
    - b. Objects of similar material are used to avoid giving clues by texture or temperature, and objects are graded to require increasing ability to discriminate.
    - c. Specific testing technique and procedure can be found in References 6 and 8.
  - 3. Ninhydrin test
    - a. An objective test of sympathetic function most helpful when testing children, patients with language problems, or malingerers.
    - b. The test identifies areas of decreased sweat secretion after peripheral nerve disruption: the Ninhydrin spray turns purple when it reacts with amino acids in sweat.
    - c. Specific technique and procedure can be found in References 17 and 18.
    - d. Frequently parallels recovery of pain and temperature (i.e., protective sensation).[6]
    - e. Does not correlate with return of sensory function.
  - 4. O'Riain wrinkle test
    - a. An objective test that identifies areas of denervation (i.e., denervated skin does not wrinkle, as does normal skin when soaked in warm water).
    - b. Specific technique and procedure can be found in References 18 and 19.
    - c. Does not correlate with return of sensory function.
- VI. Recommendations for test selection
  - A. Compression syndromes
    - 1. Tinel's sign
    - 2. Provocative tests
    - 3. PSSD (if available) to detect earliest signs of nerve compression (i.e., abnormal threshold for two-point discrimination).
    - 4. Electrodiagnostic testing
    - 5. Vibration tests
    - 6. Touch/pressure threshold tests: Semmes–Weinstein monofilaments or PSSD.
    - 7. Static and moving two-point discrimination to detect advanced sensory changes.
  - B. Nerve repair
    - 1. Examination of hand for sympathetic dysfunction.

2. Tinel's to determine level of regenerating axons.
3. Vibration (30 cps), moving touch, constant touch, and vibration (256 cps).
4. Semmes–Weinstein monofilaments to help assess level of touch return.
5. PSSD to quantify pressure threshold.
6. When return of touch reaches fingertips, static and moving two-point on fingertips, with localization of touch over entire area of dysfunction, will determine level of functional return.
7. Moberg pick-up or Dellon modification.

POSTOPERATIVE COMPLICATIONS

I. Neuroma
II. Continued decrease in sensibility.
III. Continued hypersensitivity (see protocol on desensitization).

EVALUATION TIMELINE

I. Nerve repair
   A. Baseline evaluation at 6 to 8 weeks postoperatively.
   B. Re-evaluation every 6 to 8 weeks.
   C. Begin desensitization and re-education when appropriate (as described in Chs. 8 and 9).

REFERENCES

1. Bell-Krotoski JA: Sensibility testing: state of the art. p. 109. In Hunter JM, Schneider LH, Mackin EJ, Callahan AD (eds): Rehabilitation of the Hand: Surgery and Therapy. 4th Ed. Mosby, St Louis, 1995
2. Dellon AL: Somatosensory Testing and Rehabilitation. AOTA, Silverspring, MD, 1996
3. Horch K, Hardy M, Jimenez S, Jabalay M: An automated tactile tester for evaluation of cutaneous sensibility. J Hand Surg 17A:829, 1992
4. Dellon AL: A numerical grading scale for peripheral nerve function. J Hand Ther 6:152, 1993
5. MacKinnon SE, Dellon AL: Classification of nerve injuries as the basis for treatment. p. 35. In: Surgery of the Peripheral Nerve. 1st Ed. Thieme Medical Publishers, New York, 1988
6. Dellon AL: Evaluation of Sensibility and Re-education of Sensation in the Hand. Williams & Wilkins, Baltimore, 1981
7. MacKinnon SE, Dellon AL: Sensory rehabilitation after nerve injury. p. 521. In: Surgery of the Peripheral Nerve. 1st Ed. Thieme Medical Publishers, New York, 1988
8. Callahan AD: Sensibility assessment: prerequisites and techniques for nerve lesions in continuity and nerve lacerations. p. 129. In Hunter JM, Mackin EJ, Callahan AD (eds): Rehabilitation of the Hand: Surgery and Therapy. 4th Ed. Mosby, St. Louis, 1995

9. Fess EE: Documentation: essential elements of an upper extremity assessment battery. p. 185. In Hunter JM, Mackin EJ, Callahan AD (eds): Rehabilitation of the Hand: Surgery and Therapy. 4th Ed. Mosby, St. Louis, 1995

10. Bell-Krotoski JA: Light touch-deep pressure testing using Semmes-Weinstein monofilaments. p. 585. In Hunter JM, Schneider LH, Mackin EJ, Callahan AD (eds): Rehabilitation of the Hand: Surgery and Therapy. 3rd Ed. Mosby, St. Louis, 1990

11. Tassler PL, Dellon AL: Correlation of measurements of pressure perception using the pressure-specified sensory device with electrodiagnostic testing. J Environ Med 37:862, 1995

12. Dellon AL, Edgerton MT: Evaluating recovery of sensation in the hand following nerve injury. Hopkins Med J 130:235, 1972

13. MacKinnon SE, Dellon AL: Diagnosis of nerve injury. p. 65. In: Surgery of the Peripheral Nerve. 1st Ed. Thieme Medical Publishers, New York, 1988

14. Dellon AL, MacKinnon SE, Crosby PM: Reliability of two-point discrimination measurements. J Hand Surg 12A:693, 1987

15. Crosby PM, Dellon AL: Comparison of two-point discrimination testing devices. Microsurgery 10:134, 1989

16. Levin LS, Regan N, Pearsall LG, Nunley JA: Variations in two-point discrimination as a function of terminal probes. Microsurgery 10:236, 1989

17. Moberg E: Objective methods for determining the functional value of sensibility in the hand. J Bone Joint Surg 40B:454, 1958

18. Phelps PE, Walker E: Comparison of the finger wrinkling test results to establish sensory tests in peripheral nerve injury. Am J Occup Ther 31:565, 1977

19. O'Riain S: New and simple test of nerve function in the hand. Br Med J 3:615, 1973

SUGGESTED READINGS

Bell-Krotoski JA, Buford WL: The force/time relationship of clinically used sensory testing instruments. J Hand Ther 1:76, 1988

Bell-Korotoski JA: Advances in sensibility testing. Hand Clin 7:527, 1991

Bell-Korotoski J, Weinstein S, Weinstein C: Testing sensibility, including touch-pressure, two-point discrimination, point localization, and vibration. J Hand Ther 6:114, 1993

Dellon AL: Sensory recovery in replanted digits and transplanted toes: a review. J Reconstr Microsurg 2:123, 1986

Dellon AL: "Think Nerve" in upper extremity reconstruction. Clin Plast Surg 16:617, 1989

Dellon AL: Sensibility testing. p. 135. In Gelberman RH (ed): Operative Nerve Repair and Reconstruction. Lippincott–Raven, Philadelphia, 1991

Eversmann WW: Compression and entrapment neuropathies of the upper extremity. J Hand Surg 8:759, 1983

Frykman G: The quest for better recovery from peripheral nerve injury: current status of nerve regeneration research. J Hand Ther 6:83, 1993

Greenspan JD, Lamotte RH: Cutaneous mechanoreceptors of the hand: experimental studies and their implications for clinical testing of tactile sensation. J Hand Ther 6:75, 1993

Hardy M, Jimenez S, Jabalay M, Horch K: Evaluation of nerve compression with the automated tactile tester. J Hand Surg 17A:838, 1992

Louis DS, Greene TC, Jacobson KE et al: Evaluation of normal values for stationary and moving two-point discrimination in the hand. J Hand Surg 9A:552, 1984

MacDermid JC, Kramer JF, Roth JH: Decision making in detecting abnormal Semmes-Weinstein monofilament thresholds in carpal tunnel syndrome. J Hand Ther July-Sept:158, 1994

MacKinnon SE, Dellon AL: Two-point discrimination tester. J Hand Surg 10A:906, 1985

Melzack R, Wall PD: On the nature of cutaneous sensory mechanisms. Brain 85:331, 1962

Moberg E: The unsolved problem — how to test the functional value of hand sensibility. J Hand Ther, July-Sept:105, 1991

Nishikawa H, Smith PJ: The recovery of sensation and function after cross-finger flaps for fingertip injury. J Hand Surg 17B:102, 1992

Novak CB, MacKinnon SE, Williams JI, Kelly L: Establishment of reliability in the evaluation of hand sensibility. J Plast Reconstr Surg 92:311, 1993

Omer GE: Nerve response to injury and repair. p. 515. In Hunter JM, Schneider LH, Mackin EJ, Callahan AD (eds): Rehabilitation of the Hand: Surgery and Therapy. 3rd Ed. Mosby, St. Louis, 1990

Szabo RM, Gelberman RH, Dimick MP: Sensibility testing in patients with carpal tunnel syndrome. J Bone Joint Surg 66A:60, 1984

Tubiana R: Examination of the Hand and Upper Limb. WB Saunders, Philadelphia, 1984

Waylett-Rendall J: Sequence of sensory recovery: a retrospective study. J Hand Ther 2:245, 1989

Waylett-Rendall J: From the periphery to the somatosensory cortex—a global view of nerves and their function. J Hand Ther 6:71, 1993

Weinstein S: Fifty years of somatosensory research: From the Semmes-Weinstein monofilaments to the Weinstein enhanced sensory test. J Hand Ther Jun-Mar:11, 1993

Werner JL, Omer GE: Evaluating cutaneous pressure sensation of the hand. Am J Occup Ther 24:347, 1970

Appendix 7-1

Semmes–Weinstein Monofilaments*

INTERPRETATION AND RELATIONSHIP TO FUNCTION

The interpretation of monofilament force levels was based on the review I made of 150 cases and 200 tests of patients with peripheral nerve problems at the Philadelphia Hand Center, Ltd, Philadelphia, from 1976 to 1978. Subsequent discussion of the data with von Prince and experience in use of the interpretation in patients with peripheral nerve problems over the last 15 years has continued to support the relationship of force thresholds to functional sensibility. Comparisons were made between the Semmes–Weinstein monofilaments and other tests of sensibility routinely given to patients as a test battery. The results are summarized in Fig. 9-15.

Normal touch is a recognition of light touch, and therefore deep pressure, that is within normal limits. This level is the most significant of all levels because it allows the examiner to distinguish between areas of normal sensibility and areas of sensory diminution.

Diminished light touch is diminished recognition of light touch. If a patient has diminished light touch, provided that his motor status and cognitive abilities are in play, he has fair use of his hand, his graphesthesia and stereognosis are both close to normal and adaptable, he has good temperature appreciation, he definitely has good protective sensation, he most often will have fair to good two-point discrimination, and he may not even realize he has had a sensory loss.

Diminished protective sensation is just that. If a patient has diminished protective sensation, he will have diminished use of his hands, he will have difficulty manipulating some objects, he will have a tendency to drop some objects, and he may complain of weakness of his hand, but he will have an appreciation of the pain and temperature that should help keep him from injury, and he will have some manipulative skill. Sensory reeducation can begin at this level. It is possible for a patient to have a gross appreciation of two-point discrimination at this level (7 to 10 mm).

Loss of protective sensation is again what it says. If a patient has loss of protective sensation he will have little use of his hand, he will have a

---

*(From Bell-Krotoski,[1] with permission.)

diminished, if not absent, temperature appreciation, he will not be able to manipulate objects outside his line of vision, he will have a tendency to injure himself easily, and it may even be dangerous for him to be around machinery. He will, however, be able to feel a pinprick and have deep pressure sensation, which does not make him totally asensory. Instructions on protective care are helpful to prevent injury.

If a patient is *untestable*, he may or may not feel a pinprick but will have no other discrimination of levels of feeling. If a patient feels a pinprick in an area otherwise untestable, it is important to note this during the mapping. Instructions on protective care of the hand are mandatory at this level to prevent the normally occurring problems associated with the asensory hand.

SCALE OF INTERPRETATION OF MONOFILAMENTS

		Filament Markings	Calculated Force (g)*
Green	Normal	1.65–**2.83**	0.0045–0.068
Blue	Diminished light touch	3.22–**3.61**	0.166–0.408
Purple	Diminished protective sensation	3.84–**4.31**	0.697–2.06
Red	Loss of protective sensation	**4.56–6.65**	3.63–447
Red-lined	Untestable	Greater than 6.65	Greater than 447

*Force data from Semmes J and Weinstein S: Somatosensory Changes After Penetrating Brain Wounds in Man. Harvard University Press, Cambridge, MA, 1960. Minikit monofilaments are in bold. Descriptive levels based on other scales of interpretation and collapse of data from 200 patient tests.

Appendix 7-2

Quantitative Sensory Testing

Pressure Sensory One / Two Point Device

Location	1 PT Static GM/SQmm	2 PT Static GM/SQmm	MM	1 PT Moving GM/SQmm	2 PT Moving GM/SQmm	MM
Left						
Index	40.0	30.2	10.1	36.0	49.8	10.1
Little	1.0	2.5	5.5	1.0	0.7	5.5
Thenar palm	39.3	37.2	22.0	57.0	25.5	22.0
Right						
Index	53.6			85.5	76.8	13.5
Little	1.4	2.9	6.0	0.9	2.2	6.2
Thenar palm	73.5	76.3	25.0	60.8	60.6	25.0

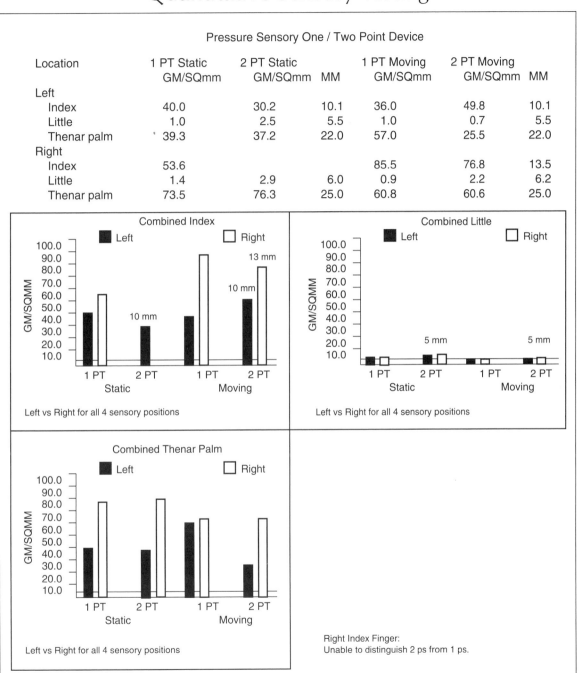

Right Index Finger:
Unable to distinguish 2 ps from 1 ps.

(Courtesy of Lee Dellon, M.D., Baltimore, MD.)

Appendix 7-3

THE UNION MEMORIAL HOSPITAL BALTIMORE, MARYLAND 21218	DATE	IMPRINT WITH PATIENT CHARGE PLATE
HAND SENSIBILITY EVALUATION		

Diagnosis: _____ Date & Type of Operation _____

_____   _____

SUBJECTIVE COMPLAINTS

_____

_____

RIGHT   LEFT

TWO-POINT DISCRIMINATION

	R MOVING	STATIC (WEBER)	L MOVING	STATIC (WEBER)
THUMB				
INDEX				
3RD				
4TH				
5TH				

COMMENTS:

KEY

xx	30 c.p.s.
**	256 c.p.s.
—	Light Movement
= =	Heavy Movement
°°	Light Touch
⬤⬤	Heavy Touch
X	Tinel's

Two-Point (Static)

2-6 mm	Normal
7-10 mm	Fair
11-15 mm	Poor
16 mm	Non-Functional

Two-Point (Moving)

2-3 mm	Normal
4-6 mm	Fair
7-9 mm	Poor

Semmes-Weinstein

1.65-2.83	Normal
3.22-3.61	Diminished Light Touch
3.84-4.31	Diminished Protective
4.56-6.65	Loss of Protective
6.65	Untestable

Therapist's Signature _____

License No. _____

SENSORY TESTING (A GENERAL GUIDELINE)

Sensory Level	Tests	Test Results	Additional Tests	Functional Level
Untestable	Pin prick or Semmes–Weinstein 6.65	Negative response	—	Nonfunctional Protective care instruction mandatory
Loss of protective	Pin prick or Semmes–Weinstein 4.56–6.56	Positive response	Vibration Temperature	Tendency to injure hand Protective care instruction helpful
Decreased protective	Semmes–Weinstein (SW)	Possible hypersensitivity 3.84–4.31 SW	—	Decreased use of hand Some manipulative skills Tendency to drop objects
Diminished light touch	Semmes–Weinstein (SW)	3.22–3.61 SW	Moberg pick-up test or Dellon modification	Fair use of hand Close to normal graphesthesia and tactile gnosis
Moving touch out to fingertips	Moving two-point discrimination	7–9 mm (poor) 4–6 mm (fair)	Moberg pick-up test or Dellon modification	Fair use of hand Good hand function and tactile gnosis May still drop objects
Constant touch out to fingertips	Static two-point discrimination	11–15 mm (poor) 7–10 mm (fair)	Moberg pick-up test or Dellon modification	Fair use of hand Good hand function
Normal sensation	Moving two-point Static two-point Semmes–Weinstein	2–3 mm 2–6 mm 2.36–2.83	— — —	Return to normal level of function

Desensitization 8

Mallory S. Anthony

Hypersensitivity often occurs after hand trauma. The patient experiences an exaggerated, painful response to a normally nonpainful stimuli, at or near the injury site. (This hypersensitivity should not be confused with the general manifestations of pain, as seen in causalgia or the shoulder–hand syndrome.) Desensitization techniques are used to diminish symptoms of hypersensitivity and are designed to gradually increase the patient's tolerance for touch to the area. Desensitization techniques are identical in concept to sensory re-education. Instead of the patient learning to associate an old name with a new pattern of transmitted impulses to identify an object he or she is touching, the patient is learning to filter out the unpleasant sensations to permit perception of the underlying meaningful sensory input.[1] This is re-education of unpleasant sensations instead of re-education of touch.

The following protocol suggests several techniques, based on the use of graded stimuli, beginning with nonirritating media and progressing to stronger types of stimulation.

DEFINITION

  I. Hypersensitivity (hyperalgesia): a condition of extreme discomfort or irritability in response to normally non-noxious tactile stimulation.
  II. Desensitization: the use of modalities and procedures designed to reduce the symptoms of hypersensitivity.

TREATMENT PURPOSE

To gradually increase the patient's tolerance to tactile stimulation in an area of hypersensitivity.

TREATMENT GOALS

To help patient achieve maximal level of function by increasing tolerance to touch in the hypersensitive area.

INDICATIONS/PRECAUTIONS FOR THERAPY

I. Indications
    A. Neuromas
    B. Sensitive amputated tips (stumps).
    C. Hypersensitive scars and surrounding areas.
    D. Nerve injuries with dysesthesia (a painful and persistent sensation induced by a gentle touch of the skin).
II. Precautions
    A. Diffuse pain
    B. Areas with open wounds.
    C. Deep pain not remediated with desensitization.

THERAPY

I. Evaluation of hypersensitivity.
    A. Evaluation of pain may be assessed with visual analog scale and/or McGill Pain Questionnaire.
    B. Measure active and passive range of motion.
    C. Assess level of tolerance of patient's hypersensitive area to textures, contact particles, and vibration (i.e., what is the most irritating stimulus the patient can tolerate?). The Three Phase Hand Sensitivity Test can be used and is the only commercially available test to date[2,3] (Appendix 8-1).
    D. Measure grip and pinch strength.
    E. Assess activities of daily living (ADL) and function.

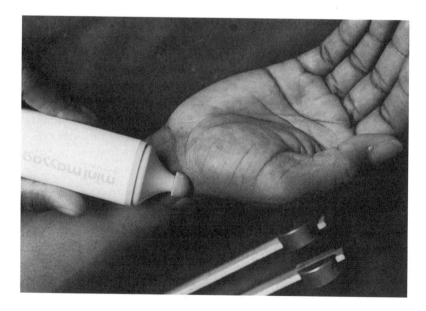

Fig. 8-1. Graded vibration can range from tuning fork to battery or electric powered vibrators.

II. Desensitization program
  A. Treatment time: 5 to 10 minutes (stop when stimulus becomes noxious), three to four times a day.
  B. Demonstrate technique on self or patient's noninvolved side.
  C. May need to protect the area initially (splint with bubble, gel sheet, elastomer, cuff of lamb's wool).
  D. The less irritating stimulus should feel comfortable before advancing to a more irritating stimulus.
III. Techniques (based on a hierarchy of least irritating stimulus to most)
  A. Vibration
    1. Graded uses of vibration can range from tuning fork to battery or electric powered vibrators with various shaped attachments and varying speeds (Fig. 8-1).
    2. Progression can range from stimulating only the periphery of the hypersensitive area, to intermittent stimulation of actual area, to continuous contact with actual area as tolerance allows.
  B. Texture
    1. Graded textures can be used to stroke and tap the hypersensitive area.
    2. The following list is a suggested guideline of progression:
      a. Cotton
      b. Lamb's wool
      c. Felt
      d. Orthopedic felt (1/8 inch)
      e. Orthopedic felt (1/4 inch)
      f. Terrycloth towel
      g. Velcro loops
      h. Velcro hook or fine grades of sandpaper (Fig. 8-2).

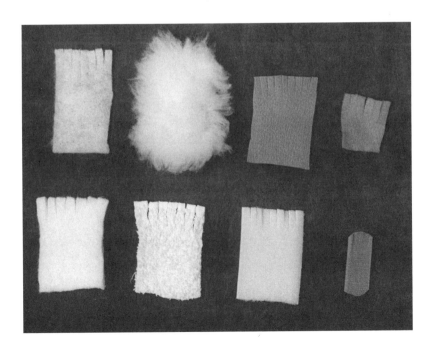

Fig. 8-2. Examples of graded textures to be used in hypersensitive areas.

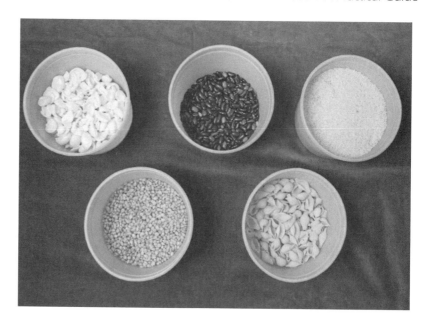

Fig. 8-3. Examples of particle media.

   C. Immersion particles
     1. Immersion of the involved hand into a number of containers filled with particles ranging from least irritating to most.
     2. The following is a suggested list of particle media (Fig. 8-3).
       a. Cotton
       b. Styrofoam pieces
       c. Sand
       d. Beans
       e. Popcorn
       f. Rice
       g. Macaroni
   D. Maintained pressure
     1. The use of continuous mild pressure with an Isotoner glove, gelsheet, or elastomer mold can also increase comfort in hypersensitive area.
     2. Progress treatment using varying degrees of pressure over area, including weight-bearing pressure as patient tolerates.
   E. Other modalities to decrease hypersensitivity
     1. Massage
     2. Tapping
     3. Transcutaneous electrical nerve stimulator (TENS) directly on or adjacent to hypersensitive area (Fig. 8-4).
     4. Fluidotherapy (Fig. 8-5)
     5. Moist heat for relaxation.
   F. Therapeutic activities to regain confidence and restore function.
     1. Theraplast and exercises for strengthening
     2. Work simulation and/or craft activities should be included as soon as tolerated (Fig. 8-6).

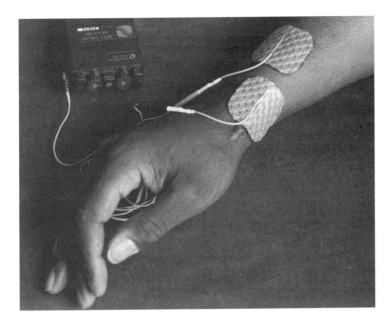

Fig. 8-4. TENS used to decrease hypersensitivity.

    3. Resume re-education if necessary, after hypersensitivity is gone.
G. Stimuli that may magnify pain symptoms (and should be avoided in early desensitization treatment):[3]
    1. Exposure to cold
    2. Emotional stress
    3. Local irritants

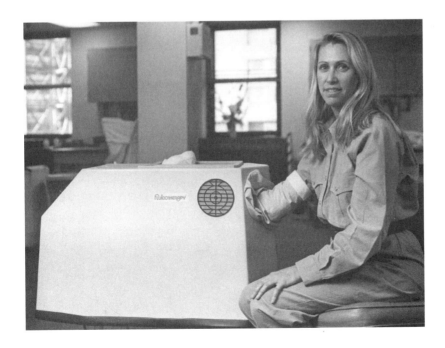

Fig. 8-5. Fluidotherapy.

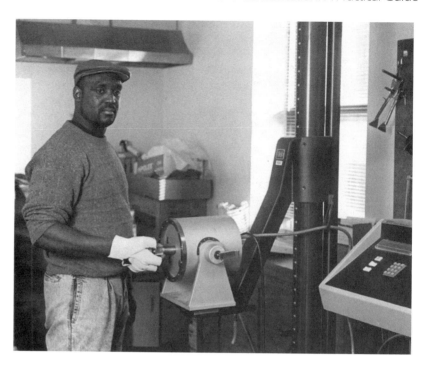

Fig. 8-6. Work simulation to regain confidence and restore function.

COMPLICATIONS THAT MAY CAUSE HYPERSENSITIVITY

    I. Nerve regeneration without an intact endoneural tube.
   II. Scar formation of regenerating axons with or without constriction.
  III. Neuroma formation.
  IV. Adherence of nerve to its bed.
   V. Constriction of blood flow causing ischemic pain.

EVALUATION TIMELINE

Initially, patient should be rechecked two to three times a week for treatment, assessment, and home program reviews. Gradually decrease frequency of visits as patient feels comfortable with home program and shows improvement. Then recheck once a month until discharge.

REFERENCES

1. MacKinnon SE, Dellon AL: Sensory rehabilitation after nerve injury. p. 521. In: Surgery of the Peripheral Nerve. 1st Ed. Thieme Medical Publishers, New York, 1988

2. Barber LM: Desensitization of the traumatized hand. p. 721. In Hunter JM, Schneider LH, Mackin EJ, Callahan AD (eds): Rehabilitation of the Hand: Surgery and Therapy. 3rd Ed. Mosby, St. Louis, 1990

3. Waylett-Rendell J: Desensitization of the traumatized hand. p. 693. In Hunter JM, Mackin EJ, Callahan AD (eds): Rehabilitation of the Hand: Surgery and Therapy. 4th Ed. Mosby, St. Louis, 1995

SUGGESTED READINGS

(Please also refer to Ch. 7—Sensory Evaluation—Suggested Readings)

Campbell JN et al: Peripheral neural mechanisms of nociception. p. 22. In Wall PD, Melzack R (eds): Textbook of Pain. 2nd Ed. Churchill Livingstone, New York, 1989

Campbell JN, Raja SN, Meyer RA, MacKinnon SE: Myelinated fibers in peripheral nerves signal hyperalgesia that follows nerve injury. Pain 32:89, 1988

Davis RW: Phantom sensation, phantom pain, and stump pain. Arch Phys Med Rehabil 74:79, 1993

Dellon AL: Techniques of sensory re-education. In: Somatosensory Testing and Rehabilitation. AOTA, Silver Spring, MD, 1996

Hardy MA, Moran CA, Merritt WH: Desensitization of the traumatized hand. Virginia Med 109:134, 1982

Hochreiter NW et al: Effect of vibration on tactile sensitivity. Phys Ther 63(6), 1983

Jensen TS et al: Phantom limb, phantom pain and stump pain in amputees during the first six months following limb amputation. Pain 17:243, 1983

Melzack R: Phantom limbs, Sci Am April:120, 1992

Melzack R: The puzzle of pain. Basic Books, New York, 1973

Merzenich NM, Jenkins WM: Reorganization of cortical representations of the hand following alterations of skin inputs induced by nerve injury, skin island transfers and experience. J Hand Ther 6:89, 1993

Sachs F: Biophysics of mechanoreceptors. Membr Biochem 6:173, 1986

Sunderland S: Nerve Injuries and Their Repair: A Critical Appraisal. p. 305. Churchill Livingstone, New York, 1991

Wilson RL: Management of pain following peripheral nerve injuries. Orthop Clin North Am 12:343, 1981

Wolpe J: Systematic desensitization. J Nerve Ment Dis 132:189, 1961

Appendix 8-1

THREE PHASE DESENSITIZATION RECORD FORM

1 NAME _John Doe_ _____ AGE _25_ SEX _M_

2 DIAGNOSIS _Median Nerve Laceration (Partial)_ _____

3 SOURCE OF PAIN: AMPUTATION _____ SCAR _____ CRUSH _____ NEUROMA _____ BURN _____ OTHER _See above_

4 DESCRIPTION OF PAINFUL AREA: INITIAL: _3/7/95_ _____

5   DISCHARGE: _____

6 DOMINANCE: RIGHT _X_ LEFT _____

7 HOW INJURY OCCURRED _____

8 DATE OF INJURY _12/5/94_ DATE OF SURGERY _12/7/94_ DATE OF 1ST RX: _12/30/94_

9 NO. OF WEEKS FROM D.O.I. OR SURGERY TO 1ST DESEN. RX: _3 weeks_

10 NO. OF WEEKS BETWEEN 1ST AND LAST RX: _____ NO. OF TREATMENTS _____ REFERRING M.D. _____

11

LEVEL A		DATE BEGUN/COMMENTS	LEVEL B		DATE BEGUN/COMMENTS	LEVEL	DATE BEGUN/COMMENTS
DOWEL TEXTURES			**CONTACT PARTICLES**			**VIBRATION**	
1	1	12/30/94	1	3	12/30 tolerated	1	1/5/95
2	2	"	2	2	1/17/95 "	2	
3	3	"	3	1		3	
4	4	"	4	4		4	
5	5	"	5	5		5	
6			6	6		6	
7			7	8		7	
8			8	9		8	
9			9	7		9	
10			10	10		10	

(Form © 1983 LMB Hand Rehab Products, Inc.)

THREE PHASE DESENSITIZATION TREATMENT PROTOCOL

Dowel Textures	Contact Particles	Vibration
1. Moleskin	1. Cotton	1. Battery/no contact
2. Felt	2. Terry cloth pieces	2. Battery/near contact
3. Quickstick	3. Dry rice	3. Low cycle/near contact
4. Velvet	4. Unpopped popcorn	4. Low cycle/intermittent contact
5. Semirough cloth	5. Pinto beans	5. Low cycle contact
6. Velcro loops*	6. Macaroni	6. Low cycle continuous
7. Hard T-foam	7. Plastic wire insulation pieces	7. High cycle/intermittent
8. Burlap	8. Small pebbles	8. High cycle/intermittent
9. Rug back	9. Larger pebbles	9. High cycle/continuous
10. Velcro hook	10. Plastic squares	10. Vibration, not irritating

(From Waylett-Rendell,[3] with permission.)

Sensory Re-education 9

Mallory S. Anthony

After peripheral nerve repair, the transmission of neural impulses is altered (due to factors discussed under postoperative complications) for sensory perception in the somatosensory cortex. When a patient attempts to interpret, at a conscious level, this altered profile of neural impulses, he or she must match the current profile to his memory of profiles stored in some "association" cortex. If no match is made, the altered profile of sensory impulses may be ignored, or the patient may not know what he or she has felt. Sensory re-education is an attempt to give the patient a new set of matching profiles.[1,2]

Re-education requires a patient who is intelligent, motivated, and willing to make a conscious effort to incorporate the involved hand into daily activities and to carry out a structured program on a daily basis. In this way, through the use of higher cortical functions (attention, learning, memory), a patient can learn to compensate for sensory deficits.[3]

The following treatment protocol is a guideline. There is no single technique for sensory re-education. Timing for the exercises is determined by the pattern of sensory recovery. It is never too late to begin sensory re-education.

DEFINITION

Sensory re-education is a method by which the patient learns to interpret the pattern of abnormal sensory impulses generated after an interruption in the peripheral nervous system.

TREATMENT PURPOSE

Following injury to sensory nerves, the pattern of recovery is variable and never returns to normal. Only some sensory fibers reach their proper end organs; therefore, the territory of reinnervation is incomplete. To help the patient with rehabilitation, the patient is trained to recognize the altered sensory feedback to the brain and interpret the sensory stimulus.

TREATMENT GOALS

I. To teach the patient who lacks protective sensation guidelines for protecting the hand against stress during everyday functional activities.
II. To guide patient in early and late re-education to maximize hand function and help patient achieve the fullest functional potential provided by nerve repair.

INDICATIONS/PRECAUTIONS FOR THERAPY

I. Indications
   A. Patient in whom protective sensation is lacking or severely decreased as evidenced by inability to perceive potentially harmful stimuli (pinprick, deep pressure, hot/cold, repetitive low-grade friction).[3]
   B. Patients who have protective sensation but lack discriminative sensation (i.e., localization, two-point discrimination, and tactile gnosis).[3]
II. Precautions
   Sensory re-education cannot be applied to a painful, hypersensitive, stiff, or swollen upper extremity.[2]

POSTOPERATIVE THERAPY

I. Home program
   A. Patient should practice re-education exercises 5 minutes, three to four times a day.
   B. Patients should not stimulate the involved hand directly with the uninvolved hand, as they will receive two sets of sensory information, one from each hand, and this will be confusing.[1]
   C. Any interested individual (spouse, other family members, friends) can be shown sensory re-education exercises to help the patient with home program.
II. Patients who lack protective sensation should be instructed in the following guidelines, suggested by Callahan,[3] to help them compensate.[4]
   A. Avoid exposure of involved area to heat, cold, and sharp objects.
   B. Be conscious of not applying more force than necessary when gripping a tool or object.

C. Note that the smaller the handle, the less distribution of pressure over the gripping surfaces. Avoid using small handles by building them up whenever possible.

D. Avoid tasks that require use of one tool for long periods of time, especially if the hand is unable to adapt by changing the manner of grip.

E. Change tools frequently at work to rest tissue areas subject to pressure.

F. Observe the skin for signs of stress (i.e., redness, swelling, warmth) from excessive force or repetitive pressure. Rest the hand if these signs occur.

G. If blisters, lacerations, or other wounds occur, treat them with the utmost care to avoid further injury to the skin and possible infection.

H. Keep skin soft. Follow a daily routine of skin care including soaking and oil (or lotion) massage to hold in moisture.

III. Early phase re-education: begin when 30 cps vibration and/or moving touch have returned to an area, for example, the palm,[1] or when protective sensation is present and there is return of touch perception out to the fingertips, within the range of 4.31 or lower as measured by Semmes-Weinstein monofilaments.[3]

A. To re-educate specific perceptions (i.e., movement vs. constant touch, sharp versus dull).

B. To re-educate incorrect localization (where is stimulus perceived in reference to site of stimulation).

C. Suggested techniques[1–5]

  1. Use fingertip or pencil eraser (blunt surface) (Fig. 9-1).

  2. Press hard enough for patient to feel stimulus.

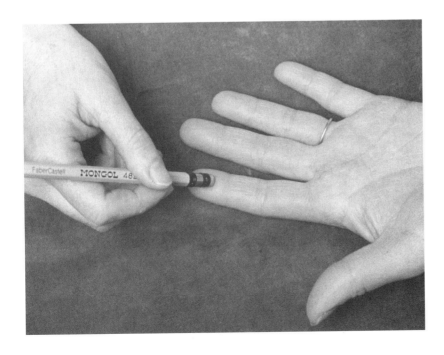

Fig. 9-1. Blunt surface used for sensory re-education in early phase.

3. Perform moving and/or constant touch to palm or finger when these submodalities reach the area.
4. The patient observes what is happening (moving versus constant, sharp versus dull, location of stimulus), shuts the eyes and concentrates on what he or she is perceiving, then opens the eyes to confirm what is happening.
5. If patient incorrectly identifies the stimulus, repeat process.

D. Evaluate progress with accuracy of response, mapping of localization, Semmes Weinstein monofilaments, and/or vibration testing (preferably vibrometer).

IV. Late phase re-education: begin when moving and constant touch, and/or 256 cps vibration can be perceived at the fingertips with good localization.

A. To guide patient in recovery of tactile gnosis.
B. Suggested techniques[1–5]
1. Exercises should be graded beginning with the discrimination of larger objects, with greater differences among them in size, shape, and texture, progressing to more subtle differences (Fig. 9-2).
2. Discrimination of various textures (Fig. 9-3), as well as object identification using a set of familiar household objects, can be used for re-education.
3. The sequence used for object (or texture) grasp is first with eyes open, then shut with concentration of perception, then eyes open for reinforcement.

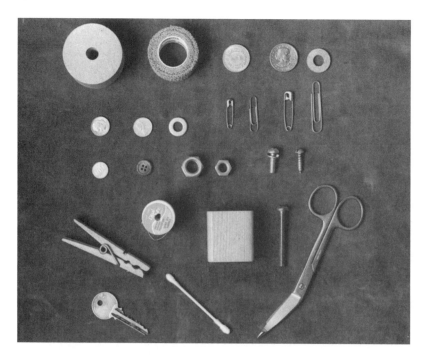

Fig. 9-2. Graded object discrimination to recover tactile gnosis.

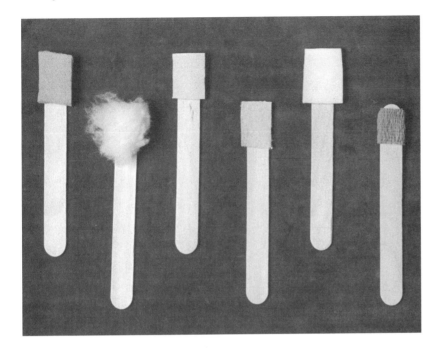

Fig. 9-3. Textures may be used for late phase re-education.

   C. Accuracy of response (i.e., number of correctly identified objects or textures) is recorded. Time to perform the task may also be recorded.

   D. Moving and static two-point discrimination should be tested periodically to assess sensory status.

V. Other techniques of re-education.

   A. Graphesthesia: therapist traces a number, letter, or geometric figure on involved area and patient tries to identify it.[3]

   B. Bilateral exercises can be used by having the patient differentiate between various textures of material or sandpaper, with vision, then vision occluded.[2]

   C. Patients can be asked to pick out and identify an object in a bowl of sand, rice, or beans with vision occluded (Fig. 9-4).

   D. Activities that duplicate or incorporate work activities should be included in patient's therapy to practice specific sensory grips and prepare patient for previous work.

POSTOPERATIVE COMPLICATIONS THAT MAY REQUIRE RE-EDUCATION

  I. Axons may regenerate to an irreversibly degenerated end organ.

  II. Axons may arrive at correct digital area, but reinnervate the wrong end organ.

  III. Axons may never re-enter distal endoneurial sheath.

  IV. Axons may be misdirected to the wrong finger.

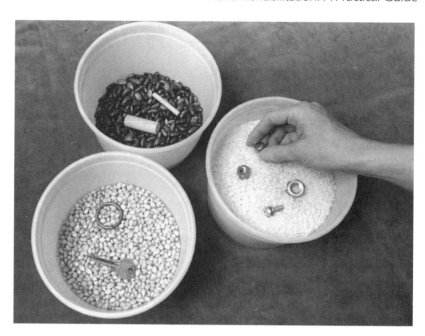

Fig. 9-4. Locating and identifying objects imbedded in various media.

EVALUATION TIMELINE

Initially, patient should be checked in the clinic once a week for several weeks, for sensory assessment and home program review. As patient feels comfortable with home program, decrease the frequency of treatment. Check patient every 6 to 8 weeks for sensory evaluation and any necessary changes in re-education program.

REFERENCES

1. Dellon AL: Evaluation of Sensibility and Re-education of Sensation in the Hand. Williams & Wilkins, Baltimore, 1981
2. MacKinnon SE, Dellon AL: Sensory rehabilitation after nerve injury. p. 521. In: Surgery of the Peripheral Nerve. Thieme Medical Publishers, New York, 1988
3. Callahan AD: Methods of compensation and reeducation for sensory dysfunction. p. 701. In Hunter JM, Schneider LH, Mackin EJ, Callahan AD (eds): Rehabilitation of the Hand: Surgery and Therapy. 4th Ed. Mosby, St. Louis, 1995
4. Carter-Wilson M: Sensory reeducation. In Gelberman RH (ed): Operative Nerve Repair and Reconstruction. Lippincott-Raven, Philadelphia, 1991
5. MacKinnon SE, Dellon AL: Appendix E: Sensory re-education protocols. p. 589. In: Surgery of the Peripheral Nerve. Thieme Medical Publishers, New York, 1988

SUGGESTED READINGS

(Please also refer to Ch. 7—Sensory Evaluation—Suggested Readings)

Anthony M: Sensory re-education. Adv Phys Ther 5:19, 1994

Brand PW: Rehabilitation of the hand with motor and sensory impairment. Orthop Clin North Am 4:1135, 1973

Brand PW: Management of sensory loss in the extremities. In Omer GE, Spinner M (eds): Management of Peripheral Nerve Problems. WB Saunders, Philadelphia, 1980

Callahan AD: Methods of compensation and reeducation for sensory dysfunction. p. 611. In Hunter JM, Schneider LH, Mackin EJ, Callahan AD (eds): Rehabilitation of the Hand: Surgery and Therapy. 3rd Ed. Mosby, St. Louis, 1990

Chassard M, Pham E, Comtet JJ: Two-point discrimination tests versus functional sensory recovery in both median and ulnar nerve complete transections. J Hand Surg 18B:790, 1993

Dellon AL: Techniques of sensory re-education. In: Somatosensory Testing and Rehabilitation. AOTA, Silver Spring, Md, 1996

Dellon AL, Jabaley ME: Reeducation of sensation in the hand following nerve suture. Clin Orthop 163:75, 1982

Dellon AL, Curtis RM, Edgerton MT: Reeducation of sensation in the hand after nerve injury and repair. Plast Reconstr Surg 53: 297, 1974

Imai H, Tajima T, Natsumi Y: Interpretation of cutaneous pressure threshold (Semmes-Weinstein monofilament measurement) following median nerve repair and sensory reeducation in the adult. Microsurgery 10:142, 1989

Imai H, Tajima T, Natsumi Y: Successful reeducation of functional sensibility after median nerve repair at the wrist. J Hand Surg 16A:60, 1991

Merzenich MM, Jenkins WM: Reorganization of cortical representations of the hand following alterations of skin inputs induced by nerve injury, skin island transfers and experience. J Hand Ther 6:89, 1993

Nakada M: Localization of a constant-touch and moving touch stimulus in the hand: a preliminary study. J Hand Ther 6:23, 1993

Omer GE: Sensation and sensibility in the upper extremity. Clin Orthop Relat Res 104:30, 1974

Rosen B, Lundborg G, Dahlin LB et al: Nerve repair: correlation of restitution of functional sensibility with specific cognitive capacities. J Hand Surg 19B:452, 1994

Tajima T, Imai H: Results of median nerve repair in children. Microsurgery 10:145, 1989

Waylett-Rendall J: Sequence of sensory recovery: a retrospective study. J Hand Ther 2:4, 1989

Extensor Tendon Repair 10

Barbara Steinberg

Both immobilization and early passive motion therapeutic apporoaches to extensor tendon injuries are described. For the uncomplicated extensor tendon injuries in zones V, VI, and VII, the immobilization approach is used most often. If the surgeon requests the metacarpophalangeal (MCP) joint to be splinted statically at 20 to 30 degrees of flexion to retain the integrity of the collateral ligaments, it is appropriate to use early passive motion method to prevent extensor lag.[1] The early passive motion method also facilitates a better outcome in the complicated extensor tendon injury, which is defined as including injury to the periosteum of bone, extensor retinaculum, or adjacent soft tissue.[1]

When progressing a patient using either method, it is important to have a "feel" of the tendon. When there is a developing MCP extensor lag, a longer course of MCP extension splinting is indicated to be balanced with MCP flexion as permitted by tendon healing. Conversely, if the problem is decreased MCP flexon and/or extrinsic extensor tendon tightness, dynamic MCP flexion splinting may be indicated when the extensor tendon is strong enough to tolerate this.

Two methods of extensor tendon rehabilitation are described. It is important to keep abreast of further research in tendon healing and post-operative treatment to facilitate the best outcome for each patient.

DEFINITION

Primary repair of complete rupture or laceration of any digital extensor tendon in zones V, VI, or VII, thumb extensors in zones T-III, T-IV, or T-V, and wrist extensors in zone VII (Fig. 10-1).

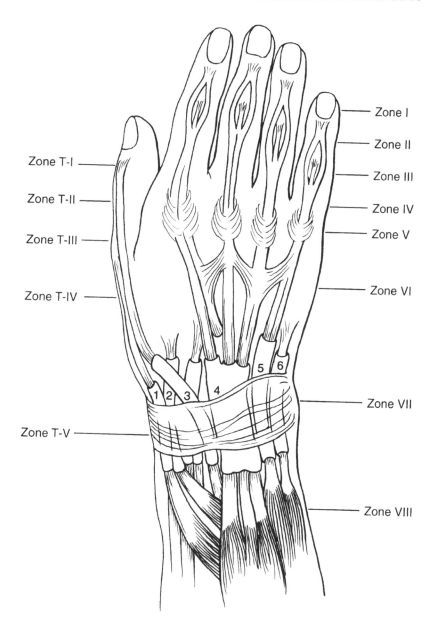

Zone T-I

Zone T-II

Zone T-III

Zone T-IV

Zone T-V

Zone I

Zone II

Zone III

Zone IV

Zone V

Zone VI

Zone VII

Zone VIII

Fig. 10-1. Extensor tendon zones and dorsal compartments through which extensors travel.

SURGICAL PURPOSE

To restore continuity and maintain gliding of the extensor mechanism from the metacarpal phalangeal joints proximally toward the wrist level. Tendon gliding is critical beneath the retinacular ligaments covering the fibrosseous compartments at the wrist. Scarring over the dorsal surface of the hand is a problem because of scant soft tissue protection between the skin's surface and the underlying skeletal structures. Tendon suturing techniques may vary depending on the zone where the actual juncture is placed. The zone of tendon division may not coincide with the actual skin laceration. Other than lacerations, extensor tendon continuity may be lost secondary to attrition from sharp bone fragments after fracture, rheumatoid arthritis, tendinitis, and developmental absence.

TREATMENT GOALS

   I. Prevent tendon rupture.
  II. Promote tendon healing.
 III. Encourage tendon gliding while minimizing tendon gapping and extensor lag.
 IV. Restore active range of motion (AROM) and passive range of motion (PROM).
  V. Edema control.
 VI. Pain control.
VII. Scar management.
VIII. Maintain full range of motion (ROM) of all uninvolved joints of the affected upper extremity.
 IX. Return to previous level of function.

POSTOPERATIVE INDICATIONS/ PRECAUTIONS FOR THERAPY

  I. Indications
     Surgical repair of finger extensor tendons in zones V, VI, VII, thumb extensors in zones T-III, T-IV, T-V, and/or wrist extensor Zone VII.
 II. Precautions
   A. Infection
   B. Combined flexor tendon repair
   C. Fractures
   D. Extreme pain
   E. Severe edema

POSTOPERATIVE THERAPY

  I. Finger extensors: zones V, VI, VII
   A. Immobilization method[1]
     1. 0 to 21 days postoperative
       a. Splinting—volar—wrist 30 to 45 degrees extension, MCPs and interphalangeal (IPs) 0 degrees extension (Fig. 10-2)
         i. Variations
           A. Simple injury of extensor indices proprius (EIP) or extensor digiti minimis (EDM)—Only repaired tendon/digit needs to be immobilized.

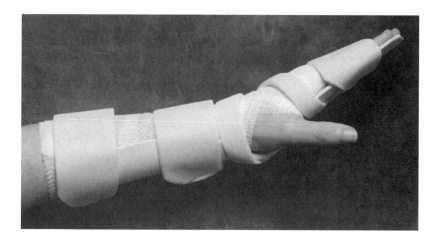

Fig. 10-2. Immobilizing postoperative splint for fingers.

B. Simple injury of single extensor digitorum communis (EDC).
  (1) Repair site *proximal* to interconnecting juncturae tendinum—All fingers splinted in extension.
  (2) Repair site *distal* to interconnecting juncturae tendinum—Affected digit full MCP/IP extension; adjacent digits 30 degrees MCP flexion with IPs free.

b. Therapy
  i Wound care
  ii Edema control
  iii. MCP joint protective ROM: therapist supports wrist and IPs in full extension, while gently moving the *index* and *middle* finger MCPs from slight hyperextension to 30 degrees flexion, and the *ring* and *small* finger MPs from slight hyperextension to 40 degrees flexion.
  iv. Proximal interphalangeal/distal interphalangeal (PIP/DIP) joint protective ROM: therapist supports wrist and MCPs in full extension, while passively moving each individual PIP and DIP joint through complete range of motion. If PIP and/or DIP motion is limited, the immobilizing splint is cut away, allowing full PIP and DIP motion while maintaining wrist and MCPs in full extension. A removable volar component may be applied sleeping and/or intermittently during day to prevent PIP joint flexion contracture and/or extensor lag.

2. 3 weeks postoperative.
  a. Splinting—volar—wrist 20 degrees extension, MCPs 0 degrees extension. With PIP extension lag or flexion contracture, use removable volar component. With MP joint flexion less than 30 to 40 degrees with a "hard" end

feel—initiate dynamic MP flexion splinting to achieve 30 degrees flexion at *index* and *middle* and 40 degrees flexion for *ring* and *small* fingers.[1] IP static extension splints can be used during active MCP joint exercises.

    b. Therapy

        i. MCP AROM and active assistive range of motion (AAROM) with tenodesis: MCP extension with wrist in neutral to slight flexion. MCP flexion (40 to 60 degrees) with wrist in full extension.

        ii. IP AROM, AAROM, PROM through complete range, while wrist and MCPs are supported in full extension.

  3. 4 weeks postoperative.

    a. Splinting—dynamic MCP flexion as needed.

    b. Therapy

        i. Composite MCP/IP flexion with wrist extension.

        ii. Individual finger extension.

        iii. Isolated EDC extension.

  4. Between 4 and 5 weeks postoperative.

    a. Splinting—combination of MCP and IP traction may be initiated to decrease extrinsic extensor tightness.

    b. Therapy—(same as 3 and 4 weeks postoperative).

  5. 6 to 10 weeks postoperative.

    a. Splinting—only as needed.

    b. Therapy.

        i. Composite finger and wrist flexion, initiated when no extension lag present.

        ii. Mild progressive strengthening including wrist flexion/extension and forearm pronation/supination.

  6. 10 to 12 weeks postoperative: Strong resistive exercise.

B. Early passive motion method.[1]

  1. 24 hours to 3 days postoperative.

    a. Splinting (Fig. 10-3)—two part dynamic splint.

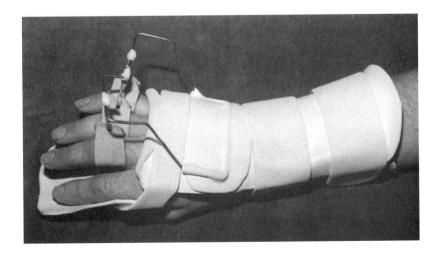

Fig. 10-3. Splint for dynamic treatment of finger extensor repairs in zones V, VI, and VII.

     i. *Dorsal component*: Wrist—30 to 45 degrees static extension; MCPs and IPs—0 degrees dynamic extension.

    ii. *Interlocking volar component*: Wrist—same as dorsal component; MCPs—permits active flexion of 30 degrees for index and middle and 40 degrees for ring and small.

  b. Therapy

     i. Wound care

    ii. Edema control

   iii. Splint adjustments

   iv. Controlled passive IP motion (see immobilization method, PIP/DIP joint protective ROM—0 to 21 days postoperative).

    v. Each waking hour.

While maintaining IP extension, patient actively flexes digits at MCP joints until fingers touch volar splint. Patient releases digits, allowing extension loops to passively extend MCPs to 0 degrees. For Zone VII—while loops support other digits in extension, patient individually flexes index finger MCP to splint, small finger MCP to splint, and then middle and ring fingers together to splint. Patient relaxes digits to allow extension outrigger to passively extend MP joints to 0 degrees

   vi. Wrist tenodesis.

Zones V and VI—simultaneous wrist extension with 30 degrees index and middle MCP flexion and 40 degrees ring and small MCP flexion followed by simultaneous wrist flexion to 20 degrees with all digital joints held at 0 degrees

Zone VII *without* wrist tendon involvement—as above except when digits are placed in 0 degrees, wrist is no less than 10 degrees of extension

Zone VII *with* wrist tendon involvement—as above except when digits are placed in 0 degrees, wrist is no less than 20 degrees extension

2. 3 weeks postoperative

  a. Splinting

     i. Day: volar block splint removed. Continue with dorsal dynamic splint.

    ii. Night: wear volar static splint (adjusted to 30 to 45 degrees wrist extension and 0 degrees MCP/IP extension).

  b. Therapy

     i. Begin gradual active motion of MCP and IP joints within dynamic extension splint.

    ii. Modalities, dynamic splinting and exercise the same as management by immobilization from the 3 week period onward.

3. 4 to 5 weeks postoperative: Initiate composite finger flexion with wrist in extension. Splinting continues.

4. 6 to 12 weeks postoperative: Same as immobilization method.

II. Wrist extensors *without* finger extensor involvement (Zone VII).

A. Splinting

1. Wrist 30 to 45 degrees extension with MCPs and IPs free.

2. Continue protective splinting up to 8 weeks.

B. Therapy

1. 3 weeks postoperative—Gravity eliminated active motion from 0 degrees to full wrist extension.

2. 5 to 8 weeks postoperative—slowly add increments of wrist flexion, radial and ulnar deviation.

3. 8 to 12 weeks postoperative—progressive strengthening.

III. Thumb extensors (Zones T-III, T-IV, T-V).

A. Immobilization method[1]

1. 0 to 21 days postoperative.

a. Splinting—volar protective (Fig. 10-4). Wrist 30 degrees extension; carpometacarpal (CMC) slight abduction; MCP and IP 0 degrees.

b. Therapy

i. Wound care.

ii. Edema control.

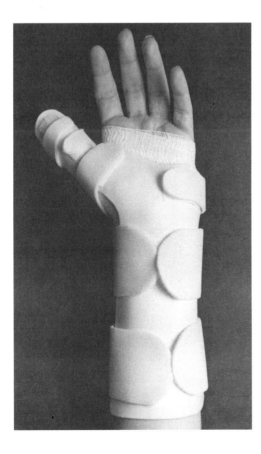

Fig. 10-4. Immobilizing postoperative splint for thumb.

        iii. MCP joint protective ROM: therapist supports wrist and IP in full extension, while gently moving MCP from full extension to 30 degrees flexion. Check splint to be sure thumb MCP is not hyperextended.

        iv. IP joint protective ROM: therapist supports wrist and MCP in full extension, while gently moving thumb IP from full extension to 60 degrees flexion.

  2. 3 to 4 weeks postoperative

    a. Splinting—All the time except for exercise and showering. Shorten splint to allow active flexion and extension of IP joint

      i. Variations

        A. IP extensor lag—add removable volar component.

        B. MCP extension contracture—intermittent gentle dynamic MCP flexion splinting while supporting wrist and first metacarpal in extension.

    b. Therapy

      i. Initiate supervised thumb abduction and MCP/IP flexion.

      ii. Home program

        MCP mobility—supporting wrist and IP in full extension, gently move MCP from full extension to 30 degrees flexion.

        IP mobility—supporting wrist and MCP in full extension, gently move thumb IP from full extension to 60 degrees flexion.

  3. 5 weeks postoperative.

    a. Splinting—combination of thumb abduction, MCP and IP flexion may be initiated.

    b. Therapy—add combination of thumb abduction, MCP and IP flexion to home program.

  4. 6 to 10 weeks postoperative.

    a. Splinting—as needed.

    b. Therapy

      i. Composite thumb and wrist flexion.

      ii. Mild progressive strengthening including wrist flexion/extension and forearm supination/pronation.

  5. 10 to 12 weeks postoperative.

    a. Therapy—strong resistive exercise.

B. Early passive motion method.[1]

  1. 0 to 21 days postoperative.

    a. Splinting (Fig. 10-5).

      i. Dorsal—wrist—30 degrees static extension; MCP/IP—0 degrees dynamic extension.

      ii. Volar—static splint allowing 60 degrees of IP motion.

    b. Therapy

      i. By patient—active flexion to volar splint with passive extension via dynamic traction.

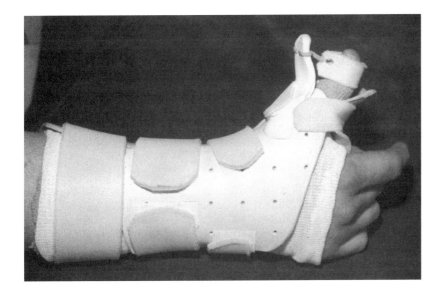

Fig. 10-5. Splint for dynamic treatment of thumb extensor repair in zones T-IV and T-V.

     ii. By therapist—maximal wrist extension with simultaneous MCP joint flexion to 30 degrees.

     iii. Wrist tenodesis—wrist to 0 degrees extension with simultaneous thumb CMC, MP, IP extension alternating with full wrist extension with thumb CMC, MP, IP relaxed.

2. 3 to 4 weeks postoperative.
   a. Splinting—all the time except for exercise and showering.
   b. Therapy—add therapist exercises of first 3 weeks to home program.

3. 5 to 12 weeks postoperative—splinting and exercise essentially the same as early immobilization method from 5 to 12 weeks.

POSTOPERATIVE COMPLICATIONS

  I. Tendon rupture.
  II. Excessive scar formation.
  III. Active extensor tendon lag.
  IV. Extrinsic extensor tendon tightness limiting composite flexion.

EVALUATION TIMELINE

  I. 4 weeks: AROM MCP and IP joints.
  II. 5 weeks: AROM wrist.
  III. 7 weeks: PROM and AROM wrist, MCP and IP joints.
  IV. 10 weeks: Strength; re-evaluate ROM and strength measurements every 4 weeks.

REFERENCE

1. Evans RB: An update on extensor tendon management. p. 565. In Hunter JM, Mackin EJ, Callahan AD (eds): Rehabilitation of the Hand: Surgery and Therapy. 4th Ed. Mosby, St. Louis, 1995

SUGGESTED READINGS

Browne EZ, Ribik CA: Early dynamic splinting for extensor tendon injuries. J Hand Surg 14A:72, 1989

Evans RB, Burkhalter WE: A study of the dynamic anatomy of extensor tendons and implications for treatment. J Hand Surg 11A:774, 1986

Newport ML, Blair WF, Steyers CM, Jr: Long-term results of extensor tendon repair. J Hand Surg 15A:961, 1990

Rosenthal EA: The extensor tendons: Anatomy and management. p. 519. In Hunter JM, Schneider LH, Mackin EJ, Callahan AD (eds): Rehabilitation of the Hand. 4th Ed. Mosby, St. Louis, 1995

Flexor Tendon Repair   11

Barbara Steinberg

Immobilization, early passive motion (EPM), and early active motion (EAM) treatment approaches are described for Zones I through V. These address the primary goals of preventing tendon rupture, encouraging tendon gliding and preventing flexion contractures.

Treatment for flexor pollicus longus repairs is essentially the same as for digital tendon lacerations except that the position of the rubber band (if used) should be directed toward the ulnar side of the wrist.[1]

DEFINITION

Primary and delayed primary repair of complete rupture or laceration of digital flexor tendons in Zones I through V. See introduction for changes to treatment approach following repair of flexor pollicus longus.

SURGICAL AND TREATMENT PURPOSE

To restore maximum active flexor tendon gliding to ensure effective finger joint motion. The two most common impediments to this goal are rupture of the tendon repair or scarring with adhesions. The surgical technique requires gentle tendon handling; strong, effective suture material with grasping stitches; and meticulous postoperative management. The zone of tendon injury may not coincide with the level of skin laceration because of finger position when the cut occurs. The zone within which the tendon is repaired dictates to some extent the therapy methods to be used (Figs. 11-1 and 11-2). The thumb flexor tendon lies alone in the digital sheath, whereas two intimately related tendons—profundus and superficialis—are in each digital sheath of the fingers. This fact will alter some of the therapy requirements for the fingers compared with those of the thumb. The causes of flexor tendon injury are most commonly traumatic; however, rheumatoid arthritis may also bring it about.

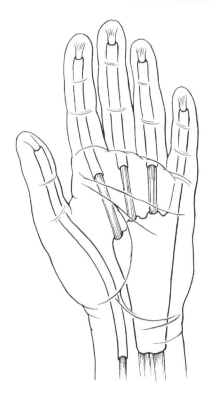

Fig. 11-1. Volar skin creases and their relationship to tendons in an extended position.

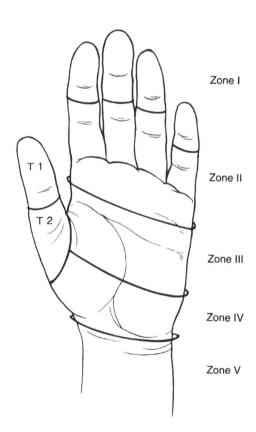

Fig. 11-2. Tendon zones.

TREATMENT GOALS

    I. Prevent tendon rupture.
    II. Prevent flexion contractures.
    III. Promote tendon healing.
    IV. Encourage tendon gliding.
    V. Restore active range of motion (AROM) and passive range of motion (PROM).
    VI. Maintain full range of motion (ROM) of all uninvolved joints of affected upper extremity.
    VII. Return to previous level of function.

POSTOPERATIVE INDICATIONS/ PRECAUTIONS FOR THERAPY

    I. Indications: Surgical repair of flexor tendons to fingers and/or thumb.
    II. Precautions
        A. Infection
        B. Combined extensor tendon repair
        C. Fractures
        D. Nerve repair
        E. Vessel repair
        F. Extreme pain
        G. Severe edema

POSTOPERATIVE THERAPY

    I. Immobilization method (Zones I through V)[2,3]
        A. 0 to 3 weeks postoperative
            1. Splint—dorsal thermoplastic or plaster cast
                a. Wrist—10 to 30 degrees flexion
                b. Metacarpophalangeals (MCPs)—40 to 60 degrees flexion.
                c. Interphalangeals (IPs)—full extension.
            2. Therapy
                a. By patient
                    i. ROM of uninvolved joints (as instructed by therapist).
                    ii. Elevation
                b. By therapist in structured therapy sessions.
                    i. Protected PROM
                        A. Proximal interphalangeal (PIP) motion—passive wrist, MCP, distal interphalangeal (DIP) flexion while passively flexing and extending each PIP joint.
                        B. DIP motion—passive wrist, MCP, PIP flexion while passively flexing and extending each DIP joint.
                    ii. Wound care.

      iii. Edema control.
      iv. Scar management.
B. 3 weeks postoperative.
  1. Splint
    a. Wrist—neutral.
    b. MCPs — 40 to 50 degrees flexion.
    c. IPs—0 degrees.
  2. Therapy
    a. Patient removes splint hourly for exercise
      i. Protected PROM (with wrist at 10 degrees extension).
      ii. Tendon gliding[4,5]
        A. *Tenodesis.*
        B. Hook fist with wrist in slight flexion.
        C. Flat fist with wrist in 10 degrees extension.
        D. Full fist with wrist in 10 degrees extension.
        E. *Place and hold with tenodesis.*
        F. *Place and hold (without resistance)*—grasp and release various diameter cones, dowels, etc.
C. 3 1/2 weeks postoperative.
  1. Evaluate tendon glide
    a. If *more* than 50 degrees difference between total active motion (TAM) and total passive motion (TPM), program continues to progress.
    b. If *less* than 50 degrees difference between TAM and TPM, above therapy is continued until 6 weeks postoperative.
D. 3 1/2 to 6 weeks postoperative.
  1. Splint
    a. Protection—dorsal blocking splint discontinued except sleeping and crowds.
    b. *Extrinsic flexor muscle-tendon tightness*—wrist and fingers in maximal *comfortable* extension. Serially adjusted to accommodate increased extension.
  2. Therapy
    a. Protected PROM.
    b. Tendon gliding (passive and then place and hold).
    c. *Gentle* blocking for isolated flexor digitorum superficialis (FDS)/flexor digitorum profundus (FDP)
    d. Place and hold, non-resisted grasp and release using cones and/or dowels.
E. 4 1/2 to 7 weeks postoperative.
  1. Evaluate tendon glide.
    a. If active flexion is improving, do *not* upgrade program.
    b. If *no* increase in active motion, add
      i. Towel walking.
      ii. Light grasp and release.
      iii. *Gentle* putty squeezing (no more than 10 repetitions of lightest putty).
F. 5 1/2 to 8 weeks postoperative.
  1. Evaluate tendon glide.
    a. If active tendon glide is improving, do *not* upgrade program.

      b. If *no* increase in active motion, add

        i. Sustained grip, (i.e., light sanding with adapted sander).

        ii. Hand helper with *one* rubberband.

        iii. Putty scraping.

        iv. Use of heavier putty (progress from very light to light or medium).

        v. Lifting (begin with 1 pound and increase slowly up to 10 pounds with physician clearance).

    G. 10 to 12 weeks postoperative.

      1. Therapy—progress to

        a. Heavy putty.

        b. Lifting over 10 pounds.

        c. Job simulation (manual labor).

II. Early passive motion methods (zones II to V).[1,3–10]

    A. 0 to 3 or 4 weeks postoperative.

      1. Splint (dorsal)

        a. Wrist—10 to 30 degrees flexion.

        b. MCPs—50 to 70 degrees flexion.

        c. IPs

          i. Without rubberband/elastic traction (modified Duran).[3,6,7]

            A. 0 degrees.

            B. Strapped in extension with Velcro strap between exercise sessions and while sleeping.

          ii. With rubberband/elastic traction.

            A. All digits (four finger method)[3,6–8]

              (1) Plaster cast or circumferential splint (ends at PIP joint allowing full PIP and DIP extension).

              (2) "Thick" rubberband to all four digits (regardless of how many involved). Palmar pulley used and all four rubberbands attached to a removable ring at proximal volar forearm (Fig. 11-3).

              (3) A hand-based thermoplastic volar splint, maintaining IPs at 0 degrees, is added to circumferential cast/splint while sleeping (without rubberband traction (Fig. 11-4).

            B. Only involved digit(s) (modified Washington method).[3,11,12]

              (1) Dorsal splint to end of digits while allowing full PIP and DIP extension.

              (2) Nylon fishing line from fingernail(s) through palmar pulley, each attached to two rubberbands (one thick and the other cut in half to form less resistive single strand or use elastic thread). Both rubberbands attached to proximal volar forearm strap (Figs. 11-5, 11-6).

              (3) While sleeping: loosen rubberband traction or remove rubberband or elastic traction

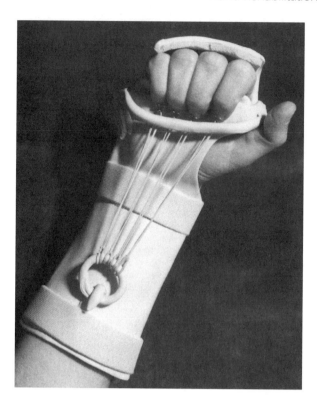

Fig. 11-3. Four finger method splint showing palmar pulley, "thick" rubber bands to all 4 digits attached to removable ring.

and strap IPs in extension via Velcro strap or removable volar thermoplastic splint.

2. Therapy: 10 to 15 repetitions per hour
   a. By patient: *Modified Duran* (without rubberband traction)[3,6,7]
      i. Protected PIP and DIP PROM (described under immobilization method)
      ii. Passive modified hook, flat and full fists each alternating with active IP extension while passively blocking MCPs into greater flexion to maximize PIP and DIP extension.
      iii. *Modified Kleinert* (four finger method or Washington regimen with rubberband/elastic traction)[3,11,12] — Passive IP joint flexion of all four digits alternating with full active IP extension of all four digits by either removing rubberbands from proximal hook (Fig. 11-7) or removing heavy rubberband while leaving lighter rubberband or elastic thread in place (Fig. 11-6). If indicated (i.e., beginning of PIP flexion contracture) protected PIP/DIP PROM may be added to program (described under immobilization method).

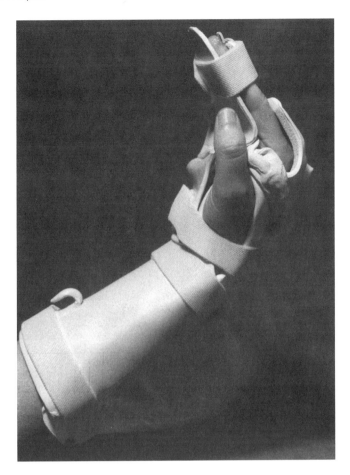

Fig. 11-4. Volar splint maintains IPs at 0 degrees.

    b. By therapist (optional)—*Tenodesis* (passive): splint is removed. Passive full fist with wrist at 10 to 30 degrees extension alternating with passive wrist and MCP flexion along with active IP extension. Passive flat fist with wrist at 10 to 30 degrees extension alternating with passive wrist and MCP flexion along with active IP extension. Passive modified hook fist with wrist hyperflexed, MCPs at 0 to 30 degrees passive flexion and IPs fully flexed (passively) alternating with passive wrist and MCP flexion along with active IP extension.

B. 3 weeks postoperative.
  1. Splint: wrist to neutral with or without rubberband/elastic traction.
  2. Therapy: therapist evaluates tendon glide by performing protected PIP/DIP PROM, passive tendon gliding with tenodesis (see immobilization method) and then place and hold tendon gliding with tenodesis.

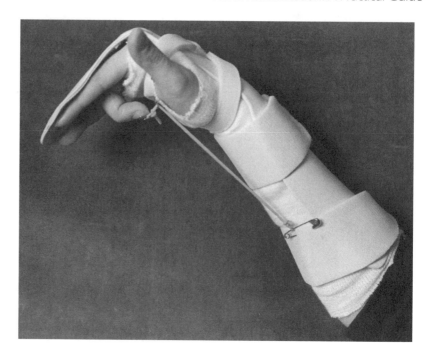

Fig. 11-5. Splinting with elastic traction to digital palmar crease and then to proximal forearm maintains IPs in full flexion at rest.

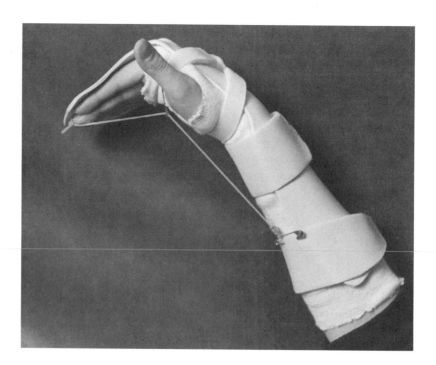

Fig. 11-6. Traction splint should allow full extension to limit of splint via lighter weight rubber band or elastic thread.

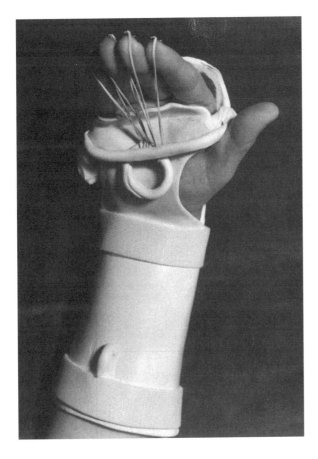

Fig. 11-7. Ring holding all 4 rubber bands removed, allowing full IP extension.

    a. If more than 50 degree difference between full fist TAM and TPM, program is upgraded to add place and hold tenodesis to home program as well as nonresisted place and hold grasp and release (see immobilization method).

    b. If less than 50 degree difference between TAM and TPM, home program is not upgraded. Place and hold tenodesis only done in supervised therapy sessions with partial place and hold fisting after passive motion performed.

  C. 4 weeks postoperative.

    1. Splints

      a. Splint worn only sleeping and in crowds or wrist band with elastic traction used (Fig. 11-8).

      b. Extrinsic flexor muscle-tendon tightness (see immobilization method).

    2. Therapy: upgrade following guidelines in immobilization method.

III. Zone I early passive motion method[13]

  A. 0 to 21 days postoperative.

    1. Splints

      a. Dorsal static protective extending to fingertips.

        i. Wrist—30 to 40 degrees flexion.

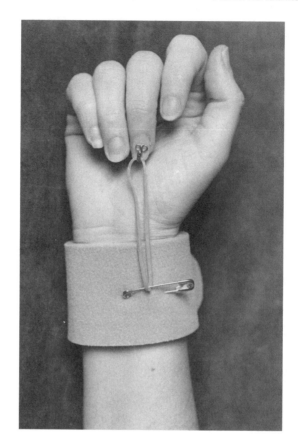

Fig. 11-8. Wristlet with rubber band traction.

ii. MCPs—30 degrees flexion.
iii. PIPs—0 degrees.
b. Affected DIP static splint.
   DIP: 40 to 45 degrees flexion. (Splint extends from proximal portion of middle phalanx to the tip of the finger and is taped *only* to the middle phalanx.)
2. Therapy
   a. Wound care.
   b. Edema control.
   c. Scar management.
   d. Exercise
      i. *By patient*: 10 to 20 repetitions per waking hour. Both splints are kept on during exercise. Distal joint is passively flexed from 40 or 45 to 75 degrees (or full flexion). All digits are passively placed in a full fist position. All digits placed in hook position. MCP joints passively hyperflexed by the uninvolved hand while PIPs are actively extended to 0 degrees. Distal strap holds unaffected fingers in extension while gentle place and hold active exercise for superficialis of involved finger is done.

      ii. *By therapist*: Therapist removes hand from dorsal protective splint, keeping the dorsal digital splint in place. While passively flexing fingers into the palm, therapist extends wrist to 10 degrees extension. With the wrist hyperflexed, therapist places fingers in a hook fist position with the MCPs at 0 degrees and the IPs in full passive flexion.

  B. 3 weeks postoperative.

    1. Splints: digital splint discontinued and dorsal protective splint wear continues.

    2. Therapy

      a. Place and hold hook and full fist (within splint) added to patient exercises of first 3 weeks.

      b. Progress by 4 weeks to: Patient removing splint during exercise sessions to perform: place and hold tenodesis full fist, flat fist, and hook fist. Gentle blocked profundus exercise.

  C. 4 1/2 weeks postoperative.

    1. Splints: if indicated, static digit extension splinting may be initiated.

    2. Therapy: upgrade following guidelines in immobilization method.

IV. Early active motion methods

  A. Factors to consider

    1. Strength and quality of repair.

    2. Time from repair.

    3. Ability and motivation of patient to cooperate.

    4. Knowledge and skill of therapist.

  B. Indiana method[14,15]

    1. Indications

      a. Suture: four strand Tajima and horizontal mattress repair (or equivalent four strand repair) with a running peripheral epitendinous suture.

      b. Within 48 hours of repair.

      c. Patient with ability and motivation to reproduce the therapy program as demonstrated by the therapist.

      d. Edema: minimal to moderate with no restrictions to passive flexion.

      e. Wound: minimal complications.

    2. 24 to 48 hours postoperative

      a. Splints

        i. Traditional dorsal blocking splint.

          A. Wrist—20 degrees flexion.

          B. MCPs—50 degrees flexion.

          C. IPs—0 degrees.

        ii. Forearm based tenodesis dorsal hinged splint.

          A. Wrist hinge—allows full wrist flexion to 30 degrees extension (Figs. 11-9 and 11-10).

          B. Hand—MCPs—60 degrees flexion; IPs—0 degrees.

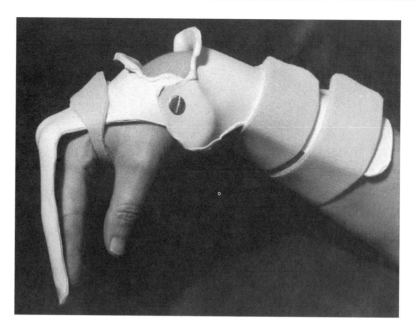

Fig. 11-9. Tenodesis splint allows full wrist flexion.

b. Therapy
  i. Wearing dorsal block splint: 15 repetitions per hour of individual passive flexion and extension to the PIP and DIP joints followed by composite PIP/DIP PROM.
  ii. Hinged tenodesis splint applied: tenodesis place and hold performed 25 times per hour while wearing the tenodesis splint. Patient passively flexes digits while simultaneously actively extending the wrist. This position is then very gently actively held for 5 seconds. After 5 seconds, the patient relaxes and allows their wrist to drop into flexion. This allows digits to straighten within the limits of the tenodesis splint.
  iii. Dorsal block splint reapplied.
3. 4 weeks postoperative

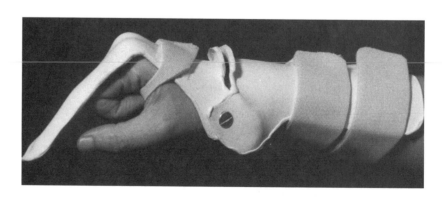

Fig. 11-10. Tenodesis splint blocks wrist extension at 30 degrees.

a. Splints: hinged tenodesis splint discontinued. Static dorsal block splint worn at all times except during exercise until 6 weeks postoperative.

b. Therapy: dorsal block splint removed. The following performed 25 repetitions every 2 hours.

    i. Tenodesis place and hold without splint.

    ii. Active flexion and extension exercises of the digits and wrist with a light muscle contraction. The patient is instructed *NOT* to simultaneously extend the wrist and digits to avoid potential gapping or elongation at the repair site.

4. 6 weeks postoperative

    a. Splint: dorsal block splint discontinued.

    b. Therapy: blocking exercises for index, middle, and ring finger may be added if digital active flexion is greater than 3 cm from the distal palmar crease.

       NOTE: No blocking is initiated to the small finger profundus because of the diameter and vascular supply of this tendon, both of which are deficient as compared to the other digits.

5. 7 weeks postoperative.

    a. Therapy—passive extension may be added.

6. 8 weeks postoperative.

    a. Therapy—gentle strengthening initiated.

7. 12 to 14 weeks postoperative.

    a. Return to normal, unrestricted activity.

C. Minimum active muscle tendon tension (MAMTT) method.[16]

1. Indications

    a. Therapist must factor in

       i. Strength of suture (must include epitenon running suture).

       ii. Amount of edema.

       iii. Significant increase in flexion forces during active combined wrist and finger flexion or active full fisting at the end of the flexion range even with wrist in extension.

       iv. Time from repair (should be initiated within 24 to 48 hours of repair).

2. Guidelines

    a. Splint: removable dorsal block splint with or without elastic traction.

    b. Therapy: (essentially same as EPM method except for the following):

       i. *By patient:* follow guidelines under early passive motion methods. No place and hold by patient without therapist supervision.

       ii. *By therapist:* begun 24 to 48 hours postoperative. Therapist performs appropriate PROM (as described in immobilization method). Therapist removes splint and positions wrist in 20 degrees extension while passively flexing MCPs to 80 degrees, PIPs to 75 degrees, and DIPs to 40 degrees. The patient then holds this position using no more than 20 grams of force. Patient relaxes. Therapist passively flexes wrist and MCPs while patient actively extends IP joints.

D. Four finger active method[17]
  1. Indications
    a. Suture: modified Kessler core suture and a new "cross-stitch" epitenon suture (or other suture with equal strength).
    b. Timing: within 48 hours of repair.
  2. 24 to 48 hours postoperative.
    a. Cast or circumferential splint.
      i. Wrist: neutral.
      ii. MCPs, IPs: rubberband traction and volar night splint same as four finger early passive motion method.
    b. Therapy: exercise same as EPM four finger method, except the patient actively holds full fist (after passive full fist) for 2 to 3 seconds. Program is progressed the same as four finger early passive motion.

POSTOPERATIVE COMPLICATIONS

  I. Tendon rupture.
  II. Minimal tendon gliding.
  III. Flexion contractures.
  IV. Excessive scar formation.
  V. Extreme pain.
  VI. Severe edema.
  VII. Infection.

EVALUATION TIMELINE

  I. First postoperative therapy session.
    A. General assessment of
      1. Wound
      2. Edema
      3. Pain
      4. Sensibility
      5. Passive flexion and active PIP/DIP joint extension in protective splint.
  II. 6 weeks (or as early as 3 weeks with adherent tendons): AROM and PROM.
  III. 10 weeks: Strength.
  IV. 12 weeks: Work assessment.

REFERENCES

1. von Strien G: Postoperative management of flexor tendon injuries. In: Hunter JM, Schneider LH, Mackin EJ, Callahan AD (eds): Rehabilitation of the Hand. 3rd Ed. Mosby, St. Louis, 1990

2. Collins DC, Schwarze L: Early progressive resistance following immobilization of flexor tendon repairs. J Hand Ther 4:118, 1991

3. Stewart KM, von Strien G: Postoperative management of flexor tendon injuries. In: Hunter JM, Mackin EJ, Callahan AD (eds): Rehabilitation of the Hand: Surgery and Therapy. 4th Ed. Mosby, St. Louis, 1995

4. Wehbe MA, Hunter JM: Flexor tendon gliding in the hand I: in vivo excursions. J Hand Surg 10A:570, 1985

5. Wehbe MA, Hunter JM: Flexor tendon gliding in the hand II: differential gliding, J Hand Surg 10A:575, 1985

6. Duran R, Houser R: Controlled passive motion following flexor tendon repair in Zones 2 and 3. In: AAOS Symposium on Tendon Surgery in the Hand. Mosby, St. Louis, 1975

7. Duran RJ, Coleman CR, Nappi JF: Management of flexor tendon lacerations in Zone 2 using controlled passive motion post operatively. In Hunter JM, Schneider LH, Mackin EJ, Callahan AD (eds): Rehabilitation of the Hand. 3rd Ed. Mosby, St. Louis, 1990

8. May EJ, Silfverskiold KL, Sollerman CJ: Controlled mobilization after flexor tendon repair in zone II: a prospective comparison of three methods. J Hand Surg 17A:942, 1992

9. Silfverskiold KL, May EJ, Törnvall AH: Flexor digitorum profundus excursions during controlled motion after flexor tendon repair in Zone II: a prospective clinical study. J Hand Surg 17A:122, 1992

10. Silfverskiold KL, May EJ, Törnvall AH: Tendon excursions after flexor tendon repair in zone II: results with a new controlled motion program. J Hand Surg 18A:403, 1993

11. Chow J, Thomes LJ, Dovelle S et al: A combined regimen of controlled motion following flexor tendon repair in "no man's land." Plast Reconstr Surg 79:447, 1987

12. Dovelle S, Heeter P: The Washington regimen: rehabilitation of the hand following flexor tendon injuries. Phys Ther 69:1034, 1989

13. Evans R: A study of the zone I flexor tendon injury and implications for treatment. J Hand Ther 3:133, 1990

14. Cannon N: Post flexor tendon repair protocol. Indiana Hand Center Newsletter 1:13, 1993

15. Strickland JW: Flexor tendon repair: Indiana method. Indiana Hand Center Newsletter 1:1, 1993

16. Evans RB, Thompson DE: The application of force to the healing tendon. J Hand Ther 6:266, 1993

17. Silfverskiold KL, May EJ: Flexor tendon repair in zone II with a new suture technique and an early mobilization program combining passive and active flexion. J Hand Surg 19A:53, 1994

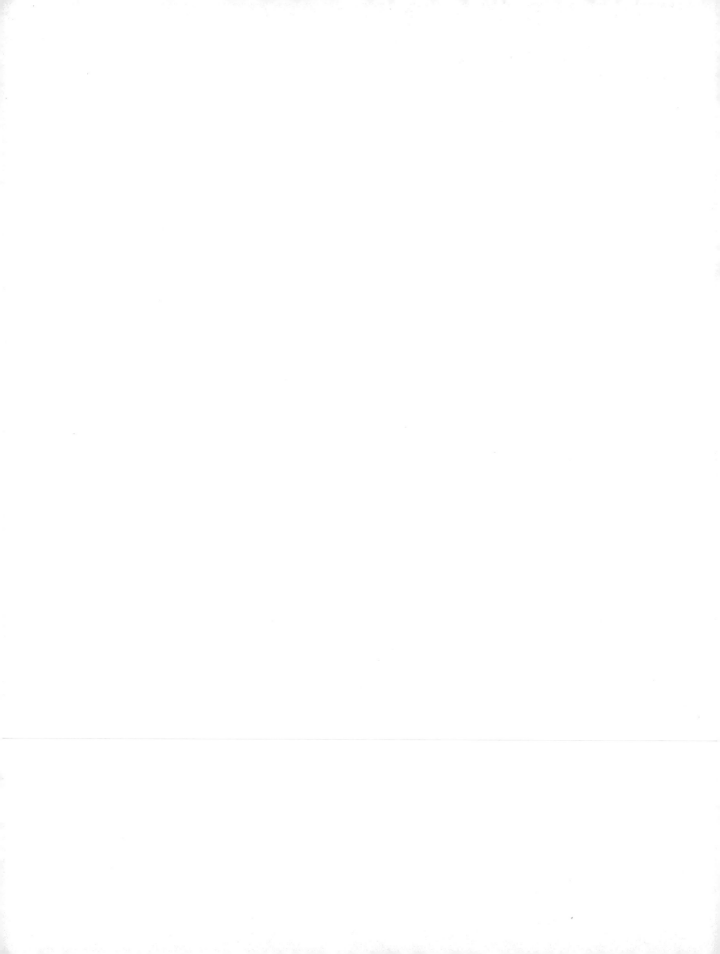

Flexor Tenolysis 12

Barbara Steinberg

Flexor tenolysis is an elective surgical procedure that may be performed after primary tendon repair, grafting, or staged tendon reconstruction. It may be indicated when despite appropriate surgery and postoperative therapy with a highly motivated and compliant patient, active range of motion (AROM) is significantly less than passive range of motion (PROM) secondary to scar adhesions.[1]

Close surgeon—therapist communication is indicated before initiation of treatment to understand the condition of the tendon intraoperatively and to be made aware of any ancillary procedures. If the therapist is able to observe the surgery, this communication is greatly facilitated.

After surgery, two different treatment approaches may be used during the first 4 to 6 weeks. Both approaches involve early mobilization. With a good quality tendon and good quality pulleys (as noted by the surgeon intraoperatively), the more progressive approach may be used.[1,2] The "frayed tendon protocol"[1] is used with a poor quality tendon and/or after pulley reconstruction. If an auditory or palpable crepitation is noted while using the more progressive approach on an apparently good quality tendon without pulley reconstruction, it is important to move to the frayed tendon guideline, as this may be a sign of impending rupture.[1] The frayed tendon guideline is used to decrease demands on the involved tendon or pulley while maintaining the tendon excursion achieved during surgery.

DEFINITION

Flexor tenolysis is a secondary surgical procedure in which adhesions or other obstacles that impede normal flexor tendon gliding are released (Fig. 12-1).

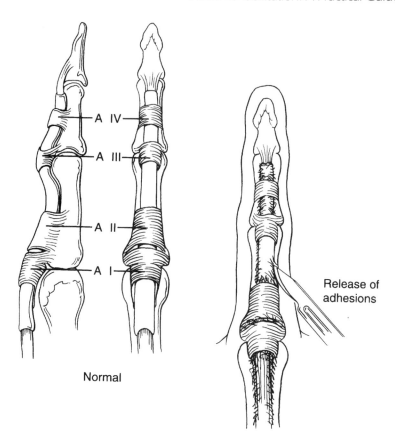

Normal

Fig. 12-1. Adhesions are released in tenolysis surgery.

SURGICAL AND TREATMENT PURPOSE

To restore flexor tendon function to a finger or fingers when tendon gliding has been compromised or lost because of scar adhesions. The surgical approach may be very localized or very extensive depending on the preoperative and intraoperative assessment. Sharp dissection is used and great care is taken to preserve the critical portions of the digital pulley systems. Intraoperative assessment can be made by pulling on the tendons themselves or by carrying out the operation under local anesthesia to observe active motion. Early therapy is instituted frequently to reduce the opportunities for re-scarring. Tendon rupture is a real and serious complication because tenolysis may render the structure avascular. Careful and attentive postoperative care is required to achieve an optimal goal.

PURPOSE OF POSTOPERATIVE TREATMENT

I. Week 1
   A. Achieve intraoperative active/passive range of motion (A/PROM) before binding adhesions can form.
   B. Prevent flexion contracture via splinting.[3]

II. Weeks 2 to 3
   A. Maintain AROM as collagen bands begin to form.
   B. Control edema.
   C. Initiate functional use of involved hand.
   D. Achieve independence in activities of daily living (ADLs).[3]
III. Weeks 4 to 6
   A. Maintain A/PROM as collagen bands continue to form and gain in strength.
   B. Scar management to continue to remodel collagen.
   C. Increase grip and pinch strength as tendon integrity allows.[3]
IV. Weeks 7 to 8
   A. Maximize strength.
   B. Initiate job simulation in preparation for return to work at 8 to 12 weeks, depending on job demands.
   C. Initiate heavy resistance at week 8.[3]

POSTOPERATIVE INDICATIONS/ PRECAUTIONS FOR THERAPY

I. Indications
   Digit(s) having undergone flexor tenolysis surgery
II. Precautions
   A. Pulley reconstruction.
   B. Capsulectomy.
   C. Poor quality or badly scarred tendon as reported by surgeon following procedure.
   D. An auditory or palpable crepitation in the digit during early mobilization may indicate impending rupture.

POSTOPERATIVE THERAPY

I. Consult with surgeon regarding intraoperative A/PROM, condition of the tendon, status of the pulley system, as well as any additional procedure performed such as pulley reconstruction and/or capsulectomy.
II. Pulley reconstruction protection[4]
   A. Identify areas of pulley reconstruction.
   B. Protect by circumferential Velcro/thermoplastic ring until edema is under control and then thermoplastic ring (Fig. 12-2).
   C. Continue protection 6 months postoperatively.
III. Program for good quality tendons
   A. 12 to 24 hours through first postoperative week (inflammation phase of wound healing)
   1. Splint
      a. Forearm based progressive extension or static extension (Fig. 12-3) worn day and night for 2 weeks to help prevent flexion contractures. Remove only for exercise and wound care.

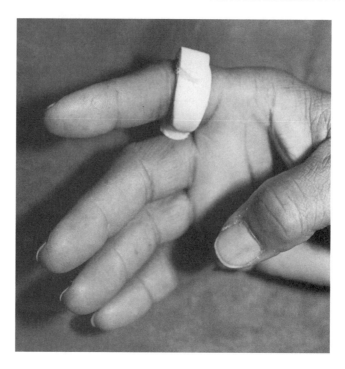

Fig. 12-2. Pulley reconstruction is protected by circumferential thermoplastic ring.

2. Exercise
    a. Active: 5 to 10 repetitions each exercise hourly.
        i. Place and hold as defined in Exercises Defined I.
        ii. Finger blocking as defined in Exercises Defined IV.
        iii. Finger extension
    b. Passive: 5 to 10 repetitions three times a day[3,4] or as often as every hour if passive motion is limited.[1] Gentle, PROM all joints.
3. Edema control

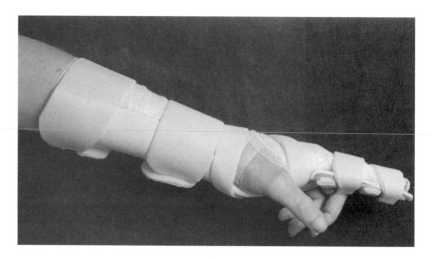

Fig. 12-3. A forearm based static extension splint is used postoperatively.

B. 2 to 3 weeks postoperative (initiation of proliferative phase of wound healing)

1. Splint
   a. Static or progressive extension: decrease use in day as AROM achieved intraoperatively is maintained pain free. Continue use at night to prevent/decrease flexion contracture.
   b. Dynamic extension for flexion contractures may be used with surgeon's approval, for short periods during the day (Fig. 12-4).

2. Exercise
   a. Continue exercises as above.
   b. Add active tendon gliding (3 to 10 repetitions per hour) as defined in Exercises Defined II.

3. Activities of daily living (ADL)
   a. Light ADL
   b. Nonresistive grasp and release

C. 4 to 6 weeks postoperative (proliferative phase of wound healing ending as scar remodeling phase begins)

1. Splint
   a. Static or progressive extension. Wear in daytime only if needed. Continue night use for 6 months postoperatively.
   b. Dynamic extension to assist with extension as needed. May leave on for most of the day. Patient may exercise into flexion against resistance of splint.

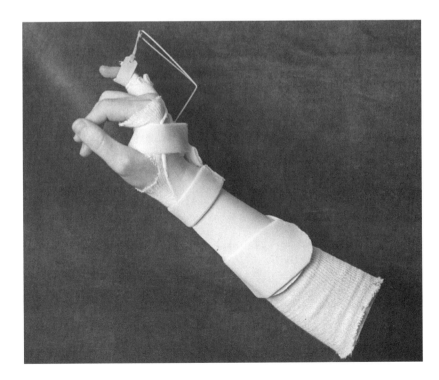

Fig. 12-4. Dynamic extension for contractures may be used with doctor's approval.

       2. Exercise
         a. Continue exercises above as needed.
         b. Graded isometric grip strengthening with physician approval. Monitor closely.
       3. ADL
         a. ADL
         b. Graded ADL
    D. 8 to 12 weeks postoperative (scar remodeling continues)
       1. Gradually increase resistive exercises and activities to no restrictions at 12 weeks.
IV. "Frayed tendon program"[1,2,5]
    A. Indications
       1. Surgical finding of poor quality tendon.
       2. Pulleys reconstructed.
       3. Tendons with auditory or palpable crepitation during uncomplicated early mobilization program.
    B. First 4 to 6 weeks postoperative
       1. Splint: same as uncomplicated
       2. Exercise
         a. Protected PROM as defined in Exercises Defined III, 10 repetitions, three times a day.
         b. Place and hold.
    C. 7 to 12 weeks postoperative: same as good quality tendon program

POSTOPERATIVE COMPLICATIONS

    I. Pain
   II. Edema
  III. Bleeding
  IV. Infection
   V. Patient's inability to tolerate postoperative therapy
  VI. Excessive scar formation
 VII. Auditory or palpable crepitation
VIII. Tendon rupture
  IX. Flexion contractures
   X. Reconstructed pulley rupture
  XI. Minimal gain or actual loss of motion

EXERCISES DEFINED

  I. Place and hold technique[1]
    A. Passively manipulate the digit into the fully flexed position with the uninvolved hand.
    B. Patient actively maintains the digit in this position.

C. Manipulation hand is released and lysed tendon(s) are maintained in flexion with their own muscle power, confirming active muscle contraction. This is followed by actively extending the digit(s).

D. Additional protection can be achieved by maintaining some element of wrist flexion, although full excursion of tendon is not achieved in this position.

E. The patient's discomfort level determines the beginning number of repetitions, maintaining frequency of every waking hour, working up to 10 repetitions per hour.

II. Tendon gliding

A. *Hook fist:* begin with the fingers in full extension. With metacarpophalangeal (MCP) joints in extension, actively flex proximal interphalangeal (PIP) joints and distal interphalangeal (DIP) joints. Flexor digitorum superficialis [FDS] and flexor digitorum profundus [FDP] independently glide over each other most in this position.[6]

B. *Full fist:* beginning in hook fist position, flex MCPs, PIPs, and DIPs fully, touching distal palmar crease. (FDP reaches its maximum excursion with respect to bone in this position.) End with fingers in full extension.[6]

C. *Straight fist:* begin with fingers in full extension. Actively flex MCPs and PIPs while maintaining DIPs in extension. (FDS reaches its maximum excursion in respect to bone in this position.)[6]

D. Wrist flexion with finger flexion.[7]

E. Wrist extension with finger extension.[7]

III. Protected PROM technique

Passively flex other digits and wrist while passively extending and flexing in turn the MCP, PIP, and DIP joints.

IV. Finger blocking technique

A. Block MCP and PIP joints into extension, allowing isolated active DIP flexion.

B. Block MCP into extension, allowing isolated PIP flexion.

EVALUATION TIMELINE

I. 1 to 2 weeks preoperative

A. AROM and PROM (blocked and full excursion)

B. Fingertip to distal palmar crease (active and passive)

C. Strength

D. Circumferential measurements

II. First postoperative therapy session (12 to 24 hours postoperative)

A. Assessment

1. Wound

2. Edema

3. Pain

4. Sensibility

    B. Measurement
       1. AROM and PROM
       2. Fingertip to distal palmar crease (active and passive)
III. A/PROM and scar re-evaluated weekly first 8 weeks and then every 4 weeks.
IV. Strength measurements at 4 to 6 weeks with good quality tendons and surgeon approval, at 8 weeks, then at 4-week intervals.
V. Sensibility re-evaluated at 4 weeks, then at 4-week intervals.

REFERENCES

1. Cannon NW, Strickland JW: Therapy following flexor tendon surgery. Hand Clin 1:147, 1985
2. Strickland JW: Flexor tenolysis: a personal experience. p. 216. In Hunter JM, Schneider LH, Mackin EJ (eds): Tendon Surgery in the Hand. Mosby, St. Louis, 1987
3. Schneider LH, Mackin EJ: Tenolysis: dynamic approach to surgery and therapy. p. 417. In Hunter JM, Schneider LH, Mackin EJ, Callahan AD (eds): Rehabilitation of the Hand. 3rd Ed. Mosby, St. Louis, 1990
4. Mackin EJ: Benefits of early tendon gliding after tenolysis. In Hunter JM, Schneider LH, Mackin EJ (eds): Tendon Surgery in the Hand. Mosby, St. Louis, 1987
5. Strickland JW: Flexor tenolysis. Hand Clin 1:121, 1985
6. Wehbe MA: Tendon gliding exercises. Am J Occup Ther 41:164, 1987
7. Cannon NW: Enhancing flexor tendon glide through tenolysis … and hand therapy. J Hand Ther 2:122, 1989

SUGGESTED READINGS

Schneider LH: Flexor tenolysis. In Hunter JM, Schneider LH, Mackin EJ (eds): Tendon Surgery in the Hand. Mosby, St. Louis, 1987
Verdan C: Tenolysis: p. 137. In Verdan C (ed): Tendon Surgery of the Hand. Churchill Livingstone, New York, 1979

Primary Tendon Grafts

13

Barbara Steinberg

Although primary flexor tendon repair is generally the best postinjury treatment choice, there are times when this is neither possible nor indicated. These include, but are not limited to, the following situations: the wound or the patient's general condition may disallow direct repair,[1] a flexor tendon injury may be missed at the time of injury,[1] or there may be a late referral for definitive care that may make it impossible for the surgeon to perform an end to end repair.[1]

Three basic postsurgical treatment approaches are described: (1) early mobilization similar to zone II primary flexor tendon repairs,[2] (2) 3 to 4 weeks of immobilization,[2] and the situation in which the flexor digitorum profoundus is repaired in a digit with a noninjured flexor digitorum superficialis.[3]

As with primary tendon repairs, it is necessary to adjust the progression of treatment according to the "feel" of the tendon graft as it is healing. When early recovery of active range of motion (AROM) is seen and the tendon is gliding well, protective splinting is continued longer and treatment progresses more slowly, as the risk of tendon rupture is greater in the "soft healers."[1]

Conversely, where little active tendon glide is noted when AROM is initiated, progression may need to be faster (in consultation with physician) to decrease the effect of tendon adhesions while preventing tendon rupture.

Judgment must also be used in educating the more active or impulsive patient, as well as the more reluctant to facilitate patient compliance in achieving the best result with the fewest complications.

DEFINITION

Removal of injured tendon and replacement with palm to fingertip tendon graft (Fig. 13-1).

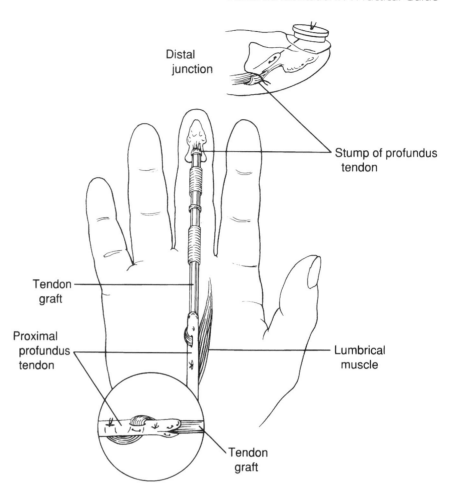

Fig. 13-1. Injured tendon is removed and replaced with a tendon graft.

SURGICAL PURPOSE

After flexor or extensor tendon injuries or conditions that cause scarring that prevents tendon gliding, tendon grafting is sometimes indicated. The tendon graft is used to bridge a gap between the muscle unit and the insertion of the tendon into bone. It is most commonly used for the flexor tendons that have been interrupted between the origin of the lumbrical muscles and their distal insertion.

TREATMENT GOALS

I. Loss of both flexor digitorum superficialis (FDS)/flexor digitorum profundus (FDP) function
   A. Preoperative
      1. Full passive range of motion (PROM) proximal interphalangeal (PIP) and distal interphalangeal (DIP) joints
      2. Soft, pliable tissues

    3. Patient education regarding
       a. Preoperative therapy
       b. Postoperative therapy
  B. Postoperative
     1. Prevent rupture at proximal and distal tendon junctures.
     2. Minimize adhesion formation.
     3. Prevent flexion contractures.
     4. Prevent hyperextension deformity at PIP joint, which can
        occur with absent superficialis.
     5. Promote tendon healing.
     6. Encourage tendon gliding.
     7. Restore AROM and PROM.
     8. Maintain full AROM of all uninvolved joints of affected
        upper extremity.
     9. Return to previous level of function.
II. FDS intact/FDP absent.
    Preoperative and postoperative goals are the same as above,
    except add:
  A. Preoperative: normal FDS AROM and PROM.
  B. Postoperative: regain active superficialis function while protect-
     ing profundus graft.

PREOPERATIVE INDICATIONS FOR THERAPY

  I. Indications
     A. Decreased range of motion (ROM)
     B. Adherent scar
     C. Weak proximal muscle units

PREOPERATIVE THERAPY

  I. Patient education regarding complexity of rehabilitation and nec-
     essary patient compliance.
 II. Scar management
III. PROM
 IV. AROM of PIP joint if FDS uninvolved
  V. Strengthening
     A. Proximal flexor motor units
     B. Extrinsic/intrinsic extensors

POSTOPERATIVE INDICATIONS/ PRECAUTIONS FOR THERAPY

  I. Indications
     Digit has undergone free tendon grafting procedure.

II. Precautions
  A. Avoid strengthening until 9 to 10 weeks following graft due to avascular nature of free tendon grafts.[2]
  B. Protect reconstructed pulleys if indicated.

POSTOPERATIVE THERAPY

I. Both FDS/FDP absent preoperatively
  A. Two approaches
    1. Early mobilization
      a. Weeks 0 to 8: same as primary flexor tendon guideline except delay in strengthening.
      b. Weeks 9 to 10: initiate graded strengthening.
      c. Weeks 12 to 14: normal unrestricted use of hand.
    2. Early immobilization
      a. Weeks 0 to 3 or 4
          Splint: posterior plaster or thermoplastic with wrist 20 degrees to 30 degrees flexion, MCP joints 60 degrees to 70 degrees of flexion and IP joints in extension.
      b. Weeks 3 to 4
        i. Splint: worn between exercise programs for 1 to 2 additional weeks.
        ii. Exercise: AROM initiated.
      c. Weeks 4 to 14: same as early mobilization
II. FDS intact with FDP absent preoperatively[3]
    Weeks 0 to 8: same as above (Postoperative Therapy I) except active isolated FDS flexion begun first week postoperative with wrist and MCPs flexed while holding unaffected digits (PIPs/DIPs) in passive extension.

POSTOPERATIVE COMPLICATIONS

  I. Tendon rupture
  II. Adhesions limiting tendon gliding
  III. Flexion contracture
  IV. Extreme pain
  V. Severe edema
  VI. Infection
  VII. Pulley ruptured or attenuated
VIII. Suboptimal graft length

EVALUATION TIME LINE

I. Preoperative
  A. Wound and skin condition
  B. Edema

    C. Pain

    D. Sensibility

    E. PROM

    F. AROM

    G. Strength

II. Postoperative

    A. First postoperative visit gross assessment

       1. Wound and skin condition

       2. Edema

       3. Pain

       4. Sensibility

       5. Passive flexion

    B. Week 6: active and passive motion

    C. Week 12: strength

REFERENCES

1. Schneider LH, Hunter JM: Flexor tendons—late reconstruction. p. 1969. In Green DP (ed): Operative Hand Surgery. Vol. 3. Churchill Livingstone, New York, 1988
2. Cannon NM: Therapy following flexor tendon surgery. p. 147. Hand Clin 1:156, 1985
3. McClinton MA, Curtis RM, Wilgis EFS: One hundred tendon grafts for isolated flexor digitorum injuries. J Hand Surg 7:224, 1982

Staged Tendon Reconstruction

14

Barbara Steinberg

Staged tendon reconstruction is a salvage procedure. Therapy for this procedure consists of three parts: preoperative, postoperative stage I, and postoperative stage II.

At the preoperative phase, patient education is a major component. The purpose of patient education is twofold. The first is to educate the patient regarding the surgical and rehabilitative requirements of these procedures. The second purpose of patient education is to monitor the patient's compliance with preoperative therapy to help assess the patient's willingness and ability to follow through with postoperative therapy.

Therapist–surgeon communication regarding surgical details is indicated after stage I and II procedures. After stage I, the therapist should be made aware of any other procedures such as pulley reconstruction or joint releases. After stage II, the therapist should be made aware of the amount of tension on the graft and the predicted active motion of the digit.

DEFINITION

Staged tendon reconstruction is a two-stage tendon graft procedure with implantation of Silastic rod at stage I to establish a smooth walled channel.[1,2] This is followed by removal of the implant and placement of a free tendon graft within the neosheath at stage II[1-3] (Figs. 14-1 and 14-2).

SURGICAL PURPOSE

Staged tendon reconstruction is used most often for the flexor units, although the technique may be used for the extensors. It is used when there is a scarred bed through which the tendons may be required to

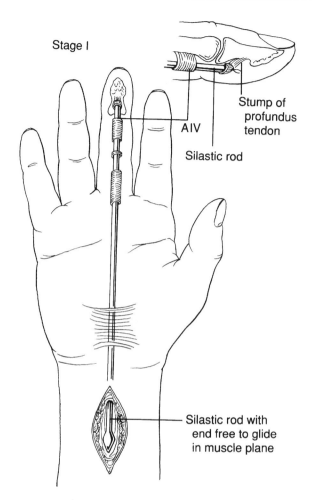

Stage I

Stump of
profundus
tendon

A IV

Silastic rod

Silastic rod with
end free to glide
in muscle plane

Fig. 14-1. Digit with Silastic rod
during stage I.

glide. Concomitantly pulley reconstructions may be necessary. A passive
tendon prosthesis of silicone is placed in the finger and palm to create a
new tendon sheath through which an autologous tendon is passed later.
The method is primarily used for salvage operations when other alternatives are not available.

TREATMENT GOALS

   I. Preoperative
     A. Restoration of passive range of motion (PROM) with fingertip
       passively touching distal palmar crease.
     B. Maintain or re-establish supple soft tissues.
     C. Maintain or re-establish strength of proximal muscles.
     D. Promote balanced flexion–extension system.
  II. Postoperative stage I
     A. Continue with goals A through D above.

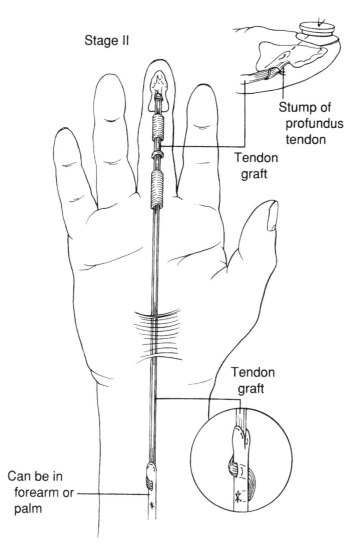

Fig. 14-2. Digit with graft within neosheath at stage II.

B. Facilitate proximal portion of sheath formation in as lengthened a position as possible via splinting.[4]

III. Postoperative stage II
   A. Prevent rupture at proximal and distal tendon junctures.
   B. Minimize adhesion formation.
   C. Prevent flexion contractures.
   D. Prevent hyperextension deformity at proximal interphalangeal (PIP) joint, which can occur with absent superficialis.
   E. Promote tendon healing.
   F. Encourage tendon gliding.
   G. Restore active range of motion (AROM) and PROM.

H. Maintain full AROM of all uninvolved joints of affected upper extremity.

I. Return to previous level of function.

INDICATIONS FOR PREOPERATIVE THERAPY

I. Decreased range of motion (ROM)
II. Adherent scar
III. Weak proximal muscle units

PREOPERATIVE THERAPY

I. Exercise
   A. PROM
   B. "Finger trapping"[2]
II. Splinting
   A. Flexion limited
      1. Buddy taping (Fig. 14-3).
      2. Intrinsic stretch splinting (Fig. 14-4)
      3. PIP/distal interphalangeal (DIP) joint flexion straps (Fig. 14-5)
   B. Extension limited
      1. Three-point extension splint (Fig. 14-6)

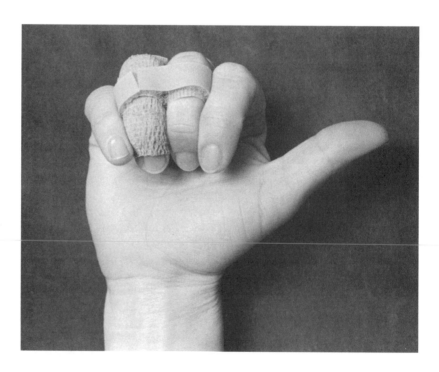

Fig. 14-3. Buddy taping to facilitate increased flexion.

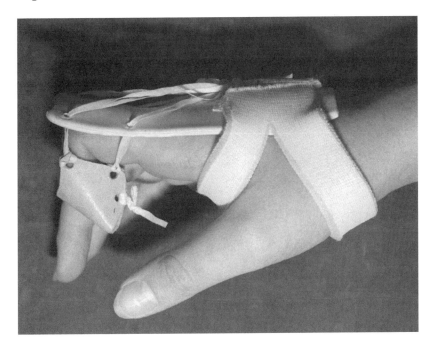

Fig. 14-4. Intrinsic stretch splinting to increase flexion.

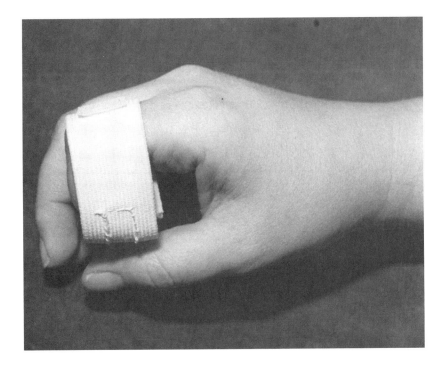

Fig. 14-5. PIP/DIP flexion strap for improving flexion.

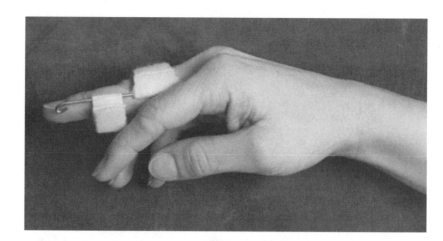

Fig. 14-6. Three-point extension splint to increase extension.

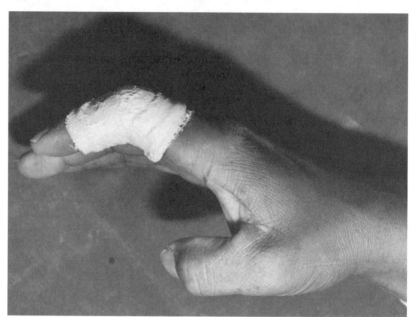

Fig. 14-7. Serial casts can help increase extension.

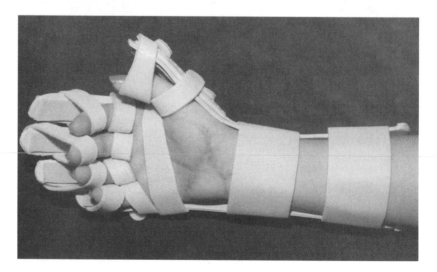

Fig. 14-8. Serially applied thermoplastic splints can increase extension.

2. Serial casts (Fig. 14-7)
3. Serially applied thermoplastic splints (Fig. 14-8)
III. Strengthening

INDICATIONS/PRECAUTIONS FOR POSTOPERATIVE THERAPY

I. Indications
   Digit has undergone stage I or stage II tendon reconstruction.
II. Precautions
   A. Stage I postoperative
      1. Avoid overexercising, which can lead to synovitis.
      2. Avoid attenuation of extensor tendon at DIP joint.
      3. Protect reconstructed pulleys if present.
   B. Stage II postoperative
      Monitor pain at insertion, which could be precursor of rupture.

POSTOPERATIVE THERAPY

I. Stage I
   A. Immediately postoperative
      Splint: dorsal protective splint with wrist in 30 degrees flexion, metacarpophalangeal (MCP) joints in 60 degrees to 70 degrees flexion, and interphalangeal (IP) joints in full extension (Fig. 14-9).
   B. Day 1 to 3 weeks postoperative
      1. PROM
      2. Wound care
      3. Edema control
      4. Scar management
   C. 3 weeks to 6 weeks
      1. Splint
         a. Protective splint discontinued unless signs of synovitis are present.
         b. Initiate splints to facilitate full PROM.
         c. Figure-of-eight splint for PIP joint if "swan-neck" deformity is present or developing (Fig. 14-10). Continue until volar plate is strong enough to support PIP joint or until stage II surgery is performed.[4]
      2. Exercise, wound care, edema control, and scar management continue.
   D. 6 weeks
      1. Return to normal activities.
      2. Treatment continued until stage I goals are met.

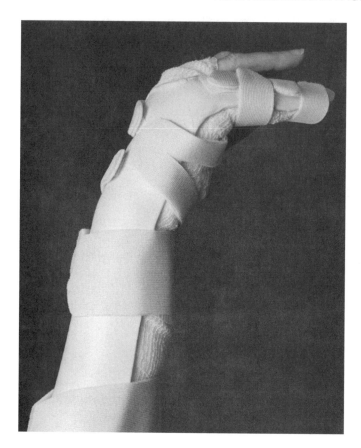

Fig. 14-9. Dorsal protective splint following stage I surgery.

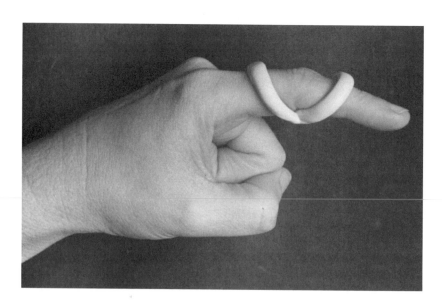

Fig. 14-10. Figure-of-eight splint is used if "swan-neck" deformity is present or develops.

II. Stage II

Same as zone II primary flexor tendon graft: see appropriate guideline.

POSTOPERATIVE COMPLICATIONS

I. Stage I
   A. Synovitis
   B. Swan-neck deformity
   C. Limited ROM/attenuation of extensor tendon
   D. Skin breakdown at distal insertion of implant
   E. Implant "kinking" or disruption
   F. Pain
   G. Edema
   H. Hematoma
   I. Infection
II. Stage II
   A. Tendon rupture
   B. Adhesions limiting tendon gliding
   C. Flexion contracture
   D. Extreme pain
   E. Severe edema
   F. Infection
   G. Suboptimal graft length

EVALUATION TIMELINE

I. Preoperative
   A. Wound and skin condition
   B. Edema
   C. Pain
   D. Sensibility
   E. PROM
   F. AROM
   G. Strength
II. Stage I postoperative
   A. Wound
   B. Edema
   C. Pain
   D. Sensibility
   E. Passive flexion
   F. Active PIP/DIP extension with wrist and MCP flexed
III. Stage II postoperative
   A. First postoperative visit general assessment of
      1. Wound and skin condition
      2. Edema

3. Pain
4. Sensibility
5. Passive flexion/protected active/passive extension
B. Week 6: active flexion and passive extension
C. Week 12: strength

REFERENCES

1. Cannon NM, Strickland JW: Therapy following flexor tendon surgery. Hand Clin 1:156, 1985
2. Mackin EJ, Hunter JM: Pre- and Post-Operative Hand Therapy Program for Patients with Staged Tendon Implants (Hunter Design). Hand Rehabilitation Foundation, Philadelphia, 1986
3. Hunter JM, Singer DI, Mackin EJ: Staged flexor tendon reconstruction using passive and active tendon implants. p. 427. In Hunter JM, Schneider LH, Mackin EJ, Callahan AD (eds): Rehabilitation of the Hand, 3rd Ed. Mosby, St. Louis, 1990
4. Stanley BG: Flexor tendon injuries: late solution therapist's management. Hand Clin 12:140, 1986

SUGGESTED READINGS

Hunter JM, Blackmore SM, Callahan AD: Flexor tendon salvage and functional redemption using the Hunter tendon implant and the superficialis Finer operation. J Hand Ther 2:107, 1989

Hunter JM, Daniel IS, Jaeger SH et al: Active tendon implants in flexor tendon reconstruction. J Hand Surg 13A:849, 1988

Lister MBG: Pitfalls and complications of flexor tendon surgery. Hand Clin 1:133, 1985

Schneider LH, Hunter JM: Flexor tendons—late reconstruction. p. 1967. In Green DP (ed): Operative Hand Surgery. Vol. 3. Churchill Livingstone, New York, 1988

Wehbe MA: Staged tendon reconstruction: technique and repair. p. 260. In Hunter JM, Schneider LH, Mackin EJ (eds): Tendon Surgery in the Hand. Mosby, St. Louis, 1987

Wehbe MA: Tendon gliding exercises. Am J Occup Ther 41:164, 1987

Mallet Finger **15**

Arlynne Pack Brown

Mallet finger injury is a traumatic disruption of the terminal tendon resulting in a loss of active extension of the distal interphalangeal (DIP) joint. This may or may not be associated with a fracture of the articular surface. Names synonymous with mallet finger injury are baseball finger[1] and drop finger.[2]

The primary goal of rehabilitation is to promote healing of the tendon so as to maximize function and range of motion (ROM) of the injured DIP joint.

Ruptures and lacerations may be treated closed with noninvasive splint immobilization or open with Kirschner wire (K-wire) fixation. Avulsion fractures are commonly secured into bone using the button technique with interosseus wire.

Whether immobilized closed with splints or open with K-wires or the button technique, the first 6 weeks of treatment are the same. During this initial period, the involved joint is immobilized full time while exercises are performed to maintain the ROM of the uninvolved joints. At the conclusion of the initial immobilization, the splints or internal fixators are removed and the integrity of the terminal tendon evaluated. If the tendon is unable to maintain extension and the joint droops into flexion, a splint is reapplied and tested periodically thereafter for healing and strength. When the tendon is "healed" enough, active flexion and extension are begun, monitored for overstretching, and progressed or digressed in ROM and strengthening exercises as indicated.

DEFINITION

I. Traumatically induced loss of active extension of the DIP joint caused by avulsion, rupture, laceration of the terminal tendon,[3] or fractured base of distal phalanx with tendon insertion attached (Fig. 15-1).

143

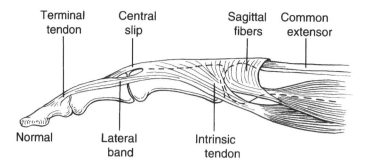

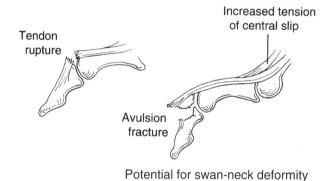

Potential for swan-neck deformity

Fig. 15-1. Normal anatomy and two variations of mallet finger injury.

II. Injury may be classified according to the amount of articular surface involved in the associated fracture.[4]
   A. Type A: fracture of less than one-third of the articular surface
   B. Type B: fracture of one-third to two-thirds of the articular surface
   C. Type C: fracture of greater than two-thirds of the articular surface
   D. Note additional category of fracture dislocation DIP joint.
III. Other names for mallet finger injury
   A. Mallet finger deformity[3]
   B. Baseball finger[1]
   C. Drop finger[2]

TREATMENT AND SURGICAL PURPOSE

To restore extension to the DIP joint where there has been disruption of the terminal portion of the extensor tendon. When the injury is closed and the tendon continuity is lost, splinting of the DIP joint is preferred. If there has been a laceration of the tendon, a surgical repair by suture may be indicated. An avulsion fracture of the distal phalanx without DIP dislocation may be treated by splinting with the joint in extension. When there is an avulsion fracture with volar subluxation of the distal phalanx, open reduction and internal fixation is considered. The results of these treatment regimens frequently provide a good result; however, a permanent extension lag at the DIP joint may be anticipated. In some patients a concurrent hyperextension posture of the proximal interphalangeal (PIP) joint can be noted.

TREATMENT GOALS

I. Promote healing of terminal tendon and associated fracture.
II. Maintain full ROM of all uninvolved joints of the upper extremity.
III. Prevent swan-neck deformity and DIP joint flexion contracture.
IV. Avoid pin tract infection if applicable.
V. Maximize ROM of DIP joint and PIP joint. In particular, maximize active DIP joint extension.
VI. Return to previous level of function.
VII. Prevent re-injury.

NONOPERATIVE INDICATIONS/ PRECAUTIONS FOR THERAPY

I. Indications
  A. Mallet finger injury without fracture
  B. Mallet finger injury associated with nondisplaced fracture
II. Precautions
  A. Extreme pain
  B. Extreme edema
  C. Tape allergy[5]

NONOPERATIVE THERAPY

I. Management of closed treatment
  A. Weeks 0 to 6: continuous splinting in 0 degrees or slight hyperextension (see Splints below). Change adhesive tape and check skin regularly.
  B. Weeks 6 to 7: Continue day and night splint. Begin active flexion up to 20 degrees to 25 degrees.[6] May use a volar template to limit flexion during exercise.
  C. Weeks 7 to 8: Continue day and night splint. If no extension lag, begin active flexion to 35 degrees.[6]
  D. Weeks 8 to 12: If no extension lag, discontinue day splint but continue night splint. If extension lag persists, balance splinting and exercise to minimize lag.
  E. Week 12: begin unrestricted use.
II. Splints[5–8]
  A. Position DIP joint at 0 degrees or slight hyperextension. Hyperextend DIP joint without blanching dorsal skin.[2,6]
  B. Splints may be on dorsal or volar surface.
    1. Dorsal
      a. Advantages: does not interfere with PIP joint flexion; allows for sensibility of tip.
  C. Splint types
    1. Alumifoam (Fig. 15-2)
    2. Stack (Fig. 15-3)
    3. Sugar tong alumifoam (Fig. 15-4)

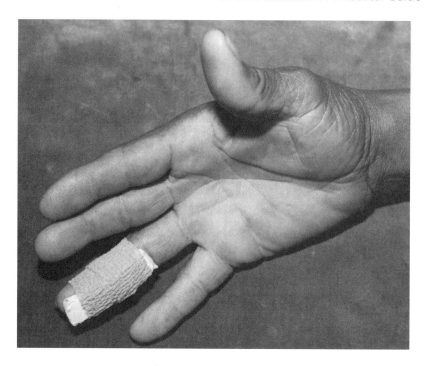

Fig. 15-2. Alumifoam splint.

    4. Custom thermoplastic (Fig. 15-5)
D. Splint fasteners
    1. Adhesive tape
    2. Velcro: may not provide enough security against axial rotation and distal slippage of splint
    3. Coban

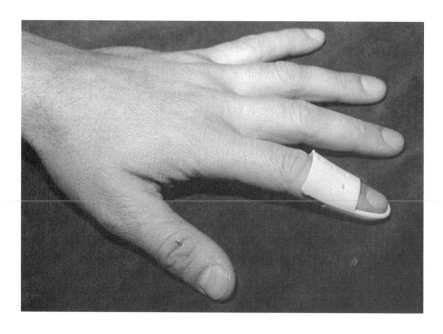

Fig. 15-3. Stack splint.

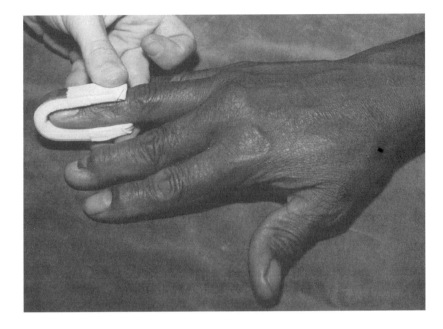

Fig. 15-4. Sugar tong alumifoam splint.

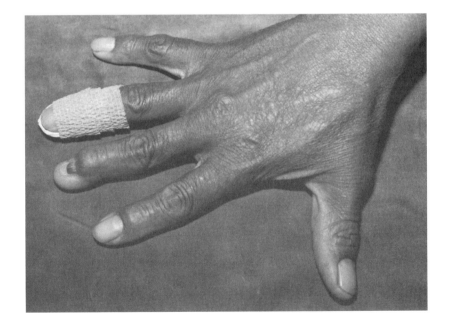

Fig. 15-5. Custom thermoplastic splint.

NONOPERATIVE COMPLICATIONS

    I. Maceration or necrosis of skin[4,5,7]
    II. Maceration or necrosis of nailbed[7]
    III. Swan-neck deformity[4]
    IV. Tape allergy[5]
    V. Extension lag at DIP joint[2]

POSTOPERATIVE INDICATIONS/ PRECAUTIONS FOR THERAPY

I. Indications

Avulsions, ruptures, or lacerations of the terminal tendon with associated intra-articular DIP joint fractures managed with K-wires or buttons

II. Precautions

A. Infection

B. Extreme pain

C. Extreme edema

POSTOPERATIVE THERAPY

I. Week 0 to 6

A. K-wire or button intact

B. ROM of uninvolved joints

C. Pin site care

II. Week 6

A. K-wire removed.

B. Begin active ROM (AROM) and follow closed treatment as described above (See Nonoperative Therapy).

POSTOPERATIVE COMPLICATIONS

I. Infection

II. Necrosis of nailbed[7]

III. DIP joint extension lag

IV. Swan-neck deformity[4]

EVALUATION TIMELINE

I. Week 1

A. AROM and passive ROM (PROM) of all upper extremity joints except involved DIP joint

B. Sensibility

II. Week 6

Active extensive DIP joint

III. Week 8

Active flexion DIP joint

IV. Week 10

A. Grip and pinch strength

B. Passive flexion at DIP joint

REFERENCES

1. Wilson RL: Management of acute extensor tendon injuries. p. 337. In Hunter JM, Schneider LH, Mackin EJ (eds): Tendon Surgery of the Hand. Mosby, St. Louis, 1987
2. Clement RC, Wray RC Jr: Operative and nonoperative treatment of mallet finger. Ann Plast Surg 16:136, 1986
3. Elliott RA: Splints for mallet and boutonniere deformities. Plast Reconstr Surg 52:282, 1973
4. Wehbe MA, Schneider LH: Mallet fractures. J Bone Joint Surg 66:658, 1984
5. Stern PJ: Complications and prognosis of treatment of mallet finger. J Hand Surg. 13A:329, 1988
6. Evans RE: Therapeutic management of extensor tendon injuries. p. 492. In Hunter JM, Schneider LH, Mackin EJ, Callahan AD (eds): Rehabilitation of the Hand. Mosby, St. Louis, 1990
7. Hunter JM, Schneider LH, Mackin EJ, Callahan AD (eds): Rehabilitation of the Hand. Mosby, St. Louis, 1990
8. Patel MR, DeSai SS, Bassini-Lipson L: Conservative management of chronic mallet finger. J Hand Surg 11A:570, 1986

Swan-neck Deformity 16

Dale Eckhaus

Swan-neck deformities occur through extrinsic, intrinsic, and articular abnormal anatomic factors.[1] The etiology of these factors include rheumatologic disease, extensor terminal tendon injuries, spastic conditions, injuries that cause volar plate laxity, fractures to the middle phalanx that heal in hyperextension, and generalized ligamentous laxity.[2] The deformity may also occur secondary to surgical procedures such as a flexor digitorum profundus (FDP) graft where the flexor digitorum superficialis (FDS) is absent. The deformity is one in which function decreases as the proximal interphalangeal (PIP) joint loses its flexibility. The lateral bands become dorsally displaced and tension to extend the distal interphalangeal (DIP) joint is reduced (Fig. 16-1). Treatment of the condition depends on the etiologic status of the PIP joint and its related anatomic structures. Classification of the deformity may help determine treatment method. Four classifications have been described as follows: (1) PIP flexion remains supple in all positions, (2) PIP flexion is limited by intrinsic tightness, (3) PIP flexion is limited in all positions by articular factors and the joint remains good radiographically, (4) PIP flexion is limited in all positions by intra-articular factors as noted radiographically.[3]

Successful treatment of swan-neck deformity depends on careful examination and determination of contributing factors.

DEFINITION

Deformity in which the PIP joint is hyperextended and the DIP joint is flexed (Fig. 16-2).

151

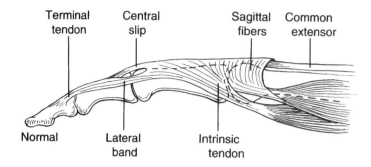

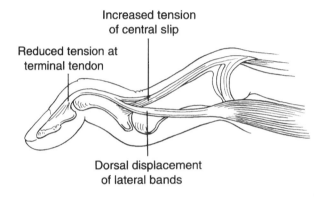

Fig. 16-1. Normal finger anatomy/dorsal subluxation of the lateral bands.

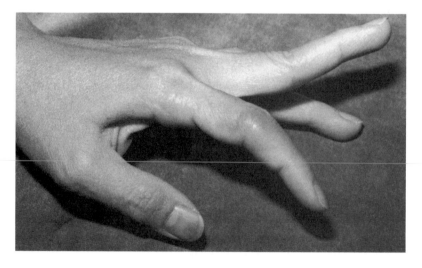

Fig. 16-2. Swan-neck deformity.

SURGICAL PURPOSE

To prevent hyperextension posture of the PIP joint with accompanying flexion of the DIP joint. Nonoperative splinting may be used temporarily to restore extensor tendon balance and to prevent fixed contractures. Surgical correction may be obtained by tendon transfers for active dynamic restoration of this balance. Such transfers may involve using the superficialis tendons or a wrist extensor prolonged with tendon grafts into the extensor mechanism. The passive restoration of balance includes a tenodesis of the PIP joint using local tendons or using a tendon graft to bridge the PIP joint.

TREATMENT GOALS

I. Nonoperative
   A. Promote balance of the extensor mechanism.
   B. Reduce intrinsic tightness.
   C. Maximize joint range of motion (ROM).
   D. Maintain ROM of wrist and uninvolved digits.
II. Postoperative
   A. Promote wound healing.
   B. Control edema.
   C. Control scar formation.
   D. Prevent attenuation or rupture of surgical procedure.
   E. Limit PIP extension and encourage full DIP extension.
   F. Promote full active flexion.
   G. Maintain ROM of uninvolved digits.

NONOPERATIVE INDICATIONS/ PRECAUTIONS FOR THERAPY

I. Indications
   Supple deformities where prevention of PIP hyperextension restores DIP extension
II. Precautions
   A. Volar plate laxity.
   B. Intrinsic tightness.
   C. Dynamic imbalance originating at other joints or due to systemic or neurologic conditions.

NONOPERATIVE THERAPY

I. Active and passive joint ROM
II. Intrinsic stretch exercises
III. Splint to balance finger extension. A tripoint splint prevents PIP joint hyperextension and restores DIP joint extension. This type of splint places dorsal pressure proximal and distal to the PIP joint and volar pressure at the PIP joint. It allows full active flexion (Fig. 16-3).

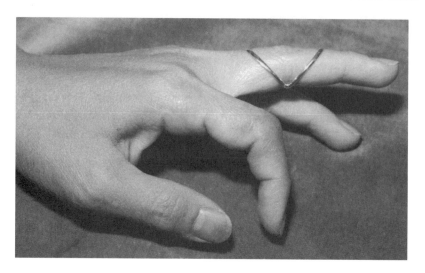

Fig. 16-3. Tripoint splint.

POSTOPERATIVE INDICATIONS/ PRECAUTIONS FOR THERAPY

I. Indications
   A. Following surgical procedures designed to relieve the deformity.
II. Precautions
   A. Excessive exercise that could cause attenuation or rupture of tenodesis procedures.
   B. Procedures that involve joint fusions.
   C. Procedures involving joint arthroplasty.
   D. Surgical treatment requiring capsulectomy.
   E. Surgical treatment requiring tenolysis.
   F. Procedure requiring intrinsic release or metacarpophalangeal (MCP) joint surgical treatment.

POSTOPERATIVE THERAPY

I. General care
   A. Edema control
   B. Wound care
   C. Scar management
   D. Pain management
   E. Maintain ROM of uninvolved digits
II. Treatment following tenodesis procedures of PIP joint
   A. Immediately postoperative wrist is splinted in slight extension[1] with MCP joint in slight flexion. The PIP joint is held in 20 degrees to 30 degrees of flexion and the DIP joint is positioned at 0 degrees.
   B. Active motion allowing full flexion and limiting extension of PIP 20 degrees to 30 degrees begins 1 to 4 weeks postoperative.[1–3] A Kirschner wire (K-wire) or splint may be used to hold DIP in

extension so that maximal flexion occurs at PIP joint.[1] Extension splint for DIP joint can continue for 6 weeks postoperative.

   C. Forearm based splint is replaced at 3 to 4 weeks by a hand based splint that allows ROM as noted above.
   D. Splinting to improve PIP flexion may be initiated if necessary at 3 weeks postoperative.
   E. At 6 to 10 weeks postoperative, PIP joint extension is permitted to gradually increase. Splint is adjusted to allow increased active extension or patient is permitted to decrease use of splint. Passive extension exercises for PIP joint are rarely necessary. PIP joint extension increases gradually over several months. A slight limitation in PIP extension is acceptable and expected. Dynamic extension splinting may be initiated at 6 weeks for PIP extension limitation greater than 20 degrees. Strengthening for flexion may begin at 6 weeks.

 III. Other procedures

   Swan-neck deformity in rheumatoid arthritis commonly requires treatment by PIP joint arthroplasty. Details concerning the rehabilitation of this procedure are noted in the appropriate guideline.

COMPLICATIONS

   I. Nonoperative
      A. Continuation of deformity
      B. Reducible deformity becomes fixed
      C. Reduction of hand function
  II. Operative
      A. Infection
      B. Excessive edema
      C. Pain
      D. Rupture of tenodesis
      E. Attenuation of tenodesis
      F. Excessive scarring
      G. Limited ROM

EVALUATION TIMELINE

   I. Nonoperative
      A. Initial evaluation
         1. Active ROM (AROM) and passive ROM (PROM): determine limiting factors if present.
         2. Strength
      B. Re-evaluate in 4 weeks.
  II. Operative: following tenodesis procedures
      A. Initial postoperative visit
         1. Condition of surgical sites
         2. Edema

     3. Sensation
     4. Pain
     5. Management of activities of daily living (ADL)
  B. Weeks 1 to 4
     1. Active flexion and extension to limit of splint
     2. Passive flexion of PIP joint and MCP joint
  C. Week 6
     1. Passive flexion and extension all joints
     2. Grip strength/pinch strength

REFERENCES

1. Tubiana R: The swan neck deformity. p. III:125. In Tubiana R (ed): The Hand. Vol. III. WB Saunders, Philadelphia, 1988
2. Burton RI: Extensor tendons—late reconstruction. p. III:2073. In Green DP (ed): Operative Hand Surgery. 2nd Ed. Vol. 3. Churchill Livingstone, New York, 1988
3. Nalebuff EA: The rheumatoid swan neck deformity. p. V:203. In Feldon P: Rheumatoid Arthritis. In Peterson BL (ed): Hand Clinics. Vol. 5. WB Saunders, Philadelphia, 1989

Boutonniere Deformity 17

Lauren Valdata Eddington

The boutonniere or "buttonhole" deformity occurs when the common extensor tendon that inserts on the base of the middle phalanx is damaged, and a volar sliding or subluxation of the lateral extensor bands occurs. These lateral extensor bands sublux volarly to the axis of the proximal interphalangeal (PIP) joint when the spiral fibers and transverse fibers are ruptured. The PIP joint then herniates, forms a buttonhole, and assumes a flexed position. With progression of the deformity, proximal retraction of the extensor apparatus will occur; this can put the metacarpophalangeal (MCP) joint into hyperextension. The distal phalanx is also involved when the oblique retinacular ligament contracts and the distal phalanx is held in hyperextension[1-3] (Fig. 17-1).

The boutonniere deformity can result from injuries caused by division, rupture, avulsion, laceration, or closed trauma to the central extensor tendon inserting on to the middle phalanx. Dorsal burns, rheumatoid arthritis, Dupuytren's contracture, and congenital disease are other causes.[1,2,4,5]

Several authors have classified different clinical stages of the boutonniere deformity. Tubiana classifies the boutonniere deformity into four stages: stage 1, minimal deficiency of extension; stage 2, proximal contracture of the middle extensor tendon; stage 3, contracture of retinacular ligaments; and stage 4, fixed contracture of the PIP joint.

"Littler and Eaton have explained this as a three stage process: (1) loss of the central slip results in unopposed PIP flexion by the superficialis tendon; (2) volar migration of the lateral bands secondary to transverse retinacular ligament and triangular ligament laxity; and (3) intrinsic tendon pull is now directly solely at the distal interphalangeal (DIP) joint with resultant hyperextension movement."[3]

157

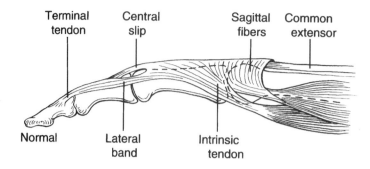

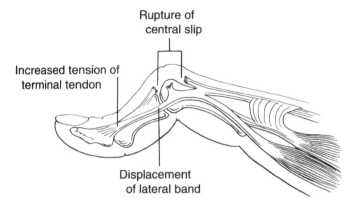

Fig. 17-1. Normal anatomy and anatomy of boutonniere deformity.

Despite different classifications and numerous surgical techniques for correction of the boutonniere deformity, it appears that most authors' treatment of choice is conservative long-term hand therapy to increase PIP extension and DIP active full flexion with external splinting. Only when an acute, open injury occurs should immediate surgery be performed. The boutonniere deformity is evaluated as an acute, closed injury; an acute, open injury; or a chronic injury.

DEFINITION

Deformity of a digit in which it assumes a posture of conjoint PIP flexion and DIP hyperextension (Fig. 17-2).

SURGICAL PURPOSE

To restore extensor tendon balance where there has been a laceration or tear of the central slip near its insertion into the middle phalanx at the PIP level. Nonsurgical treatment is directed toward splinting, either dynamic or static, which allows the central slip to heal yet permits DIP

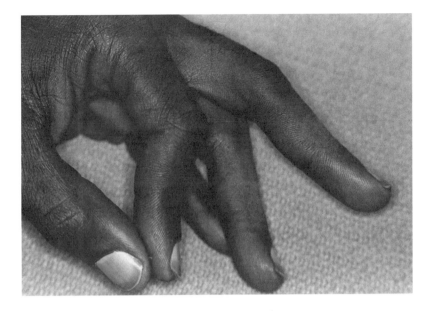

Fig. 17-2. Posture of boutonniere deformity.

joint motion to prevent a hyperextension contraction at that level. This form of treatment must be monitored carefully. Many surgical repairs and reconstructive methods are described. All are designed to restore the extensor mechanism around the PIP joint. Full passive mobility of the PIP and DIP joints is paramount to ensure a surgical success.

TREATMENT GOALS

    I. Prevent extensor tendon complete rupture.
    II. Reduce swelling and pain.
    III. Prevent PIP joint flexion contracture.
    IV. Prevent lateral band subluxation.
    V. Prevent oblique retinacular ligament contracture.
    VI. Restore active and passive range of motion (A/PROM) of MCP, PIP, and DIP joints.
    VII. Maintain range of motion (ROM) of uninvolved joints of the upper extremity.
    VIII. Return to previous level of function.

NONOPERATIVE INDICATIONS/ PRECAUTIONS FOR THERAPY

    I. Indications
       A. Lack of PIP joint extension
       B. Subluxing lateral bands
       C. Lack of DIP flexion—oblique retinacular tightness

II. Precautions
   A. Rheumatoid arthritis
   B. Burns
   C. Diabetes
   D. Steroid use

NONOPERATIVE THERAPY

I. Acute, closed injuries
   A. 0 to 4 to 6 weeks: PIP joint held in 0 degrees extension with splint, and DIP and MCP joints held free. Exercises as per Burton to increase PIP extension and DIP active flexion. Prevention of DIP joint hyperextension is necessary so as to keep oblique retinacular ligaments supple[2,2a,3] (Fig. 17-3). The splint is not removed for 4 to 6 weeks and is held in 0 degrees extension at the PIP joint at all times. Static dorsal splints are preferred to provide good immobilization, allows motion of adjacent joints and preserves the volar, tactile surface.[3] Volar (Fig. 17-4) or cylindrical splints can also be used. Modalities to decrease pain and decrease edema of the affected finger.
   B. 4 to 8 weeks: Gentle AROM exercises can begin for flexion and extension of the PIP joint. MCP and DIP flexion exercises continue. Splinting the PIP joint in full extension (0 degrees) must continue between exercises. Dorsal static splints are preferred to maintain PIP in position, although a wire splint (Fig. 17-5) or a dynamic extension splint (Fig. 17-6) may be worn.

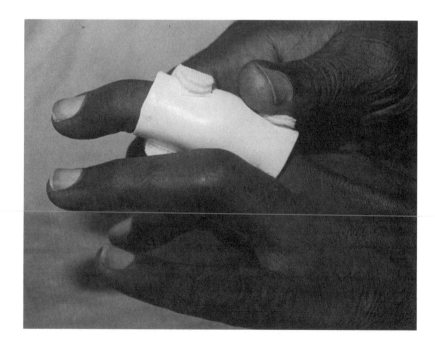

Fig. 17-3. Cylindrical splint may be worn during exercise to stretch oblique retinacular ligament.

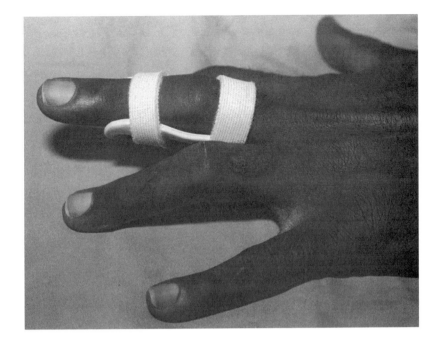

Fig. 17-4. Volar splint.

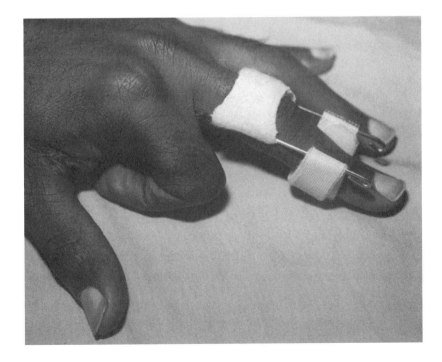

Fig. 17-5. Wire splint.

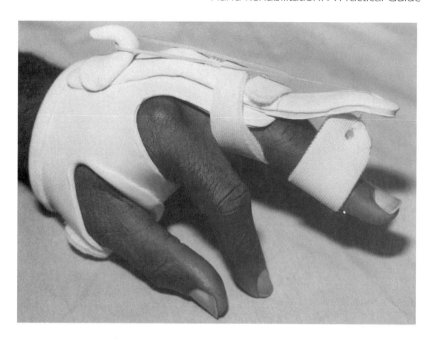

Fig. 17-6. Dynamic extension splint.

C. 8 weeks to 4 to 5 months: Continued splinting of PIP joint in 0 degrees extension with active extension of PIP joint and A flexion of DIP joint exercises continuing. Active blocked DIP flexion with the PIP held in full extension should continue. 10 to 12 weeks: Gentle strengthening may begin for full fist, and blocked exercises for MCP, PIP, and DIP joints.

II. Chronic deformity

A. All efforts to decrease pain and edema and increase ROM are attempted to avoid surgical intervention. A/PROM exercises with resisted exercise occur three to five times a day. A splinting program continues to attempt to increase PIP passive extension. Static, dorsal, serial (Fig. 17-7), or dynamic extension splints are used to attain as much motion as possible. Active DIP exercises, as described by Burton, also continue.[3]

B. Once full extension is attained, a static splint with the PIP joint in full extension, allowing DIP active and passive flexion, is worn to attempt to prevent surgery. This static splint is worn for 8 to 12 weeks, with the patient coming out of the splint only to exercise for flexion and extension of the PIP and DIP joints. Otherwise the splint is worn at all times. If PIP contracture persists after all attempts at hand therapy, surgical intervention is indicated, first for a volar capsulectomy of the PIP joint. Reconstructive surgery for boutonniere deformity cannot occur unless the PIP joint is able to attain 30 degrees or less of extension with DIP flexion (see Postoperative Therapy, II)

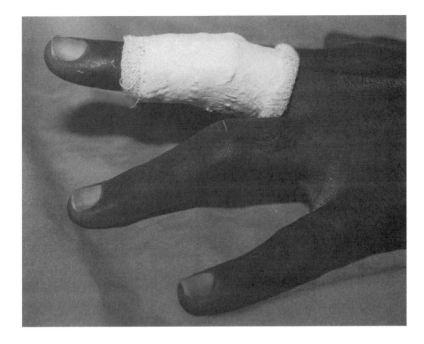

Fig. 17-7. Serial cast.

NONOPERATIVE COMPLICATIONS

   I. Deformities of PIP joint greater than 40 degrees
  II. Fixed DIP hyperextension deformity

OPERATIVE INDICATIONS AND PRECAUTIONS

   I. Indications
     A. Open lacerations with or without bone avulsion
     B. Failure of conservative treatment for longer than 6 months
  II. Precautions
     A. Dirty wounds
     B. Infection
     C. Fractures
     D. Maximal pain
     E. Severe edema
     F. Previous failed surgical attempt
     G. PIP joint contracture greater than 40 degrees

POSTOPERATIVE INDICATIONS/ PRECAUTIONS

   I. Indications
     A. Protect PIP with Kirschner (K) wire held in extension and with external extension splint

B. Wound care
C. Edema reduction
D. Restore DIP flexion

POSTOPERATIVE THERAPY

I. Acute, open injuries
   A. 0 to 6 weeks: PIP joint is held with an oblique K-wire in 0
      degrees extension; the central tendon is repaired, and if there is
      skin loss, a local rotation or transposition flap is used.[6] Immobi-
      lization in a static finger splint with the PIP joint in 0 degrees
      extension continues for 3 weeks.[7] During static splinting, DIP
      active flexion is initiated unless the lateral bands are repaired. If
      the lateral bands are repaired, the DIP joint is immobilized for
      at least 3 weeks. Initiation of active motion can vary between 3
      and 6 weeks. A static extension splint or a dynamic extension
      assist splint is worn between exercise sessions. Exercises are ini-
      tiated to attain full extension and gradual and progressive flex-
      ion. Flexion exercises are gentle and if an extension lag begins,
      extension splinting is increased.
   B. 6 to 8 weeks: MCP and DIP active exercises continue, fol-
      lowed by active gentle flexion and extension of the PIP joint.
      After 5 to 6 weeks, PIP exercises concentrate on gradually
      increasing full finger flexion with full active extension. For
      PIP extension, a static or dynamic splint (capener or wire
      splint may be worn but watched so as not to compromise
      healing or increase swelling of the digit) is worn between
      exercise sessions.
   C. 8 to 12 weeks: Active flexion and extension program continues
      for MCP, PIP, and DIP joints, with gentle resisted exercises
      beginning 8 to 10 weeks after surgery. If an extensor lag at the
      PIP joint starts to occur, PIP extension splinting continues.
      Gradual weaning of daytime extension splint occurs after 8 to
      10 weeks, with buddy taping initially to allow the involved PIP
      joint to extend fully during the day. Nighttime splinting for the
      PIP joint can continue for 4 to 5 months until the treatment
      program can be discontinued.
II. Chronic injuries
   A. Depending on the stage of deformity as described by Curtis et
      al.[8] and Burton,[2a] postoperative treatment may vary. If the
      patient has full passive extension, then only a freeing of the
      extensor tendon from the dorsal capsule is necessary. A dorsal
      splint for PIP extension is worn at all times except when the
      patient gently does active assisted and active ROM exercises.
      DIP is free and continues with active flexion and extension
      exercises. Splinting continues from 6 to 8 weeks and, if the
      patient is gradually weaned during the day, with night splinting
      only. If any droop of the PIP is noted, splinting is continued dur-

ing the day. Occasionally, the DIP joint may droop in flexion; if this is noted, the DIP initially should be splinted in extension between exercises.

B. If at surgery a central tendon reconstruction is necessary to increase PIP joint extension, a plaster cast is used with wrist in extension, MCP joints in 70 degrees flexion, and PIP and DIP joints in extension. (Operation performed should be discussed with physician before initiation of exercise program.) This cast is worn for 3 to 4 weeks or is replaced with a forearm-based dynamic PIP extension splint with MCP block (discuss with your physician). After 4 weeks, the PIP joint is still held in an extension splint, and now the MCP and DIP joints can be held free. Gentle active flexion and extension exercises begin. If a droop is noted at the DIP joint, it is included in the splint in 0 degree extension when not exercising.

C. Splinting and exercise continue daily for 2 to 4 months and occasionally to 6 months to achieve a satisfactory result.

POSTOPERATIVE COMPLICATIONS

  I. Infection
 II. Severe edema
III. Maximal pain
IV. Rupture of the repair

EVALUATION TIMELINE

  I. Nonoperative—acute
    A. 0 to 4 to 6 weeks—Initial ROM measurements are performed at 4 to 6 weeks (when physician allows PIP to begin active flexion and extension).
    B. 10 to 12 weeks—Progress ROM and strength measurements may be performed.
    C. Re-evaluate ROM and strength every 4 weeks until patient is discharged.
 II. Nonoperative—chronic
    A. A/PROM and strength measurements are performed at initial evaluation. Swelling and pain should also be noted.
    B. Re-evaluation should continue every 4 weeks.
III. Postoperative—acute
    A. 0 to 4 weeks: Initial AROM measurements can be performed when cast or dynamic PIP extension splint is removed 3 to 6 weeks after surgery.
    B. 8 to 10 weeks: A/PROM measurements can be performed.
    C. 10 to 12 weeks: A/PROM and strength measurements are performed.
IV. Postoperative—chronic

A. Depending on the surgery performed, measurements can be performed beginning at 3 to 4 weeks for extensor tendon release from the dorsal capsule.

B. For other surgeries performed, A/PROM measurements are performed 8 weeks after surgery.

C. 10 to 12 weeks: A/PROM and strength measurements can be performed.

D. Every 4 weeks until discharge, A/PROM and strength measurements should be performed.

REFERENCES

1. Tubiana R: The boutonniere deformity. p. 106. In Tubiana R (ed): The Hand. Vol. III. WB Saunders, Philadelphia, 1988

2. Schneider LH, Hunter JM: Swan-neck deformity and boutonniere deformity. p. 2041. In Green DP (ed): Operative Hand Surgery. 2nd Ed. Churchill Livingstone, New York, 1988

2a. Burton RI: Extensor tendons—late reconstruction. p. 2100. In Green DP (ed): Operative Hand Surgery. 2nd Ed. Churchill Livingstone, New York, 1988

3. Froehlich JA, Akelmand E, Hendon JH: Extensor tendon injuries at the proximal interphalangeal joint. Hand Clin 4:25, 1988

4. Wynn Parry CB, Salter M, Millar D, Fletcher I: Rehabilitation of the Hand. Butterworth, London, 1981

5. Ferlic D: Boutonniere deformities in rheumatoid arthritis. Hand Clin 5:215, 1989

6. Jupiter JB (ed): Tendon injuries and tendon transfers. Section 3, p. 256. In Flynn's Hand Surgery. 4th Ed. Williams & Wilkins, Baltimore, 1991

7. Evans RB: An update on extensor tendon management, p. 565. In Hunter JM, Mackin EJ, Callahan AD (eds): Rehabilitation of the Hand: Surgery and Therapy. 4th Ed. Mosby, St. Louis, 1995

8. Curtis RM, Reid RL, Provost JM: A staged technique for the repair of the traumatic boutonniere deformity. J Hand Surg 8:167, 1983

SUGGESTED READINGS

Caroli A, Zanasi S, Squarzina PB et al: Operative treatment of the post-traumatic boutonniere deformity. J Hand Surg 15B:410, 1990

Rosenthal EA: The extensor tendons: anatomy and management. p. 519. In Hunter JM, Mackin EJ, Callahan AD (eds): Rehabilitation of the Hand: Surgery and Therapy. 4th Ed. Mosby, St. Louis, 1995

Semple JC: Editorial: The Boutonniere injury. J Hand Surg 15B:393, 1990

Wrist and Hand Tendinitis 18

Bonnie Aiello

The tendons of the normal wrist and hand move freely in their sheaths. If there is swelling of the tendon, the synovial tissue, or the sheath itself, the movement may be painful and inhibited. Overuse, repetitive tasks, and arthritis are the most common predisposing factors. DeQuervain's tendinitis is diagnosed with a positive Finkelstein's test. Trigger finger by a click or locking of the digit in flexion or extension and wrist tendinitis by pain on palpation and resisted motion.

DEFINITION

I. DeQuervain's: Stenosing tenosynovitis of the first dorsal compartment of the wrist involving the extensor pollicis brevis (EPB) and abductor pollicis longus (APL) tendons as they pass through the osteoligamentous tunnel of the radial styloid and transverse fibers of the dorsal carpal ligament (Fig. 18-1A). It may be delineated from intersection syndrome in which the tendons of extensor carpi radialis brevis and extensor carpi radialis longus cross under the abductor pollicis longus and extensor pollicis brevis. Pain and swelling are 4 cm proximal to the first dorsal compartment.[1]

II. Trigger finger: Pathologic thickening of the sheath of the flexor tendons and/or swelling of the tendon itself (especially affecting the flexor digitorum superficialis [FDS]) at the A_1 pulley, causing pain and eventually popping as the nodule passes through the pulley (Fig. 18-1B).

III. Wrist tendinitis: Inflammation of the wrist motor tendon and/or synovial tissue surrounding it as it crosses the wrist (Fig. 18-1C).

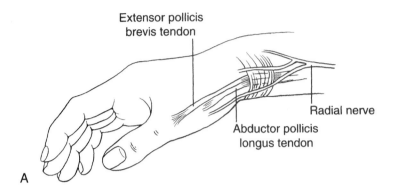

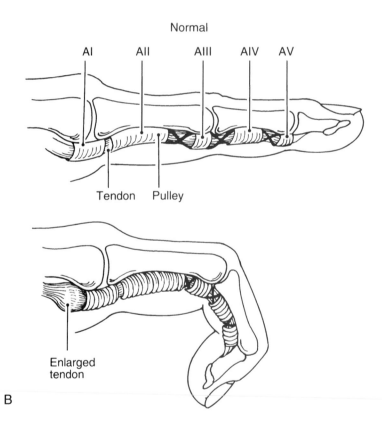

Fig. 18-1. (**A**) Anatomy of first dorsal compartment. (**B**) Anatomy of trigger finger. *(Continues.)*

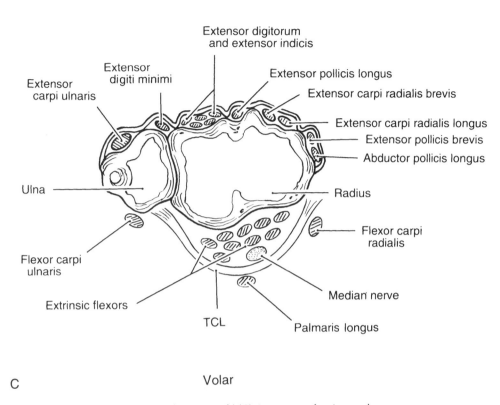

Dorsal

Fig. 18-1. *(Continued.)* **(C)** Anatomy of wrist tendons.

TREATMENT PURPOSE

DeQuervain's tendinitis, stenosing tenosynovitis (trigger finger), and tendinitis at the wrist occur when tendons become inflamed as they enter and travel through fibro-osseous sheaths. When nonoperative methods fail to relieve this inflammation, then surgery may be indicated. The surgical purpose is to release this fibrous sheath to allow more space for tendon gliding, and thus reduce the inflammatory response. It must be recognized, however, that some of the mechanics of pulley function of the involved sheath will be compromised and in turn alter the efficiency of that tendon unit.

TREATMENT GOALS

I. Restoration of normal, painless use of the involved hand.
II. Resolution of the chronic inflammatory process.
III. Prevention of recurrence.

NONOPERATIVE INDICATIONS/
PRECAUTIONS FOR THERAPY

I. Indications
    A. DeQuervain's.
        1. Pain or localized tenderness on the radial side of the wrist, aggravated by thumb motion.[2]
        2. History of chronic overuse of the wrist and hand.
        3. Positive Finkelstein's test: Instruct the patient to make a fist, tuck the thumb inside of the digits and ulnarly deviate the wrist. If a sharp pain is felt over the tunnel, the test is positive (Fig. 18-2).
        4. Wet leather sign: crepitus with motion of the involved tendons.[2]
        5. If ganglions or triggering of the involved tendons occurs.
    B. Trigger finger.
        1. Tenderness or pain over the tendon sheath increases with active range of motion (AROM) or passive stretch.
        2. Tendon nodule and clicking or locking of the digit.
    C. Wrist tendinitis.
        1. Pain over specific tendon on palpation.
        2. Pain on resisted exercise or passive stretch for the specific muscle/tendon unit.
II. Precautions
    A. Allergy to nonsteroidal anti-inflammatory drugs (NSAIDs).
    B. Contraindications to pertinent modalities.
    C. Diabetes mellitus.
    D. Rheumatoid arthritis.

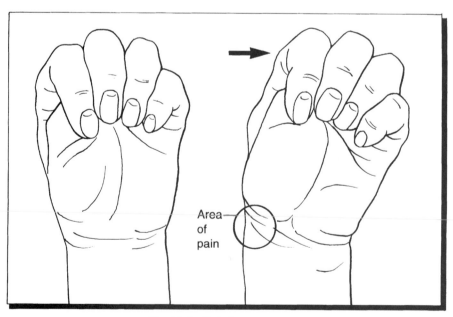

Fig. 18-2. Finkelstein's test.

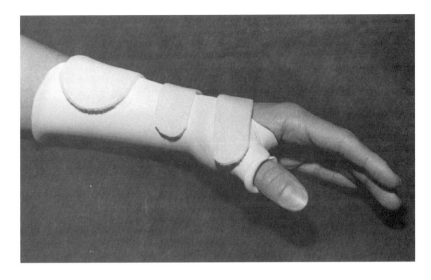

Fig. 18-3. Thumb spica splint.

NONOPERATIVE THERAPY

I. DeQuervain's
   A. Splinting: thumb spica (thumb immobilized in abduction, wrist in extension continually for 3 weeks) (Fig. 18-3).
   B. Local steroid injections.
   C. Anti-inflammatory modalities.
   D. NSAIDs
   E. Transverse friction massage.
   F. Moist heat (chronic).
   G. Ice (acute)
II. Trigger thumb and finger[3]
   A. Splinting: 7 to 21 days[4,5] (Fig. 18-4)

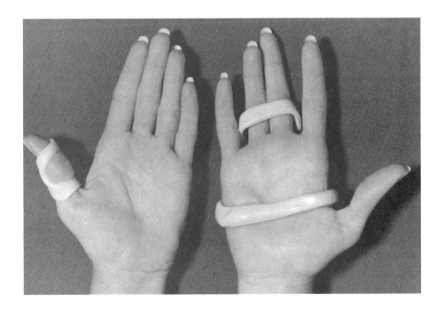

Fig. 18-4. Splint for trigger thumb or finger.

   1. Interphalangeal joint only is immobilized in neutral with passive range of motion (PROM) two to three times a day.
   2. Metacarpophalangeal (MCP) joint only is immobilized in neutral.[6]
 B. NSAIDs
 C. Anti-inflammatory modalities.
 D. Steroid injections.
III. Wrist tendinitis
 A. Splint wrist in neutral for 4 to 6 weeks.
 B. Anti-inflammatory modalities.
 C. NSAIDs
 D. Steroid injections.
 E. Deep friction massage.
 F. Progress to patient tolerance with isometric to eccentric exercises after 6 weeks. Work for endurance and increased strength.

NONOPERATIVE COMPLICATIONS

 I. Continued pain
 II. Potential tendon rupture
 III. Joint stiffness

POSTOPERATIVE INDICATIONS/ PRECAUTIONS

 I. Indications: Continued pain or triggering not relieved by conservative treatment.
 II. Precautions
 A. Diabetes mellitus or other physical neuropathies.
 B. Rheumatoid arthritis.

POSTOPERATIVE THERAPY

 I. DeQuervain's tendinitis
 A. Immobilize 10 to 14 days in thumb spica splint.
 B. Range of motion (ROM) as tolerated after that.
 C. Scar management.
 D. Resisted motion at 6 weeks.
 II. Trigger finger
 A. Active (AROM) and passive (PROM) range of motion day 1.
 B. Scar management.
 C. Strengthening 4 to 6 weeks.
 III. Wrist tendinitis
 A. Cast/splint in neutral for 10 days to 3 weeks (this may include the elbow to eliminate supination/pronation).
 B. A/PROM postimmobilization as tolerated.
 C. Strengthening may start 6 to 8 weeks.

POSTOPERATIVE COMPLICATIONS

I. DeQuervain's
   A. Neuromas or sensory deficits (superficial radial nerve).
   B. Scar hypertrophy and adherence to underlying tendons.
   C. Volar subluxation of tendons.
   D. Persistent symptoms if all tendons are not released (specifically the EPB may be in its own compartmental sheath).
II. Trigger finger
   A. PIP joint flexion contracture.
III. Wrist tendinitis
   A. Continued pain.
   B. Scar adherence.

EVALUATION TIMELINE

I. DeQuervain's (nonoperative)
   A. AROM and PROM evaluation at day 1.
   B. Sensory evaluation at day 1 to distinguish from radial tunnel and nerve laceration.
   C. Pain evaluation at day 1.
   D. Strength measurements at time of painlessness. The above measurements are done every 2 weeks.
II. Trigger finger (nonoperative)
   A. PROM day 1.
   B. AROM week 2.
   C. Strength when pain/triggering resolved.
III. Wrist tendinitis
   A. AROM and PROM day 1.
   B. Pain day 1.
   C. Strength week 4 to 6.
IV. DeQuervain's (postoperative)
   A. Pain evaluation at day 1, to rule out proximal compression.
   B. Sensory evaluation at day 1 to distinguish from radial tunnel and nerve laceration.
   C. ROM evaluation at days 10 to 14.
   D. Scar evaluation at days 10 to 14.
   E. Strength measurements at time of painlessness.
V. Trigger finger (postoperative)
   A. AROM and PROM day 1.
   B. Scar evaluation day 1.
   C. Strength measurements 4 to 6 weeks.
VI. Wrist tendinitis (postoperative)
   A. Pain/scar evaluation day 1.
   B. AROM and PROM 10 to 21 days.
   C. Strength 6 to 8 weeks.

REFERENCES

1. Green D (ed): Operative Hand Surgery. 2nd Ed. pp. 2117, 2132. Churchill Livingstone, New York, 1988
2. Alegado R, Meals R: An unusual complication following surgical treatment of DeQuervain's disease. J Hand Surg 4:185, 1979
3. Newport M, Lane L, Stuchin S: Treatment of trigger finger by steroid injection. J Hand Surg 15A:748, 1990
4. Rhoades C, Gelberman R, Manjarris J: Stenosing tenosynovitis of the fingers and thumb. Clin Orthop Relat Res 190:236, 1994
5. Phalen G: Hand Surgery. 3rd Ed. p. 489. Lippincott-Raven, Philadelphia, 1956
6. Kirkpatrick W, Lisser S: Rehabilitation of the Hand: Surgery and Therapy. 4th Ed. p. 1007. Mosby, St. Louis, 1995

SUGGESTED READING

Anderson B, Kaye S: Treatment of flexor tenosynovitis of the hand ("trigger finger") with corticosteroids. Arch Intern Med 151:153, 1991

Anderson M, Tichenor C: A patient with DeQuervain's tenosynovitis: a case report using an Australian approach to manual therapy. Phys Ther 74:314, 1994

Arens M: DeQuervain's release in working women: a report of failures, complications, and associated diagnoses. J Hand Surg 12A:4, 1987

Bishop A, Gabel G, Carmichael S: Flexor carpi radialis tendinitis. J Bone Joint Surg 76A:1009, 1994

Gabel G, Bishop A, Wood M: Flexor carpi radialis tendinitis. J Bone Joint Surg 76A:1015, 1994

Louis D: Incomplete release of the first dorsal compartment: a diagnostic test. J Hand Surg 12:87, 1987

Rask M: Superficial radial neuritis and DeQuervain's disease. Clin Orthop Relat Res 131:176, 1978

White GM, Weiland AJ: Symptomatic palmar tendon subluxation after surgical release for DeQuervain's release: a case report. J Hand Surg 9A:104, 1984

Epicondylitis **19**

Bonnie Aiello

Epicondylitis may occur at the lateral or medial epicondyle as a result of an acute or chronic injury. If tenderness occurs at the lateral epicondyle, the tendinous insertion of the extensors of the hand and wrist is involved. The extensor carpi radialis brevis (ECRB) is the most dorsally and laterally located extensor tendon. It is the most commonly involved tendon and is responsible for static wrist extension that may be seen in office tasks. The medial epicondyle involves the tendinous insertion of the hand and wrist flexors (Fig. 19-1) and may be associated with cubital tunnel syndrome or medial collateral ligament irritation.

Conservative management consists of anti-inflammatory modalities, rest, and maintenance of motion, which progresses to strengthening and re-education. Splinting may be used to relieve tension on the tendon's insertion into the bone.

Postsurgical therapy protects the insertion while increasing strength and endurance and educating the patient to prevent recurrence.

DEFINITION

Inflammation caused by single or multiple tears within the common tendon of origin. It may also be the result of periostitis caused by repeated sprains. Lateral epicondylitis may be referred to as tennis elbow and medial epicondylitis as golfer's elbow.

TREATMENT PURPOSE

To reduce painful inflammation at the origin of the extensor muscle attachments to the lateral epicondyle, or the flexor pronator origin to the medial epicondyle. The surgical approach is used when nonoperative

175

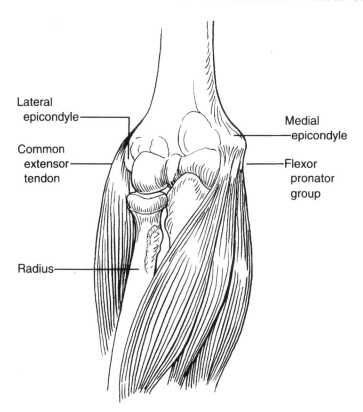

Fig. 19-1. Medial epicondylitis and surrounding tendinous insertions.

therapy has failed. Excision of scarred tendon and removal of bone overgrowth (osteophytes) along the epicondylar ridge is achieved. Some procedures enter the radial humeral joint laterally and remove a part of the annular ligament with local synovium. The goal is to reduce local pain and tenderness.

TREATMENT GOALS

I.   Restoration of normal, painless use of the involved extremity
II. Resolution of chronic inflammation process
III. Restoration of strength and extensibility of the affected muscle tendon complex
IV. Prevention of recurrence

NONOPERATIVE INDICATIONS/ PRECAUTIONS FOR THERAPY

I. Indications
   A. Lateral epicondylitis: pain on resisted wrist extension, passive wrist flexion, and palpation of the extensor muscle group origin. May be associated with radial tunnel symptoms.

B. Medial epicondylitis: pain on resisted wrist flexion, passive wrist extension, and palpation of the flexor muscle group origin. May be associated with cubital tunnel symptoms.

II. Precautions
   A. Allergy to nonsteroidal anti-inflammatory drugs

NONOPERATIVE THERAPY

I. Acute
   A. Ice several times a day
   B. Immobilization of wrist/hand in a cockup splint for 3 weeks (Fig. 19-2). May be used in combination with tennis elbow cuff.
   C. Gentle active range of motion (AROM). Wrist: flexion, pronation; elbow: extension
   D. Restrict motions: grasp, pinch, fine finger motions
   E. Gentle transverse friction massage
   F. Electrical stimulation for pain control and edema
   G. May use anti-inflammatory modalities, iontophoresis, phonophoresis
   H. Microcurrent electrical neuromuscular stimulation (MENS)
   I. Nonsteroidal anti-inflammatory drugs (NSAIDs) or steroid injections

II. Chronic
   A. Restrict repetitive grasp activities and wrist flexion and extension.
   B. Tennis elbow cuff: May be used on lateral epicondylitis and medial epicondylitis. (Be careful not to compress the ulnar nerve) (Fig. 19-2). May be used in combination with wrist splint.
   C. Ultrasound (may use phonophoresis).
   D. Deep transverse friction massage
   E. Iontophoresis
   F. Heat before and ice after activity.
   G. Stretching
      1. Lateral epicondylitis: wrist flexion, pronation; elbow extension.

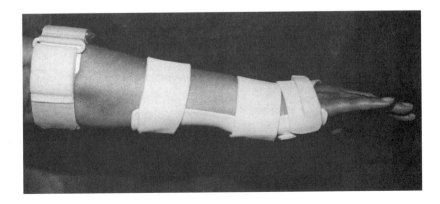

Fig. 19-2. Cockup splint with tennis elbow cuff.

      2. Medial epicondylitis: wrist extension, supination; elbow flexion.
- H. Education about posture of hand and wrist during tasks, muscle protection, and what to do if symptoms return.
- I. Strengthening when painfree to increase strength and endurance.
- J. NSAIDs or steroid injection

III. Prevention
- A. Medial epicondylitis
  1. Increase and maintain flexor strength and flexibility.
- B. Lateral epicondylitis
  1. Increase and maintain extensor strength and flexibility.
- C. Postural and positioning education.

NONOPERATIVE COMPLICATIONS

I. Continued pain

POSTOPERATIVE INDICATIONS FOR THERAPY

I. Severe pain, marked and localized tenderness over the epicondyle.
II. Failure to respond to restricted activity or immobilization of the elbow and wrist (using splints, slings, etc.).
III. Failure to respond to two injections of steroids into the epicondylar area during the period of immobilization.

POSTOPERATIVE THERAPY

I. AROM in 24 hours and increase as tolerated. May return to full athletic ability after 6 to 8 weeks with tennis elbow straps.
II. Scar management
III. Pain control with appropriate modalities

POSTOPERATIVE COMPLICATIONS

I. Infection
II. Pain
III. Recurrence of symptoms

EVALUATION TIMELINE

I. Evaluate initially
- A. AROM
- B. Pain

II. After 3 weeks
   A. Passive range of motion (PROM)
   B. Strength
III. Should be re-evaluated biweekly

SUGGESTED READINGS

Baumgart SH, Schwartz DR: Percutaneous release of epicondylar muscles for humeral epicondylitis. Am J Sports Med 10:233, 1982

Binder AF, Hodge G, Greenwood AM et al: Is therapeutic ultrasound effective in treating soft tissue lesions? Br Med J 290:512, 1985

Binder AF, Hazelman BL: Lateral humeral epicondylitis: a study of natural history and the effect of conservative therapy. Br J Rheumatol 22:73, 1983

Boyd HB, McLeod AC Jr: Tennis elbow. J Bone Joint Surg 55A:1183, 1973

Gaberech SG: Treatment of lateral epicondylitis. Br J Sports Med 94:224, 1985

Gallaway M, DeMaio M, Mangine A: Rehabilitative techniques in the treatment of medial and lateral epicondylitis. Orthopedics 15:1089, 1992

Gellman H: Tennis elbow (lateral epicondylitis). Orthop Clin North Am 23:75, 1992

Gould III J, Davis GJ: Orthopaedic and Sports Physical Therapy. Mosby, St. Louis, 1985

Green DP: Operative Hand Surgery. 2nd Ed. Churchill Livingstone, New York, 1988

Kessler RM, Hutley D: Management of Common Musculoskeletal Disorders. Harper & Row, Philadelphia, 1983

Kivi P: The etiology and conservative treatment of humeral epicondylitis. Scand J Rehabil Med 15:37, 1982

Kohn HS: Current status and treatment of tennis elbow. Wis Med J 83:18, 1984

Nirschl RP, Pettrons FA: Tennis elbow: the treatment of lateral epicondylitis. J Bone Joint Surg 61A:832, 1979

Noteboom T, Cruver R, Keller J et al: Tennis elbow: a review. J Orthop Sports Phys Ther 19:35, 1994

Wittenberg RH, Schaal S, Murh G: Surgical treatment of persistent elbow epicondylitis. Clin Orthop 278:73, 1992

Shoulder Tendinitis **20**

Bonnie Aiello

Shoulder joint mechanics and stability are dependent on the muscles surrounding the joint. An acute injury or chronic misuse can cause inflammation of the tendons, especially those attaching to the greater tuberosity of the humerus and beneath the acromial shelf (Fig. 20-1). Untreated, these may go on to calcify, rupture, and require surgery, or because of pain, limit the patient's movement, resulting in a frozen shoulder.

Conservative management consists of anti-inflammatory modalities and rest to decrease pain and progressive strengthening to prevent re-injury.

Postsurgical therapy allows for tendon healing, decompression of the injured tendon, and progressive strengthening and stretching to regain mechanics.

DEFINITION

A combination of mechanical stresses degenerates and causes ischemic changes in the tendon, with possible subsequent calcification causing it to be prone to local inflammation.

TREATMENT PURPOSE

The purpose when dealing with biceps tendinitis is to reduce the irritation of tendon gliding in the bicipital groove of the humerus. Rotator cuff tendinitis occurs over the head of the humerus beneath the acromium process (Fig. 20-2). Inflammation caused by overuse needs to be reduced for smoother, unrestricted gliding. The surgical goals are to increase the size of this space and removal of the overlying impinging bone structures.

181

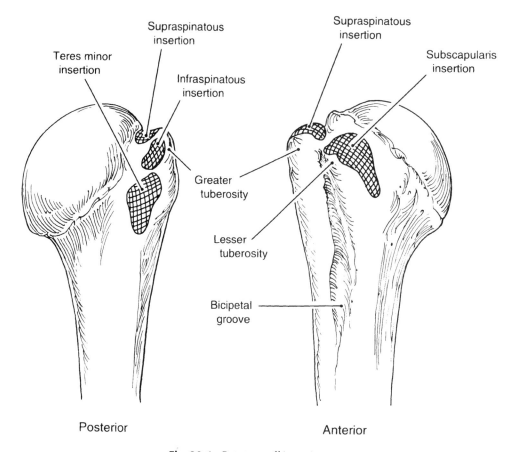

Fig. 20-1. Rotator cuff insertion.

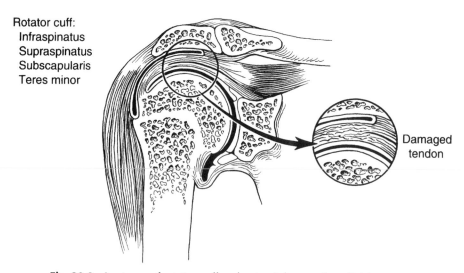

Fig. 20-2. Anatomy of rotator cuff and potential area of tendinitis.

TREATMENT GOALS

I. Restoration of normal, painless use of involved extremity.
II. Resolution of chronic inflammatory process.
III. Increase strength and extensibility to the affected muscle–tendon complex.
IV. Prevent recurrences.

NONOPERATIVE INDICATIONS/ PRECAUTIONS FOR THERAPY

I. Indications
    A. Pain on palpation of specific tendons.
    B. Pain on resisted motions for specific muscle actions.
II. Precautions
    Allergy to nonsteroidal anti-inflammatory drugs (NSAIDs).

NONOPERATIVE THERAPY

I. Acute
    A. Ice packs/massages.
    B. Rest (especially in 45 degrees of abduction to allow increased circulation to glenohumeral joint structures).
    C. Iontophoresis.
    D. Phonophoresis.
    E. Gentle transverse friction massage.
    F. Electrical stimulation for pain control and edema.
    G. NSAIDs
    H. Exercise
        1. Program of active/passive range of motion (A/PROM) to maintain range of motion.
        2. Internal and external rotator strengthening with tubing and then free weights (may need to limit external rotation if painful).
        3. Progress to strengthening mid/posterior deltoid at 90 degrees when not painful.
        4. May use closed kinetic chain exercises for scapular stabilization.
        5. Postural exercises to open the glenohumeral space.
II. Chronic
    A. Heat modalities.
    B. Steroid injections.
    C. Ultrasound (may use phonophoresis).
    D. Iontophoresis.
    E. Deep transverse friction massage.
    F. Heat before/ice after activity.

G. Stretching (especially posterior joint structures).

H. Education for prevention of recurrence.

I. Exercise
   1. Progressive program of isokinetic, eccentric, and free weights to increase strength and endurance in the rotator cuff and scapular stabilizers (including the serratus anterior).
   2. Postural exercises to increase the glenohumeral space.
   3. Use isolated exercises for specific muscle weaknesses and may use patterned exercises for combination movement (such as proprioceptive neuromuscular facilitation [PNF]).

NONOPERATIVE COMPLICATIONS

I. Continued pain
II. Calcifications of tendons
III. Tendon rupture

POSTOPERATIVE INDICATIONS/ PRECAUTIONS FOR THERAPY

I. Indication
   A. Failure to respond to conservative treatment.
   B. Severe pain and localized tenderness.
   C. Tendon calcification.
II. Precautions
   A. Tendon rupture.
   B. Repeated ossification.
   C. Shoulder decreased mobility.

POSTOPERATIVE THERAPY (DECOMPRESSION)

I. Day 2: pendulum exercises—maintenance of PROM.
II. Electrical stimulation—pain control.
III. Ice
IV. Scapular and postural exercises (isometrics if pain free).
V. Progress to active assistive/active range of motion (AA/AROM), wall walking—1 week.
VI. Strengthening—3 weeks (see conservative care).

POSTOPERATIVE COMPLICATIONS

I. Infection
II. Potential muscle tear
III. Pain

EVALUATION TIMELINE

I. Nonoperative
   A. Day 1
      1. AROM
      2. PROM
      3. Pain
   B. Week 2
      1. Strength
II. Operative (Consult physician as to surgery performed).
   A. Week 1: AROM
   B. Week 2: PROM
   C. Week 3: strengthening

SUGGESTED READINGS

Boublik M, Hawkins RL: Clinical examination of the shoulder complex. J Orthop Sports Phys Ther 18:379, 1993

Brewster C, Schwab DR: Rehabilitation of the shoulder following rotator cuff injury or surgery. J Orthop Sports Phys Ther 18:422, 1993

Brox JI, Staff PH, Ljunggren AE et al: Arthroscopic surgery compared with supervised exercises in patients with rotator cuff disease (stage II impingement syndrome). Br Med J:904, 1993

Curtis AS, Snyder SJ: Evaluation and treatment of biceps tendon pathology. Orthop Clin North Am 24:33, 1993

DePalma AF: Surgery of the Shoulder. Lippincott–Raven, Philadelphia, 1950

Ekelund AL, Rydell N: Combination treatment for adhesive capsulitis of the shoulder. Clin Orthop Relat Res 282:105, 1992

Gould III J, Davis GJ: Orthopaedic and Sports Physical Therapy. Mosby, St. Louis, 1985

Kamkar A, Irrgang JJ, Whitney SL: Nonoperative management of secondary shoulder impingement syndrome. J Orthop Sports Phys Ther 17:212, 1993

Kessler RM, Herthry D: Management of Common Musculoskeletal Disorders. Harper & Row, Philadelphia, 1983

McQueen AK: Surgical relief for the painful shoulder. Aust Fam Phys 16:768, 1987

Paine RM, Voight M: The role of the scapula. J Orthop Sports Phys Ther 18:386, 1993

Rizk TE, Christopher RP, Pinalo RS et al: Adhesive capsulitis (frozen shoulder): a new approach to its management. Arch Phys Med Rehabil 64:29, 1983

Schenk's Handbook of Orthopaedic Surgery. 9th Ed. Mosby, St. Louis, 1987

Sinki PA: Tendinitis and bursitis of the shoulder. Post Grad Med 73:177, 1983

Smith DL, Campbell SM: Painful shoulder syndromes: diagnosis and management. J Gen Intern Med 7:328, 1992

Stanish WD, Rubinovich RM, Curwin S: Ecocentric exercise in chronic tendinitis. Clin Orthop Relat Res 208:65, 1986

Wilk KE, Arrigo C: Current concepts in the rehabilitation of the athletic shoulder. J Orthop Sports Phys Ther 18:365, 1993

Zuckerman JD, Mirabello SC, Newsman D et al: The painful shoulder: Part I. Extrinsic disorders. Am Fam Physician, 43:119, 1991

Zuckerman JD, Mirabello SC, Newsman D et al: The painful shoulder: Part II. Intrinsic disorders and impingement syndrome. Am Fam Physician, 43:497, 1991

Rotator Cuff Repairs 21

Mary Schuler Murphy

The rotator cuff is important for both the mobility and stability of the glenohumeral joint, as well as for the nourishment of the articular surface of the glenohumeral joint. Studies have suggested that the rotator cuff provides 45 percent of the power in shoulder abduction and at least 90 percent of the power in external rotation.[1] The rotator cuff acts as a dynamic stabilizer, allowing the powerful deltoid to perform as the prime mover of the glenohumeral joint. Rotator cuff tears upset this delicate balance, causing varying degrees of dysfunction. A major goal of shoulder reconstruction is to preserve or restore this balance. According to Neer,[2] the most common etiologic cause of rotator cuff tears is impingement (approximately 95 percent, which occurs primarily in the over-40-year-old age group). The most common cause of impingement is decreased space beneath the anterior acromion and acromioclavicular joint.[2] Anterior acromioplasty is performed in conjunction with the rotator cuff repair to alleviate this problem. Rehabilitation of the rotator cuff requires a basic understanding of the surgical procedure and the physician's expectation of outcome. The progression of the rehabilitation program depends on the patient's age and compliance, as well as on the type of surgery performed. Only the surgeon knows the integrity of the repair and thus close communication with the surgeon is imperative to successful rehabilitation.

DEFINITION

Rotator cuff repair is the surgical repair of a partial or complete rupture of one or several of the tendons that comprise the rotator cuff (supraspinatus, infraspinatus, teres minor, and subscapularis).

Anterior acromioplasty is the surgical decompression of the rotator cuff through the enlargement of the supraspinatus outlet by beveling the anterior edge and the undersurface of the anterior third of the acromion and acromioclavicular joint.

I. Neer's cuff-tear terminology[2]
   A. Partial tear—incomplete tear that does not extend through the complete tendon thickness.
   B. Complete tear—extends through the complete thickness of the tendon.
   C. Massive tear—tear of more than one rotator cuff tendon.
   D. Degenerative tear—nutritional or metabolic factors could be indicated as well as wear or injury.
   E. Traumatic tear—implies an injury tearing a healthy tendon.
   F. Acute extension—implies an injury suddenly enlarging an impingement tear.

II. Esch's categories of rotator cuff tears (according to size):[3]
   A. Small—< 1 cm
   B. Moderate—1 to 3 cm
   C. Large—3 to 5 cm
   D. Massive—> 5 cm

SURGICAL PURPOSE

Surgery is performed for rotator cuff tears to restore the continuity of the tendon and relieve the subacromial impingement. This is often difficult to achieve, and predictability of success depends on the quality of the tendon substance, the length of time since the injury occurred, and the underlying pathology that brought on the disruption. Successful rehabilitation of these injuries requires full knowledge of these factors.

TREATMENT GOALS

I. Repair of incomplete or small tears (< 1 cm) and open and major tear repairs (1–5 cm)
   A. Short-term goals
     1. Prevent the formation of adhesions while protecting the repair.
     2. Maintain passive range of motion (PROM) within limits set by the physician.
     3. Patient education (i.e., precautions to allow for healing).
     4. Maintain full active range of motion (AROM) and strength in involved elbow, forearm, wrist, and hand.
   B. Long-term goals
     1. Restore full PROM.
     2. Restore pain-free AROM and return to functional active abduction and external rotation.
     3. Return to preinjury activity status.

II. Status post massive repairs (repairs > 5 cm) with significant loss of deltoid function, rotator cuff function, or bone
   A. Long-term goals
      1. Restore pain-free limited but functional AROM with emphasis on use of the extremity at the side.
      2. Return to as near previous level of functioning as possible.
      3. Independent home exercise program stressing stability and the avoidance of excessive mobility.

POSTOPERATIVE INDICATIONS/ PRECAUTIONS FOR THERAPY

I. Indications
   A. Exercise program for small deltoid splitting repairs, status post open repairs and for major tear repairs when the surgeon indicates that the rotator cuff quality and the glenohumeral joint stability are adequate.
II. Precautions
   A. Communication with the surgeon is of paramount importance. The therapist must know the type and quality of the repair. Severe loss of deltoid muscle function, rotator cuff, or bone requires a limited goal program with lesser ROM and increased stability.

POSTOPERATIVE THERAPY

I. Incomplete or small tear repair (< 1 cm)
   A. Day 1 to 3
      1. Pendulum exercises.
      2. Distal AROM and grasp strengthening exercises.
      3. PROM of shoulder, external and internal rotation begin in 0 to 20 degrees abduction.
      4. Pain management (including use of a sling for 1 week if painful).
   B. Day 3 to 3 weeks
      1. Progress to assistive active range of motion (A/AROM).
      2. AROM except flexion (flexion begins week 2).
      3. External rotation in the plane of the scapula.
   C. Week 3 to 6—Begin resistive external and internal rotation in the plane of the scapula.
   D. Week 6 to 10—Continue shoulder strengthening to include resistive exercise in all planes.
II. Open and major tear repair (1–5 cm)
   A. Day 1 to 10
      1. Immobilization in a sling, remove for bathing and exercises.
      2. Control pain/inflammation.
      3. Pendulum exercises (typically performed at day 3 to 7).

4. Gentle shoulder PROM exercise (restricted to 160 degrees of elevation in the plane of the scapula and 60 degrees of external rotation and commonly initiated day 3 to 7).
5. Distal upper extremity AROM of the involved side.
6. Grasp strengthening.
7. Instructions in one-handed activities of daily living (ADLs) and the use of adaptive equipment as needed.

B. Day 10 to 4 weeks
1. Gradually wean from the sling.
2. Continue above exercises.
3. Full PROM and initiate A/AROM exercises (wait 3 weeks for major tear repairs).
4. Submaximal isometric shoulder exercises throughout the painfree range.
5. Scapular stabilization exercise (Fig. 21-1).

C. Week 4 to 6
1. Shoulder AROM (wait 6 weeks for major tear repairs).
2. Initiate light functional activities (e.g., cones, pegs).

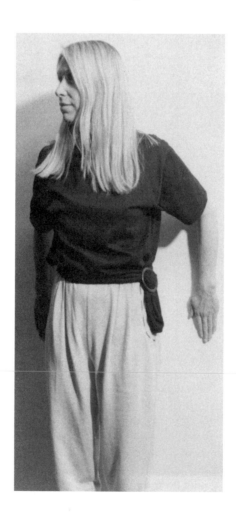

Fig. 21-1. Scapular stabilization exercise.

   D. Week 6 to 8
      1. Shoulder resistive exercises (e.g., surgical tubing, rubber tubing, one pound free weight).
      2. Scapular strengthening exercise (Fig. 21-2).
      3. Stretch tight structures.
   E. Week 8 to 10
      1. Continue to increase resistive exercise.
III. Massive tear limited goal exercise program—This exercise program avoids early overhead AROM exercises and exercises extending into full rotation. The program stresses use of the arm at the side and stability.
   A. Day 2 to 1 month
      1. Proximal immobilization with a sling, an abduction pillow or brace may be used for the first 4 to 8 weeks for the protection of the repair.
      2. Passive forward flexion is performed on a daily basis, which may be limited to 100 degrees depending on the repair and treatment goals.
      3. Distal strengthening
      4. Instructions in one-handed ADLs and the use of adaptive equipment as needed.
   B. Month 1 to 3
      1. Continued passive elevation, initiate passive external rotation with the arm at the side (this may be limited to 20 degrees depending on the repair and treatment goals).
      2. Pendulum exercises
      3. Use of the sling between exercise.
      4. A/AROM, progress to AROM (overhead AROM is delayed until 5 1/2 to 6 months).
   C. Month 2 to 3: discontinue sling
   D. Month 3 to 4: submaximal isometric shoulder strengthening
   E. Month 5: progressive resistive exercises
   F. Month 6: activities as tolerated

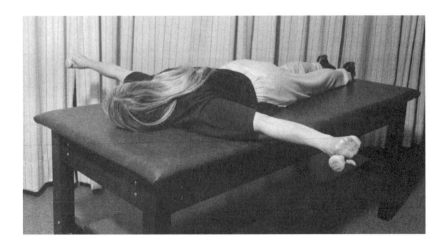

Fig. 21-2. Scapular strengthening exercise.

POSTOPERATIVE COMPLICATIONS

 I. Infection
 II. Failed rotator cuff repair with residual impingement
 III. Decreased AROM/deltoid weakness
 IV. Adhesive capsulitis
 V. Postoperative hematoma
 VI. Severe pain

EVALUATION TIMELINE

 I. Incomplete and major tear repairs
   A. 0 to 10 days—distal AROM and grip strength, and painfree PROM of shoulder flexion and abduction (typically at day 3–5)
   B. 3 to 6 weeks—PROM of shoulder, internal and external rotation
   C. 6 weeks—isometric shoulder strength testing
 II. Massive tear repairs
   A. Day 1 to 1 month—distal strength and ADL skills
   B. 1 to 3 months—passive shoulder elevation to 100 degrees and external rotation to 20 degrees
   C. 4 months—isometric shoulder strength testing

REFERENCES

1. Matsen FA, Arntz CT: Rotator cuff tendon failure. p. 647. In Rockwood CA, Matsen FA: The Shoulder. Vol. II. WB Saunders, Philadelphia, 1990
2. Neer CS: Cuff tears, biceps lesions and impingement. p. 41. In Neer CS: Shoulder Rehabilitation. WB Saunders, Philadelphia, 1990
3. Esch JC: Arthroscopic subacromial decompression and postoperative management. Orthop Clin North Am 24:161, 1993

SUGGESTED READINGS

Andrews JR, Harrelson GL: Physical Rehabilitation of the Injured Athlete. WB Saunders, Philadelphia, 1991

Brewster C, Schwab DR: Rehabilitation of the shoulder following rotator cuff injury of surgery. J Orthop Sports Phys Ther 18:422, 1993

Burkhart SL, Post WR: A functionally based neuromechanical approach to shoulder rehabilitation. p. 1655. In Hunter JM, Mackin EJ, Callahan Ad (eds): Rehabilitation of the Hand: Surgery and Therapy. 4th Ed. Vol. II. Mosby, St. Louis, 1995

Delee C, Drez D: Orthopaedic Sports Medicine: Principles and Practice. Vol. 1. WB Saunders, Philadelphia, 1994

Ellman H, Hanker G, Bayer M: Repair of the rotator cuff. J Bone Joint Surg 68A:1136, 1986

Frieman BG, Albert TJ, Fenlin JM: Rotator cuff disease: a review of diagnosis, pathophysiology and current trends in treatment. Arch Phys Med Rehabil 75:604, 1994

Gartsman GM: Arthroscopic acromioplasty for lesions of the rotator cuff. J Bone Joint Surg 72A:169, 1990

Gore DR, Murray MP, Sepic SB: Shoulder muscle strength and range of motion following surgical repair of full thickness rotator cuff tears. J Bone Joint Surg (Am) 68:266, 1986

Goss TP: Rotator cuff injuries. Orthop Rev 15:496, 1990

Jobe FW, Pink M: The athlete's shoulder. J Hand Ther 7:107, 1994

Marks PH, Warner JJP, Irrgang JJ: Rotator cuff disorders of the shoulder. J Hand Ther 7:90, 1994

Miniaci A, Fowler PJ: Impingement in the athlete. Clin Sports Med 12:91, 1993

Snyder SJ, Pachell AF, Pizza WD: Partial thickness rotator cuff tears: results of arthroscopic treatment. J Arthroscopic Relat Surg 7:1, 1991

Thoracic Outlet Syndrome

22

Mallory S. Anthony

The thoracic outlet is the triangular channel through which the nerves and vessels of the arm leave the neck and thorax. Medially, it is bounded by the anterior scalene muscle anteriorly, the medial scalene muscle posteriorly, the clavicle superiorly, and the first rib inferiorly. As one moves laterally, the thoracic outlet boundaries include the coracoid, the pectoralis minor muscle, and its tendinous insertion into the coracoid and the deltopectoral fascia. The structures at risk of compression in this area are the subclavian artery, subclavian vein, and the brachial plexus. The subclavian artery arches over the first rib behind the anterior scalene muscle, and in front of the medial scalene muscle. It then passes under the subclavius muscle and clavicle and enters the axilla beneath the pectoralis minor muscle. The subclavian vein follows the same course, except that it passes anteriorly rather than posteriorly to the anterior scalene muscle. The brachial plexus follows the route of the subclavian artery, but it lies a little more posteriorly and laterally.[1]

There are three potential spaces for compression of the brachial plexus and neurovascular structures[2] (Fig. 22-1). The first and most medial is the scalene triangle, bordered by the scalenus anterior and medius, and inferiorly by the first rib (Fig. 22-1A). The subclavian artery and brachial plexus travel within this triangle. Compression at this site would have no venous component, as the subclavian vein travels anteriorly to this space. The second space is the costoclavicular region, bordered superiorly by the clavicle and inferiorly by the first rib (Fig. 22-1B). The third potential space is the axillary region, where the anterior deltopectoral fascia, the pectoralis minor, and coracoid could all be sources of compression (Fig. 22-1C).

The causes of thoracic outlet syndrome (TOS) can be related to compressive neuropathy, postural abnormalities, or entrapment neuropathy.[2] Compression neuropathy can occur from anatomic structures such as

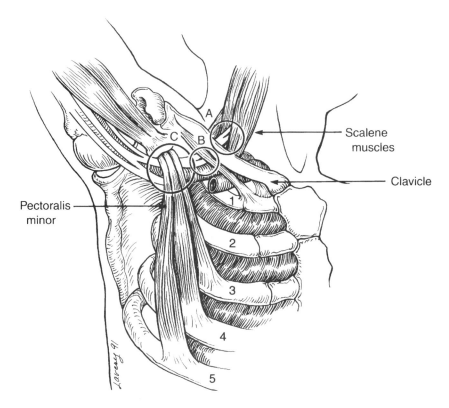

Fig. 22-1. Thoracic outlet anatomy with possible sites of compression: (**A**). Scalene triangle. (**B**). Costoclavicular region. (**C**) Axillary region.

muscle hypertrophy, adaptic shortening of surrounding fascia, or space occupying lesions (e.g., cervical rib, bifid clavicle), all of which can decrease the size of potential spaces. Postural abnormalities, which frequently involve a forward head and rounded shoulders (e.g., tight scalenes and pectoralis minor muscle) can decrease the space of the scalene triangle and axillary interval, respectively, compressing the neurovascular structures. Patients with compression problems (anatomic or postural) usually have insidious onset of pain, no history of trauma, and often early signs of repetitive stress.[2] They frequently have predictable symptom distribution over the lower trunk, which may be only nocturnal or activity related.[2] Provocative tests are helpful in identifying possible sites of compression.

A third cause of TOS is entrapment neuropathy. This is an impairment of the biomechanical aspects of the nerve's ability to glide through surrounding tissue and to tolerate tension.[2] This may be secondary to intraneural or extraneural fibrosis associated with cervical and/or shoulder trauma, or to longstanding repetitive stress activities.[2] Provocative tests are usually less reliable with these patients, and the patient usually has multiple problems such as active myofascial trigger points, cervical pathology, and glenohumeral joint pathology.

The diagnosis of TOS is based not only on a thorough upper quarter evaluation, but also on the exclusion of other pathologies (e.g., cervical disc disease, nerve root impingement, shoulder pathology, tendinitis). Patients with TOS rarely show objective test abnormalities (unless it is longstanding), because their symptoms are often intermittent and provoked by arm elevation.[3] Also, it is not uncommon to find carpal and/or cubital tunnel syndromes associated with TOS because of double or multiple crush syndromes[4,5] (i.e., a proximal source of nerve compression will render the distal nerve segment more susceptible to additional sites of compression). The progression of TOS symptoms is the same as for any peripheral nerve compression problem (see Table 7-1). The following protocol offers guidelines for both evaluation and treatment of this complex and challenging syndrome.

DEFINITION

Symptoms of arterial insufficiency, venous engorgement, or nerve dysfunction that can be produced by compression or stretching of the subclavian artery, subclavian vein, or portions of the brachial plexus as they pass from the neck to the axilla.

   I. Types of compression[6]
      A. Arterial: 1 percent of all cases. Two distinct age groups
         1. Young adults, due to external compression of the subclavian artery, usually by a cervical rib.
         2. Patients over 40 in whom localized degenerative changes of the artery may result from turbulent flow caused by extrinsic pressure.
      B. Venous: 2 percent of all cases
         1. Seen throughout adulthood.
         2. More prevalent in athletic males.
      C. Neurologic: 97 percent of all cases
         1. More prevalent in young or middle-aged adults.
         2. Females outnumber males (2 or 3:1).
  II. Cause of TOS
      A. Dynamic[1] (anatomic)
         1. Impingement at acromioclavicular joint or humeral/scapular articulation.
         2. Compression beneath the coracoid process and pectoralis minor during hyperabduction of the arm.
      B. Static[1] (postural)
         1. Muscular hypertrophy or spasm (e.g., scalenus hypertrophy or spasm, omohyoid muscle hypertrophy) may reduce anatomic space for passage of neurovascular structures.
         2. Muscular atrophy: reduction in muscle mass and tone may cause sagging of local structures. (Shoulder trauma or neurologic diseases could cause muscle weakness.)

   3. Postural abnormalities: rounded shoulders and forward head are commonly seen and can contribute to neurovascular compression, and possibly exacerbate any previously asymptomatic congenital factor. Also, guarded posturing of the upper extremity can decrease the size of the thoracic outlet.
C. Congenital[7] (anatomic)
   1. Cervical ribs (most common factor) cause compression by narrowing the intrascalene triangle.
   2. Fascial bands behind anterior scalene or abnormal insertion of middle scalene on first rib.
   3. Bifid clavicle.
   4. Bony protuberance on first rib.
   5. Enlargement of costal element of transverse process of seventh cervical vertebra.
   6. Fibrous bands extending between cervical vertebra and first ribs.
   7. Rudimentary first thoracic rib (rare condition).
   8. Scoliosis
D. Traumatic[8] (entrapment)
   1. Fibrous callous formation caused by fracture of clavicle or first rib.
   2. Shoulder dislocation
   3. Crush injury or traction injury to upper thorax (may stretch brachial plexus and/or thrombose artery or vein).
   4. Whiplash
   5. Cumulative trauma through repetitive above-shoulder level movements.
   6. Thoracoplasty surgery
E. Arteriosclerotic
F. Tumor in thoracic outlet: less common

TREATMENT PURPOSE

To increase the space in the thoracic outlet by postural exercises or by surgically removing bony or muscle structures that define the outlet to achieve the same purpose.

TREATMENT GOALS

   I. Modify postural habits and body mechanics that exacerbate the patient's symptoms.
   II. Relieve muscle tension of shoulder girdle musculature.
   III. Improve cervical and scapular alignment (restore muscle balance).
   IV. Increase nerve gliding through surrounding tissue.
   V. Return to optimal level of function.
   VI. Prevent recurrence of symptoms.

NONOPERATIVE INDICATIONS/ PRECAUTIONS FOR THERAPY

I. Indications: When symptoms of neurovascular compression are produced and *related to arm position and use. Please note:* The following is a list of other shoulder and neck conditions that may be confused with thoracic outlet syndrome:[6,8]
   A. Cervical disc abnormality
   B. Osteoarthritis
   C. Reflex sympathetic dystrophy
   D. Spinal cord tumors
   E. Arachnoiditis
   F. Multiple sclerosis
   G. Angina
   H. Blockage of subclavian artery or vein
   I. Bursitis, tendinitis, or capsulitis of the shoulder
   J. Rotator cuff injuries
   K. Acromioclavicular joint separation
   L. Median nerve compression
   M. Ulnar nerve entrapment
   N. Radial nerve entrapment
   O. Raynaud's syndrome
   P. Pancoast's tumor of the lung
II. Precautions
   A. Infection
   B. Acute fracture
   C. Extreme discomfort
   D. Marked edema

NONOPERATIVE THERAPY

I. Pretreatment evaluation
   A. History
      1. Mechanism and site of injury (possible whiplash, traction injuries, clavicle fracture).
      2. Note onset and duration of symptoms and other related injuries.
      3. Detailed description of symptoms: pain versus paresthesias, etc.
      4. Note habits, work conditions, and stressful conditions.
      5. Note which positions aggravate the symptoms (such as overhead activities) and what relieves the symptoms.
      6. Obtain results from referring physician's examination if possible.
         a. Radiographs of cervical spine
         b. Pulse volume recordings
         c. Plethysmography

   d. Angiography
   e. Phleborography
   f. Nerve conduction studies (helpful if tested in both tradi-
      tional resting position and position of provocation that
      would cause stress on lower trunk of brachial plexus).[5]
   g. Pulse palpation maneuver
   h. Social work evaluation: Minnesota Multiphasic Personal-
      ity Inventory (MMPI) results and personality factors that
      may impact on patient's response to treatment.
   i. Magnetic resonance imaging
B. Physical examination: upper quarter evaluation. Please note
   that mobility and status of lumbar spine may need to be evaluated because many activities and postures that are normally
   part of the treatment plan depend on normal lumbar motion.
   1. Visual inspection
      a. Postural assessment: rounded shoulders, uneven shoul-
         ders, forward head, head tilt, guarding posture of shoulder.
      b. Atrophy: especially in hypothenar and intrinsic mus-
         cles since C_8 and T_1 nerve roots are at greatest risk of
         compression.
      c. Color, skin condition
      d. Edema
      e. Musculoskeletal deformity
      f. Breathing pattern (i.e., diaphragmatic vs. accessory muscle
         respiration).
   2. Strength: grip and pinch measurements
   3. Manual muscle testing
      a. Identify weak and overstretched muscles (frequently
         middle/lower trapezius and cervical extensors).
      b. Identify tight muscles and hypertrophy (frequently scal-
         enes, sternocleidomastoid, upper trapezius, and pectoral
         muscles).
   4. Range of motion (ROM) evaluation
   5. Sensory evaluation (see Ch. 7)
      a. May need to perform sensory tests immediately after
         provocation of symptoms.
   6. Pain: location, type, frequency, trigger points, visual analog
      scale, McGill pain questionnaire, modified Hendler's pain
      evaluation, etc.
   7. Skin temperature (for vascular component)
   8. Supraclavicular Tinel's
   9. Compression maneuvers used to attempt to localize vascu-
      lar compression sites[1,6,7] (check bilaterally).
      a. *Adson's maneuver:* Clinician holds arm in extension and
         external shoulder rotation as the patient holds a deep
         breath and rotates head toward the affected side. Repeat
         with head turned away from the affected side. Positive
         findings result in obliteration of the radial pulse and/or
         reproduction of symptoms, presumably because of sub-

clavian artery compression by the scaleni (i.e., scalene triangle).

    b. *Costoclavicular maneuver:* Exaggerated military position with shoulders drawn downward and backward, used to check for compression occurring at costoclavicular region. Note obliteration of radial pulse and/or reproduction of symptoms.

    c. *Hyperabduction maneuver:* Arm held by clinician in fully abducted position to test for compression at pectoralis minor insertion (i.e., axillary region). Again note reproduction of symptoms and/or obliteration of radial pulse. *Note:* The above three tests should be used in conjunction with all other objective testing procedures; they are extremely technician sensitive and are frequently positive in normal, asymptomatic individuals.

10. Provocative maneuvers used to assess status of brachial plexus.

    a. *Elevated arm stress test (East)* or Roos test (also indicative of vascular manifestation): Patient assumes the "stick-up" position (i.e., shoulders abducted and externally rotated to 90 degrees and forearms flexed to 90 degrees) and then opens and closes his hands for 3 minutes or until the symptoms are provoked.[6] A modification of the Roos test can also be used. Arms are elevated overhead with elbows extended (to avoid reproducing ulnar nerve symptoms) and wrists in neutral (to avoid reproducing median nerve symptoms). This test position is maintained for 1 minute without opening and closing hands.[3]

        i. *Arterial involvement:* demonstrates pallor with empty veins.

        ii. *Venous involvement:* cyanosis and/or venous engorgement.

        iii. *Neurologic involvement:* paresthesias and heaviness.

    b. *Elvey's upper limb tension test (ULTT):* Tests mobility of brachial plexus and nerve roots. Clinician looks for provocation of symptoms by placing progressively increased tension in the nerve roots/peripheral nerve. Care must be taken to avoid placing excess traction on the plexus. Specific ULTT technique can be found in references 8 and 9.

    c. *Hunter test:* high. Tests for ulnar nerve findings (involvement of C8–T1, lower trunk). Specific technique can be found in reference 9.

    d. *Erb test:* Tests for radial nerve findings (involvement of posterior cord). Specific techniques can be found in reference 5.

    e. *Hunter test:* low. Tests for median nerve findings (involvement of C6–C7, upper trunk). Specific technique can be found in reference 9.

f. Provocative maneuvers to test for distal compression sites (i.e., cubital tunnel and carpal tunnel).

g. *Medial clavicle compression:* Manual compression superior and posterior to the medial one-third of the clavicle may also provoke symptoms.[10,11]

   Please note that some of the provocative tests as well as some movements tested during ROM evaluation may not be tolerated by a patient with severe symptoms. (Assess the irritability of tissues to determine how vigorous the evaluation should be.[12])

II. Treatment

   A. Progression[2]

      1. Stage I—decrease and control patient's symptoms; increase comfort.

      2. Stage II—treat tissues that are creating structural limitations of motion (e.g., soft tissue mobilization, nerve gliding, stretching exercises, etc.).

      3. Stage III—condition and strengthen muscles necessary to maintain postural correction; restore functional ROM of upper extremity for activities of daily living (ADL) and occupational activities.

   B. Conservative management

      1. Patient education to avoid symptom-producing postures and activities, which include occupational, recreational, and sleeping habits. (May involve splinting of involved peripheral nerve to reduce tension or compression, especially for more distal peripheral neuropathies.)

         The following is a guideline in reducing the aggravation of symptoms (unpublished protocol)[10,11]:

         a. Correct posture: patient should look in mirror, front and side (Fig. 22-2).
            i. Bring head and shoulder back to a relaxed position.
            ii. Small curve in low back.
            iii. Weight distributed equally on both feet.
            iv. Maintain correct posture when sitting, standing, or walking (Note: ideal posture must be gradually approximated over time).

         b. Sleeping
            i. Patient should avoid sleeping on affected side, in face-lying position, or with arms overhead.
            ii. A position that decreases symptoms is sidelying on the unaffected side with one pillow or cervical roll under the head and another pillow in the line of the trunk to support the upper arm (Fig. 22-3).
            iii. Another position of comfort is lying on the back with one pillow under the head and shoulders and one pillow under each arm (Fig. 22-4).

         c. Working
            i. Patient should not lean over while standing or sitting. Be as erect as possible.

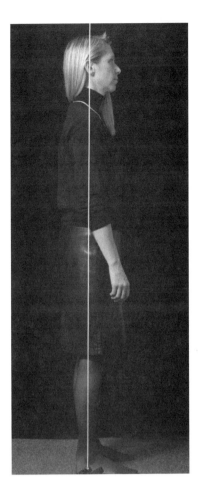

Fig. 22-2. Correct posture.

ii. When sitting at a desk or armchair, there should be a forearm-supporting surface that will not cause excessive elevation or depression of the shoulders (i.e., a slanted work surface) (Fig. 22-5).

iii. Patient should guard against working above shoulder level and should use a step stool to reach high objects.

iv. Patient should avoid carrying heavy objects with affected arm. Heavy items (briefcases, purses, grocery bags) should be carried with unaffected arm or held close to body in both arms.

d. Driving (Fig. 22-6)

i. Hands should be kept low and relaxed on steering wheel.

ii. A small pillow or arm rest should support affected side.

iii. If shoulder strap of seat belt crosses the clavicle on the affected side, the patient must not draw the strap too tightly.

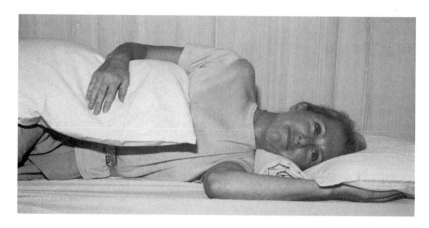

Fig. 22-3. Positioning for sidelying.

e. General precautions
   i. Stressful situations should be avoided. Stress will lead to tension of the cervical musculature.
   ii. Affected arm should not hang at side while working or standing. The hand can rest in a pocket to avoid pulling down on the shoulder.
   iii. Obesity will contribute to poor posture and continuation of symptoms.
   iv. For female patients, bra straps should not be tight, and women with large breasts should have thick bra straps, strapless bras, or underwire bras.
   v. Strenuous exercises that create labored breathing should be avoided, as this requires action of secondary respiratory muscles whose function is elevation of the ribs.
   vi. Patient should change activities or rest when symptoms arise.
   vii. Patient should have others remind him or her about correct posture.
   viii. Patients should wear several layers of light clothing during cold weather. (Heavy coats may weigh down shoulders.) Cold weather creates shivering and hypertonicity of muscles, including upper cervical musculature; hence keeping warm is important.

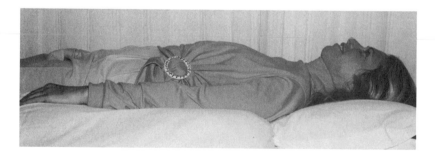

Fig. 22-4. Positioning for backlying.

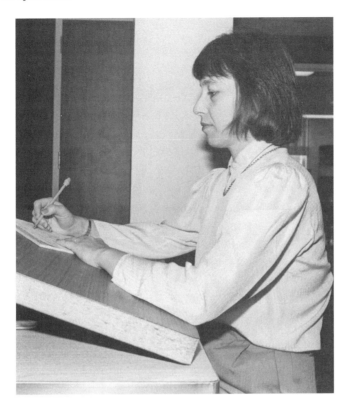

Fig. 22-5. Correct positioning for sitting at a work station.

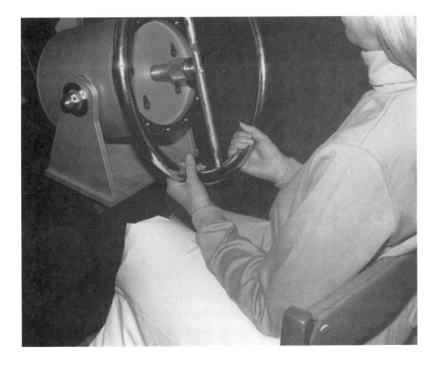

Fig. 22-6. Positioning for driving.

2. Modalities to decrease pain (e.g., transcutaneous electrical nerve stimulation [TENS], moist heat, etc.).

   Begin with pain and inflammation reducing treatments (may need sling or postural support to help maintain rest position of brachial plexus, that is, abduction and elevation of scapula, and internal rotation and adduction of shoulder).[8]

3. Management of muscle spasm and tension in shoulder girdle and cervical musculature.

   a. Moist heat
   b. Ultrasound
   c. Cold packs
   d. Massage (deep friction and relaxation)
   e. Occasionally analgesics and/or muscle relaxants are prescribed by physician

   Note: Cervical traction, either static or intermittent, should be avoided as this tends to increase rather than relieve patient's symptoms.

4. Manual therapy to restore/increase accessory joint movement.

   a. Joint mobilizations of sternoclavicular, acromioclavicular, and scapulothoracic joints.[10,13]
   b. Mobilization of the occiput on the atlas will also facilitate axial extension movement.[11]
   c. Patient must be willing to make frequent visits for therapy and must follow through with the home exercise program.
   d. Techniques of joint mobilization should be performed only by therapists with appropriate training in manual therapy.

5. Brachial plexus gliding exercises

   a. Use of the ULTT as an exercise for mobilizing the brachial plexus.
   b. Specific exercise technique can be found in references 8 and 9.

6. Postural exercises[2,7,8,11,14]

   a. Improve cervical and scapular alignment; include exercises to stretch pectoralis minor, scaleni, and cervical lateral flexors and exercises to encourage scapular adduction/depression, and paracervical extension. Shoulder/glenohumeral joint exercises and thoracic flexion/extension exercises can be added as needed.

      The following is a suggested exercise program. Exercises should be performed slowly, 10 repetitions, two times a day to start. (If patient's tolerance is low or symptoms are aggravated, decrease number and frequency of exercises and/or change exercise position to minimize stress on injured tissues, i.e., gravity-assisted positions or supine with pillow support.[3])

      i. *Shoulder girdle motion* (to emphasize shoulder retraction): sit with shoulders relaxed; arms supported. Make small circles with shoulder joints, gradually increasing in size. Work in both directions.

ii. *Stretching of scalene muscles:* stand erect; arms at sides, with shoulders internally rotated. (May also be done in supine to maximize cervical relaxation.[2]) Bend the neck, trying to touch ear to shoulder, first to right then to left. Relax and repeat. (May add shoulder depression to increase stretch) (Fig. 22-7).

iii. *Stretching of pectoral muscles:* stand facing a corner of a room with one hand on each wall; hands at head level; palms forward; elbows bent. Do a standard push-up into corner and return to original position. Inhale as body leans forward, exhale upon return. Repeat (Fig. 22-8).

iv. *Stretching of pectoralis minor:* lying supine with knees bent. Keep arms level on bed surface. Slide affected arm up into abduction, attempting to reach ear.

v. *Strengthening of scapular adductors:* sit with shoulders relaxed; arms supported in lap. Gently squeeze shoulder blades together, hold for a count of three, return to starting position and repeat (Fig. 22-9).

vi. *Strengthening of cervical extensors:* sit with shoulders relaxed; arms supported in lap; head bent forward. Slowly extend head, hold for a count of three, return to starting position and repeat.

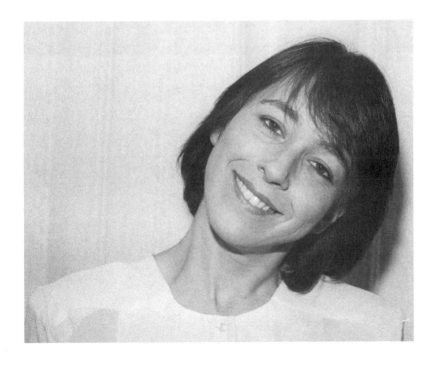

Fig. 22-7. Scalene stretch exercise.

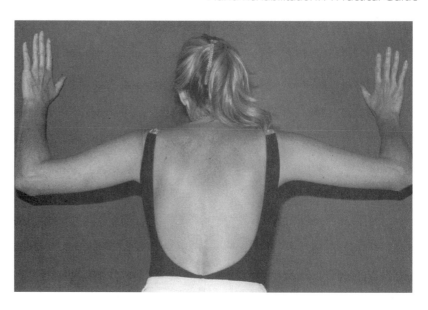

Fig. 22-8. Pectoral stretch exercise.

vii. *Diaphragmatic breathing* (to discourage overuse of accessory muscles for respiration, which elevates rib cage resulting in decreased thoracic outlet space): backlying; one hand on stomach; one hand on chest. Inhale—hand on stomach should rise; hand on chest should stay about same height. Exhale—hand on stomach should fall; hand on chest will stay same height. Perform for three inhalation/exhalation cycles.

viii. Progression

    A. Increase frequency of home exercise program slowly to patient tolerance.

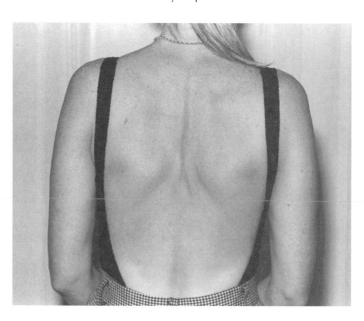

Fig. 22-9. Scapular adduction exercise.

       B. Assess progress, as often as needed (once or twice/week).

       C. Relief of symptoms should be achieved after 2 to 3 months of conservative management; otherwise an alternative method of treatment may be indicated (possible surgery).

  7. ROM exercises for cervical region and upper extremity

INDICATIONS/PRECAUTIONS FOR SURGERY

I. Indications
   A. Conservative treatment is not beneficial
   B. Patient requires narcotic medication and is unable to sleep or work
   C. Muscle atrophy
   D. Marked edema
   E. Arterial emboli or tip ulceration/gangrene
II. Precautions
   A. Malignant conditions (especially with prior irradiation)[15]
   B. Alcohol abuse
   C. Diabetes
   D. Other neurologic and vascular diseases

OPERATIVE MANAGEMENT

I. Surgical techniques
   A. Cervical rib resection
   B. Scalenectomy procedures
   C. Transaxillary approaches for fascial band release
   D. Arterial reconstructive procedures

POSTOPERATIVE THERAPY[6,8,15]

I. ROM exercises every 1 to 2 hours, as soon as possible after surgery, to maintain freedom of movement of the plexus.
   A. Elvey's ULTT is helpful for nerve gliding because the patient can perform forearm supination, wrist and finger extension, without stressing the surgical wound.[16]
   B. Cervical ROM and motion distal to the shoulder may be initiated the first postoperative day.
II. Begin gentle ROM exercises to shoulder and scapular area 1 to 2 weeks postoperatively.
III. Mild use of shoulder 4 to 6 weeks postoperatively.
IV. Full use of upper extremity 8 to 10 weeks postoperatively.

POSTOPERATIVE COMPLICATIONS

    I. Infection
   II. Persistent painful paresthesias
  III. Decreased muscle strength with atrophy
  IV. Persistent numbness
   V Decreased circulation with possible ulceration of fingertips
  VI. Nonunion of clavicle if clavicle is divided during surgery

EVALUATION TIMELINE

    I. Initial evaluation
      A. Postural assessment
      B. Edema
      C. Strength (grip and pinch measurement)
      D. Manual muscle test
      E. ROM evaluation
      F. Sensory evaluation
      G. Pain: location, type, frequency, etc. Repeat above evaluations every 4 weeks for progress assessment.

REFERENCES

1. Lord JW, Rosati LM: Clinical Symposia: Thoracic Outlet Syndromes. CIBA Pharmaceutical Co., Summit, NJ, 1971
2. Walsh MT: Therapist management of thoracic outlet syndrome. J Hand Ther April-June:131, 1994
3. Novak CB, MacKinnon SE, Patterson GA: Evaluation of patients with thoracic outlet syndrome. J Hand Surg 18A:292, 1993
4. Upton ARM, McComas AJ: The double crush in nerve-entrapment syndromes. Lancet 2:359, 1973
5. MacKinnon SE, Dellon AL: Surgery of the Peripheral Nerve. Thieme Medical Publications, New York, 1988
6. Roos DB: Thoracic outlet syndrome. p. 91. In Machleder HI (ed): Vascular Disorders of the Upper Extremity. Futura Publishing, Mount Kisco, 1983
7. Wilgis EFS: Vascular Injuries and Diseases of the Upper Limb. Little, Brown, Boston, 1983
8. Barbis JM, Wallace KA: Therapists management of brachioplexopathy. p. 923. In Hunter JM, Mackin EJ, Callahan AD (eds): Rehabilitation of the Hand: Surgery and Therapy. 4th Ed. Mosby, St. Louis, 1995
9. Totten PA, Hunter JM: Therapeutic techniques to enhance nerve gliding in thoracic outlet syndrome and carpal tunnel syndrome. Hand Clin 7:505, 1991
10. Smith KF: The thoracic outlet syndrome: a protocol of treatment. Am Phys Ther Assoc 1:89, 1979
11. Jaeger SH, Read R, Smullens SN, Breme P: Thoracic outlet syndrome: diagnosis and treatment. p. 378. In Hunter JM (ed): Rehabilitation of the Hand: Surgery and Therapy. 2nd Ed. Mosby, St. Louis, 1984

12. Maitland G: Peripheral Mobilization. Butterworth, Boston, 1977

13. Jackson P: Thoracic outlet syndrome: evaluation and treatment. Clin Management Phys Ther 7:6, 1987

14. Klinefelter HF: Postural myoneuralgia. Int Angiol 3:191, 1984

15. Whitenack SH, Hunter JM, Jaeger SH, Reed R: Thoracic outlet syndrome: a brachial plexopathy. p. 857. In Hunter JM, Mackin EJ, Callahan AD (eds): Rehabilitation of the Hand: Surgery and Therapy. 4th Ed. Mosby, St. Louis, 1995

16. Barbis J: Therapist's management of thoracic outlet syndrome. p. 540. In Hunter JM, Schneider LH, Mackin EJ, Callahan AD (eds): Rehabilitation of the Hand: Surgery and Therapy. 3rd Ed. Mosby, St. Louis, 1990

SUGGESTED READINGS

Adson AW: Surgical treatment for symptoms produced by cervical ribs and the scalenus anticus muscle. Surg Gynecol Obstet 85:687, 1947

Butler SD: Tension testing—the upper limbs. p. 141. In Butler DS (ed): Mobilization of the Nervous System. Churchill Livingstone, New York, 1991

Byron PM: Upper extremity nerve gliding: programs used at the Philadelphia hand center. p. 951. In Hunter JM, Mackin EJ, Callahan AD (eds): Rehabilitation of the Hand: Surgery and Therapy. 4th Ed. Mosby, St. Louis, 1995

Cailliet R: Neck and Arm Pain. FA Davis, Philadelphia, 1964

Cailliet R: Soft Tissue Pain and Disability. FA Davis, Philadelphia, 1977

Carroll RE, Hurst LC: The relationship of thoracic outlet syndrome and carpal tunnel syndrome. Clin Orthop Relat Res 164:149, 1982

Edwards RH: Hypothesis of peripheral and central mechanisms underlying occupational muscle pain and injury. Eur J Appl Physiol 57:275, 1988

Elvey RL: Brachial plexus tension tests and the pathoanatomical origin of arm pain. p. 116. In Glasgow EF, Twoney L (eds): Aspects of Manipulative Therapy. 2nd Ed. Churchill Livingstone, New York, 1985

Hawkes CD: Neurosurgical considerations in thoracic outlet syndrome. Neurosurg Considerations 207:24, 1986

Huffman JD: Electrodiagnostic techniques for and conservative treatment of thoracic outlet syndrome. Electrodiagn Tech 207:21, 1986

Kaltenborn FM: Manual Therapy for the Extremity Joints. Olaf Norlis Bokhandel, Oslo, 1976

Leffert RD: Thoracic outlet syndrome. J Am Acad Orthop Surg 2:317, 1994

Leffert RD, Graham G: The relationship between dead arm syndrome and thoracic outlet syndrome. Clin Orthop Relat Res 223:20, 1987

Michlovitz SL: Thermal Agents in Rehabilitation. 2nd Ed. FA Davis, Philadelphia, 1990

Novak CB: Physical therapy management of thoracic outlet syndrome in the musician. J Hand Surg April-June:74, 1992

Novak CB, Collins D, MacKinnon SE: Outcome following conservative management of thoracic outlet syndrome. J Hand Surg 20A:542, 1995

Novak CB, MacKinnon SE, Brownlee R, Kelly L: Provocative sensory testing in carpal tunnel syndrome. J Hand Surg (Br)17:204, 1992

Osterman AL: Double crush and multiple compression neuropathy. p. 1919. In Gelberman R (ed): Operative Nerve Repair and Reconstructions. JB Lippincott, Philadelphia, 1991

Roos D: Thoracic outlet syndrome: update 1987. Am J Surg 15:568, 1987

Roos DB: Thoracic outlet syndromes in musicians. J Hand Surg April-June:65, 1992

Schwartzman RJ: Neurologist's approach to brachial plexopathy. p. 837. In Hunter JM, Mackin EJ, Callahan AD (eds): Rehabilitation of the Hand: Surgery and Therapy. 4th Ed. Mosby, St. Louis, 1995

Sessions RT: Recurrent thoracic outlet syndrome: causes and treatment. South Med J 75:1453, 1982

Silliman JF: Neurovascular injuries to the shoulder complex. J Orthop Sports Phys Ther 18:442, 1993

Sommerich CM: Occupational risk factors associated with soft tissue disorders of the shoulder: a review of recent investigations in the literature. Ergonomics 36:697, 1993

Sucher BM: Thoracic outlet syndrome—a myofascial variant: Part 1. Pathology and diagnosis. J Am Osteopath Assoc:686, 1990

Travell JG, Simmons DG: Myofascial pain and dysfunction. The Trigger Point Manual. Williams & Wilkins, Baltimore, 1983

Tyson RR, Kaplan GF: Modern concepts of diagnosis and treatment of the thoracic outlet syndrome. Orthop Clin North Am 6:507, 1975

Urschel HC, Razzuk MA: The failed operation for thoracic outlet syndrome: the difficulty of diagnosis and management. Ann Thorac Surg 42:523, 1986

Whitenack SH, Hunter JM, Jaeger SH, Read RL: Thoracic outlet syndrome complex: diagnosis and treatment. p. 530. In Hunter JM, Schneider LH, Mackin EJ, Callahan AD (eds): Rehabilitation of the Hand: Surgery and Therapy. 3rd Ed. Mosby, St. Louis, 1990

Wood VE, Frykman GK: Winging of the scapula as a complication of first rib resection: a report of six cases. Clin Orthop Relat Res 149:160, 1980

Wright IS: The neurovascular syndrome produced by hyperabduction of the arms. Am Heart J 29:1, 1945

Ulnar Nerve Compression

23

Bonnie Aiello

The cubital tunnel is a bony canal formed by the ulnar collateral ligament, the trochlea, the medial epicondylar groove, and is roofed by the triangular arcuate ligament. The ulnar nerve that runs through this bony tunnel is responsible for sensation in the fifth and ulnar half of the fourth digit and supplies the ulnar intrinsics, flexor digitorum profundus fourth and fifth, and flexor carpi ulnaris[1] (Fig. 23-1).

Any irritation to the nerve at that level can cause severe pain, dysthesias, deformity, and dysfunction of grip and pinch strength, and fine motor coordination is affected. "Claw hand" or metacarpophalangeal (MCP) hyperextension with concurrent inability to fully extend proximal interphalangeal (PIP) and distal interphalangeal (DIP) joints in the ring and little fingers may also occur.

Conservative treatment consists of rest and anti-inflammatory modalities to decrease swelling in the closed space tunnel.

Surgically, the nerve is decompressed, or moved under skin or muscle out of the compressed space. Rehabilitation is directed according to the structure disrupted.

Guyon's canal is the bony canal formed by the volar carpal ligament, hook of the hamate, and the hamate. Both the ulnar nerve and artery run through this tunnel and can be affected by a space-maintaining lesion or a decrease in the actual tunnel area. (Fig. 23-2)

Motor and sensory deficits are present for all ulnar nerve innervated areas distal to the canal and may be distinguished from cubital tunnel deficits by the absence of any dorsal sensory branch symptoms. It may be caused by blunt trauma,[1] an occult tumorous condition[2,3] (e.g., lipoma, ganglion cyst), or a fracture of the hamate, ring, or little finger metacarpal bones.[1]

This deficit must be managed postsurgically after the space-maintaining lesion or fracture has been alleviated, with splinting, muscle strengthening, and sensory re-education.

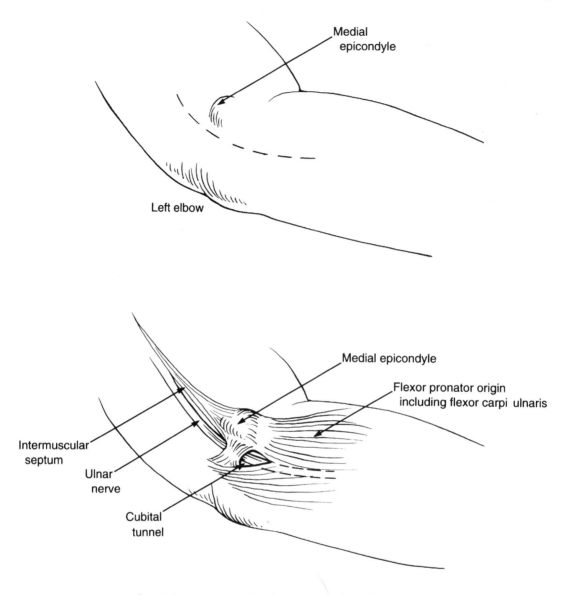

Fig. 23-1. Anatomy of the ulnar nerve in the cubital tunnel.

DEFINITION

Cubital tunnel may be defined as compression of the nerve at the elbow as it passes through the area of the cubital tunnel. Causative factors include recurrent subluxation, dislocations, rheumatoid arthritis, excessive elbow valgus, bony spurs, synovial cysts, or trauma.

Compression of the nerve in Guyon's canal may be defined as compression of the nerve at the wrist as it passes through Guyon's canal.

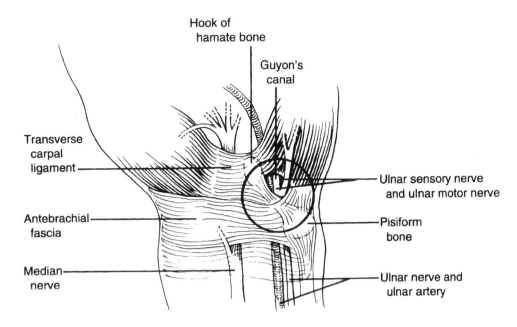

Fig. 23-2. Ulnar nerve in Guyon's canal.

SURGICAL PURPOSE

I. Cubital tunnel: To release compression of the ulnar nerve at the medial epicondyle of the elbow (Fig. 23-1). Surgical methods have a spectrum from simple ligament release, to subcutaneous or submuscular transposition of the ulnar nerve, to medial epicondylectomy. All of these techniques are designed to remove the compressive forces from the nerve.

II. Guyon's canal: To release pressure on the ulnar nerve as it passes from the wrist into the palm by dividing the supporting fibro-osseous ligaments or removing space-occupying lesions from the channel. Surgery also may correct fractures of the hook of the hamate or reconstruct thrombosis of the ulnar artery.

TREATMENT GOALS

I. Decrease painful paresthesias and hypersensitivity
II. Increase muscle strength to return to full use
III. Prevent deformity
IV. Prevent recurrence with education
V. Maintain and educate about protective and functional sensation
VI. Increase range of motion (ROM)
VII. Manage scar

NONOPERATIVE INDICATIONS/ PRECAUTIONS

I. Indications
   Symptoms may be grouped into stages.
   A. Mild: intermittent paresthesias, increased vibratory perception, complaints of clumsiness or loss of coordination, positive elbow flexion test, positive Tinel's sign.
   B. Moderate: intermittent paresthesias, decreased vibratory perception, measurable grip and pinch weakness, positive Tinel's sign, positive elbow flexion test, finger crossing may be abnormal.
   C. Severe: persistent paresthesias, decreased vibratory perception, abnormal two-joint discrimination, measurable pinch and grip weakness. Muscle atrophy is present, claw deformity may be present. Positive Tinel's sign, positive elbow flexion test, finger crossing usually abnormal, electrodiagnostic testing usually positive for moderate and severe compression. Paresthesias that radiate down the medial forearm to the ulnar 1.5 digits and compression at the elbow may be differentiated from the compression at Guyon's canal by the presence of dorsal sensory branch symptoms in the proximal compressions.
II. Precautions
   A. Diabetes
   B. Alcohol abuse associated peripheral neuropathy
   C. Other peripheral neuropathic disease
III. Nonsurgical precautions
   A. Pain caused by immobilization
   B. Persistent pain, numbness, deformity

NONOPERATIVE TREATMENT (MILD DEGREE OF COMPRESSION)

I. Cubital tunnel
   The extremity is splinted with the elbow flexed 30 to 45 degrees; wrist is dorsiflexed 0 to 20 degrees in neutral rotation for 3 months at night (Fig. 23-3). Symptomatic pain relief may be used. ROM is maintained. Postural and positional education is stressed to avoid external nerve compression (i.e., leaning on the elbow and excessive elbow flexion).

NONOPERATIVE COMPLICATIONS

I. Pain caused by immobilization
II. Persistent pain, numbness, deformity

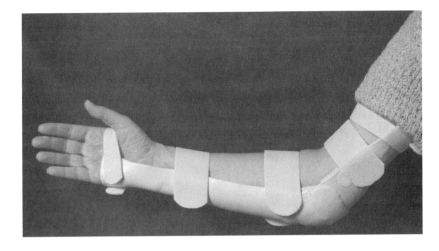

Fig. 23-3. Long arm splint.

SURGICAL TREATMENT (MODERATE TO SEVERE COMPRESSION)

  I. Decompression: The aponeurosis is divided. The arm is immobilized in a bulky dressing 10 to 14 days. ROM is then progressed as indicated and is unrestricted.
 II. Anterior transposition: The ulnar nerve is moved anteriorly beneath a skin flap; subcutaneous transposition or beneath the flexor muscle mass parallel to the median nerve; submuscular transposition.
     A. Subcutaneous transposition: splint elbow in 90 degrees flexion, forearm neutral rotation, and wrist in 20 degrees dorsiflexion for 2 weeks. Gentle active range of motion (AROM) is then started. Progress to resisted exercise at 4 weeks.
     B. Submuscular transposition: elbow splinted in 90 degrees flexion, forearm neutral rotation, and wrist in 20 degrees flexion times 8 days (with sling for 2 weeks). Day 9 elbow flexion only with wrist supported. Week 2 remove sling and begin gradual elbow extension exercise. Week 5 begin strengthening exercises.
III. Medial epicondylectomy: Medial epicondyle and distal part of the supracondylar ridge resected. Bulky soft dressing is applied immediately and AROM may start in 2 to 7 days. Week 2: passive range of motion (PROM). Progress to resisted ROM as tolerated.

POSTOPERATIVE INDICATIONS/ PRECAUTIONS FOR THERAPY

  I. Cubital tunnel
     A. Indications
        1. Moderate to severe compression
        2. Failed conservative treatment
     B. Precautions
        1. Diabetes

    2. Alcohol abuse associated peripheral neuropathy
    3. Other peripheral neuropathic disease
II. Guyon's canal
  A. Indications

    Confirmed presence of a neuropathy in the region of the wrist (especially if it is progressive); that is, the presence of combined motor and sensory neuropathy with no dorsal sensory branch symptoms.[1]

  B. Precautions
    1. Nonunited fractures
    2. Malignant conditions
    3. Alcohol abuse
    4. Diabetes
    5. Other neurologic disease

POSTOPERATIVE THERAPY

Cubital Tunnel

  I. Pain relief may be obtained via appropriate modalities.
  II. Scar management may be started as soon as wounds are healed.
  III. Splinting to prevent deformity as indicated.
  IV. Sensory re-education and education about decreased sensation must be addressed.
  V. Postural and positional education
  VI. Specific treatment
    A. Decompression
      1. Week 1
        a. Bulky dressing 10 to 14 days
        b. Sensory education
        c. Wound care
      2. Week 2: ROM as tolerated
    B. Submuscular transposition
      1. Week 1
        a. Splint in 90 degrees of flexion, neutral forearm rotation and wrist in 20 degrees flexion for 8 days
        b. Sensory education
        c. Wound care
      2. Day 9: AROM flexion of elbow with wrist supported
      3. Week 2: AROM extension
      4. Week 4: PROM
      5. Week 5: resisted ROM
    C. Subcutaneous transposition
      1. Week 1
        a. Splint 90 degree elbow flexion, neutral forearm rotation wrist in 20 degree extension 2 weeks
        b. Sensory education
        c. Wound care

2. Week 2: AROM
3. Week 3: PROM
4. Week 4: resisted ROM
D. Medial epicondylectomy
   1. Week 1
      a. Bulky dressing
      b. Sensory education
      c. Wound care
      d. AROM
   2. Week 2: PROM
   3. Week 4: resisted ROM

Guyon's Canal

I. As causes of compression of the ulnar nerve are varied, the cause must be addressed before the rehabilitation of the nerve injury (e.g., proper splintage or fixation for appropriate fractures or removal of any space-maintaining mass).
   A. Pain relief may be obtained via appropriate modalities.
   B. Scar management.
   C. After protective splinting for cause of compression (times 3 days for ganglion tumor removal, 4 weeks for fracture), claw deformity may be addressed with MCP block splint.
   D. Sensory re-education.
   E. Patient education about their decreased sensitivity must be addressed immediately.
   F. Strengthening may be started at 4 to 6 weeks for fracture (if healed), or after AROM is noted at ulnar innervated muscles.

POSTOPERATIVE COMPLICATIONS

I. Cubital tunnel
   A. Laceration of the medial antebrachial cutaneous nerve
   B. Pain caused by immobilization
   C. Persistent flexion contractures
   D. Muscle rupture
   E. Infection
   F. Persistent pain, numbness, deformity
   G. Hypersensitive scar, heavy raised scar
II. Guyon's canal
   A. Painful paresthesias and persistent dysthesias
   B. Decreased muscle strength atrophy
   C. Persistent numbness

EVALUATION TIMELINE

I. Cubital tunnel
   A. Initial

1. Pain
2. Sensation
3. Wound (for surgical patients)
B. Monthly
   1. Sensory
   2. Manual muscle test (MMT)
   3. Pain
C. Decompression
   1. 2 weeks: ROM
   2. 4 weeks: MMT, sensory, pain
D. Submuscular
   1. Day 9: AROM, flexion
   2. Week 2: PROM, extension
   3. Week 4: PROM
   4. Week 5: MMT
E. Subcutaneous
   1. 2 weeks: AROM
   2. 3 weeks: PROM
   3. 4 weeks: MMT, sensory
F. Epicondylectomy
   1. 1 week: AROM
   2. 2 weeks: PROM
   3. 4 weeks: MMT, sensory
G. Repeat monthly
II. Guyon's canal
A. Initial
   1. Sensory
   2. Pain
   3. Range of motion (ROM)
   4. Manual muscle test (MMT)
B. Monthly
   1. MMT
   2. Sensory
C. Biweekly
   ROM

REFERENCES

1. Heithoff S: Medial epicondylectomy for the treatment of ulnar nerve compression at the elbow. J Hand Surg 15A:22, 1990
2. Eversmann WW Jr: Entrapment and compression neuropathies. p. 1452. In Green DP (ed): Operative Hand Surgery. 2nd Ed. Churchill Livingstone, New York, 1988
3. Silver M, Gelberman R, Gellman H: Carpal tunnel syndrome: associated abnormalities in ulnar nerve function and the effect of carpal tunnel release in these abnormalities. J Hand Surg 5:710, 1985

SUGGESTED READINGS

Adelaar RS: The treatment of the cubital tunnel syndrome. J Hand Surg 9A:90, 1984

Baker C: Evaluation, treatment and rehabilitation involving a submuscular transposition of the ulnar nerve at the elbow. Athletic Training 23:10, 1988

Beroit BG: Neurolysis combined with the application of a Silastic envelope for ulnar nerve entrapment at the elbow. Neurosurgery 20:594, 1987

Bowers WH: The distal radioulnar joint. p. 973. In Green DP (ed): Operative Hand Surgery. 2nd Ed. Churchill Livingstone, New York, 1988

Broudy AS, Leiffert RD, Smith RJ: Technical problems with ulnar nerve transposition at the elbow: findings are results of reoperation. J Hand Surg 3:85, 1978

Clark C: Cubital tunnel syndrome. JAMA 241:801, 1979

Craven P, Green DP: Cubital tunnel syndrome treatment by medial epicondylectomy. J Bone Joint Surg 62A:986, 1980

Dellon AL: Review of treatment results for ulnar nerve entrapment at the elbow. J Hand Surg 4:688, 1989

Dellon AL, Hament W, Gittelshon A: Nonoperative management of cubital tunnel syndrome. Neurology 43:1673, 1993

Dellon A, MacKinnon S: Surgery of the Peripheral Nerve. Theime Medical Publisher, New York, 1988

Dellon A, MacKinnon S: Surgery of the peripheral nerve. p. 197. Thieme Medical Publishing, New York, 1988

Dellon AL: Operative technique for submuscular transposition of the ulnar nerve. Contemp Orthop 16:17, 1988

Dimond ML, Lister GD: Cubital tunnel syndrome treated by long-arm splintage, abstracted. J Hand Surg 10A:430, 1985

Eaton RG: Anterior transposition of the ulnar nerve using a non-compressing fasciodermal sling. J Bone Joint Surg 62A:820, 1980

Fanmir TF: Local decompression in the treatment of ulnar nerve entrapment at the elbow. R Coll Surg Edinburgh 123:362, 1978

Folberg CR, Weiss AP, Akelman E: Cubital tunnel syndrome part II: Treatment. Orthop Rev 23:233, 1994

Foster RJ: Factors related to the outcome of surgically managed compressive ulnar neuropathy at the elbow level. J Hand Surg 6:181, 1981

Fromisen AI: Treatment of compression neuropathy of the ulnar nerve at the elbow by epicondylectomy and neurolysis. J Hand Surg 5:391, 1980

Jones RE: Medial epicondylectomy for ulnar nerve compression syndrome at the elbow. Arch Neurol 139:174, 1979

Leffert RD: Anterior submuscular transposition of the ulnar nerve by the Learmonth technique. J Hand Surg 7:147, 1982

Manske PR, Johnson RJ, Pruitt DL et al: Ulnar nerve decompression at the cubital tunnel. Clin Orthop Rel Res 274:231, 1992

Moneim MS: Ulnar nerve compression at the wrist. Hand Clin 8:2:337, 1992

O'Rourke PJ, Quinlan W: Fracture dislocation of the 5th metacarpal resulting in compression of the deep branch of the ulnar nerve. J Hand Surg (Br) 18B:190, 1993

Rayan GM: Proximal ulnar nerve compression. Hand Clin 8:2:325, 1992

Rengachary S, Arjunan K: Compression of the ulnar nerve in Guyon's canal by a soft tissue giant cell tumor. Neurosurgery 8:400, 1980

Thurman RT, Jindal P, Wolff TW: Ulnar nerve compression in Guyon's canal caused by calcinosis in scleroderma. J Hand Surg 16A:739, 1991

Zahrawi F: Acute compression ulnar neuropathy at Guyon's canal resulting from lipoma. J Hand Surg 9A:238, 1984

Median Nerve Compression 24

Bonnie Aiello

The proximal median nerve may be impinged in several areas down the length of the forearm. The patient may experience pain in the volar surface of the distal arm or proximal forearm with increased activity. They may have decreased sensibility of the radial three and one-half digits, but a negative Phalen's test. Sites for impingement include:

1. Ligament of Struthers in the distal third of the humerus beneath the supracondylar process.
2. Lacertus fibrosis at the elbow joint if the median nerve is superficial to the flexor muscle mass; thereby exposing it to compression with supination and pronation.
3. In between heads of the pronator muscle; usually caused by hypertrophy of the muscle mass or by the aponeurotic fascia on the deep surface of the head of the pronator teres muscle (Fig. 24-1).
4. At the arch of flexor digitorum superficialis (FDS) as the median nerve passes deep to it.

The anterior interosseus nerve, a branch of the median nerve as it passes deep to the pronator teres, may present with nonspecific pain in the proximal forearm that increases with activity, but no sensory problems. Patients have weakness of flexor digitorum profundus of II and flexor pollicis longus (Froment's sign), and pronator quadratus.

In the carpal tunnel, the nerve is impinged beneath the transverse carpal ligament. Patients present with decreased sensation in the radial three and one-half digits, thenar clumsiness, and weakness in lumbricals 1 and 3. They may have a positive (+) Phalen's test (Fig. 24-2).

Pathologic Anatomy and Staging of Compression: In early compression the epineural blood flow is impaired, causing decreased axonal transport. Morphologic changes are absent.[1] The patient will complain

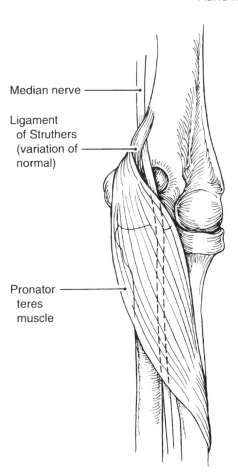

Median nerve

Ligament
of Struthers
(variation of
normal)

Pronator
teres
muscle

Fig. 24-1. Anatomy of pronator syndrome.

of intermittent symptoms, test positive only for provocative tests, and can be found to be hypersensitive to 256 cps.[2] These patients do the best with conservative therapeutic management.[2]

In moderate compression, persistent interference of intraneural microcirculation is present along with epineural and intrafascicular edema.[1] Intraneural fibrosis may be present; however, wallerian degeneration has not taken place. There is decreased vibratory sensation, positive provocative tests, and thenar weakness; and the patient complains of abnormal sensation.

In severe compression, long-standing epineural edema may be followed by endoneural edema and fibrosis.[1] There may be loss of fibers. Electromyography (EMG) shows denervation potentials in the median nerve supplied muscles. There are persistent sensory changes, abnormal static two-point discrimination greater than 4 mm, and thenar atrophy.[2]

These pathologic, histologic, and clinical findings determine which path of treatment to follow.

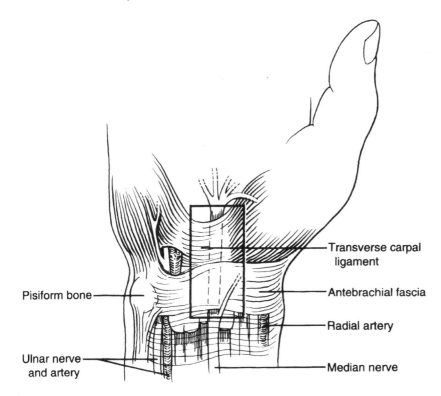

Fig. 24-2. Anatomy of carpal tunnel.

(Labels on figure:) Transverse carpal ligament; Antebrachial fascia; Radial artery; Median nerve; Pisiform bone; Ulnar nerve and artery

DEFINITION

Impingement of the median nerve in the proximal forearm, pronator teres, at the anterior interosseus level or carpal tunnel. Median nerve compression is a common cumulative trauma.

TREATMENT AND SURGICAL PURPOSE

To reduce compressive forces on the median nerve in the carpal tunnel. Nonoperative methods rely on decreasing demands on the hand and wrist to reduce inflammation of the flexor tendon synovium. This is usually accomplished by work modification, wrist splinting, and anti-inflammatory medications. Surgery is directed at enlarging the carpal tunnel by releasing the transverse carpal ligament, which allows more space for the median nerve.

TREATMENT GOALS

I. Decrease pain and paresthesias
II. Increase or maintain muscle strength

III. Maintain function of the hand
IV. Education

NONOPERATIVE INDICATIONS/ PRECAUTIONS FOR THERAPY

  I. Indications
      A. Intermittent paresthesias or pain, clumsiness.
      B. Positive provocative tests.
      C. Hypersensitive to 256 cps.[2]
 II. Precautions
      A. Metabolic disease.
      B. Alcohol abuse.

NONOPERATIVE THERAPY

  I. Proximal compression
      A. Long arm splint in 90 degrees of elbow flexion and neutral wrist position for 3 to 4 weeks followed by night wear for about the same amount of time.
      B. Nonsteroidal anti-inflammatory drugs (NSAIDs).
      C. Pnonophoresis[3]
      D. Iontophoresis[3]
      E. Cryotherapy
      F. Allow elbow and wrist active range of motion (AROM) to maintain it during the day.
 II. Distal compression
      A. Wrist splint 3 to 4 weeks in neutral position followed by night wear for approximately the same amount of time[2–8] (Fig. 24-3).
      B. Steroid injection into the carpal tunnel.[1,4–7]
      C. Vitamin B_6 therapy may be used.[2,4,8]

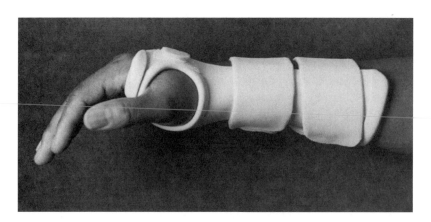

Fig. 24-3. Wrist splint for use in carpal tunnel syndrome.

D. Phonophoresis[3]
E. Iontophoresis[3]
F. Cryotherapy[3]
G. NSAIDs[6,8,9]

NONOPERATIVE COMPLICATIONS

I. Persistent pain, paresthesias.
II. Progression of thenar atrophy.
III. Progression of nerve injury.
IV. Decreased function.

POSTOPERATIVE INDICATIONS/ PRECAUTIONS FOR THERAPY

I. Indications
  A. Failed conservative treatment.
  B. Moderate to severe compression.
II. Precautions
  A. Metabolic disease.
  B. Alcohol abuse.

POSTOPERATIVE THERAPY

I. Pronator syndrome
  A. Day 3 to 5 postoperatively: bulky dressing continuing flexion/ extension, gradual increase in activity as patient permits.

OR

  B. Elbow 90 degrees for 12 days then motion exercise.[7]
II. Anterior Interosseus
  A. Sling for 8 days with digital range of motion (ROM). Then progressive ROM as the patient tolerates.

OR

  Bulky dressing supporting the elbow and wrist. Allow digital ROM and wrist flexion and extension. If the pronator teres was elevated, eliminate pronator and supination (except for 45 degrees of pronation for full pronation) for 2 to 3 weeks. Strengthening at 1 to 10 days postoperatively unless the pronator was elevated; then at 3 to 4 weeks.
  B. Scar management
III. Carpal tunnel release
  A. Days 1 to 14
    1. Patient's wrist immobilized in neutral.
    2. AROM all digits.

B. Day 15
   1. Suture removal.
   2. Wrist AROM.
   3. Continue ROM to all digits.
   4. Desensitization if needed.
   5. Scar management started.
C. Day 21: Strengthening
D. Day 28
   1. Sensory evaluation and retraining.
   2. Work hardening may begin.

POSTOPERATIVE COMPLICATIONS

I. Infection, dehiscence.
II. Neuroma.
III. Continued pain, numbness.
IV. Hypersensitive scar.
V. Reflex sympathetic dystrophy (RSD).

EVALUATION TIMELINE

I. Initial visit or preoperative.
   A. Sensory evaluation
   B. ROM
   C. Manual muscle test (MMT)
II. For nonoperative therapy: repeat above tests monthly.
III. Postoperative therapy.
   A. First visit postoperative.
      1. ROM
      2. Wound evaluation
   B. 3 weeks postoperative: MMT.
   C. 4 weeks postoperative.
      1. Sensory evaluation
      2. Repeat monthly

REFERENCES

1. Gelberman R, Szabo RM, Williamson RV: Sensibility testing in peripheral nerve compression syndromes. J Bone Joint Surg 65A:632, 1983
2. Dellon AL, MacKinnon SE: Surgery of the Peripheral Nerve. Thieme Medical Publishers, New York, 1988
3. Griffin JE: Physical Agents for Physical Therapists. 2nd Ed. Charles C Thomas, Springfield, 1982
4. Carragee E, Hentz V: Repetitive trauma and nerve compression. Orthop Clin North Am 19:157, 1988
5. Phalen G: Clinical evaluation of 398 hands. Clin Orthop Relat Res 83:29, 1972

6. Spinner R, Bachman JW, Adadio PC: The many faces of carpal tunnel syndrome. Mayo Clin Proc 64:829, 1989

7. Green D: Operative Hand Surgery. 2nd Ed. Churchill Livingstone, New York, 1988

8. Greenspan J: Carpal tunnel syndrome: a common but treatable cause of pain. Postgrad Med 84:34, 1988

9. Calliet R: Hand Pain and Impairment. 3rd Ed. FA Davis, Philadelphia, 1982

10. Robbins H: Anatomical study of the median nerve in the carpal tunnel and etiologies of the carpal tunnel syndrome. J Bone Joint Surg 45A:953, 1963

SUGGESTED READINGS

Daniels L MA, Worthingham C: Muscle Testing. 4th Ed. WB Saunders, Philadelphia, 1986

Dellon AL: Functional sensation and its re-education. Clin Plast Surg 11:95, 1984

DiBenedetto M, Mitz M: New criteria for sensory nerve conduction especially useful in diagnosis of carpal tunnel syndrome. Arch Phys Med Rehabil 67:586, 1986

Elias JM: Treatment of carpal tunnel syndrome with vitamin B6. South Med J 80:882, 1987

Eversman WW: Proximal median nerve compression. Hand Clin 8:307, 1992

Gainor BJ: Modified exposure for pronator syndrome decompression: a preliminary experience. Orthopedics 16:1329, 1993

Gelberman R, Aronson D, Weisman MH: Carpal tunnel syndrome. J Bone Joint Surg 62A:1181, 1980

Gelberman R, Rydevik B, Pess G et al: Carpal tunnel syndrome: a scientific basis for clinical care. Orthop Clin North Am 19:115, 1988

Golding R, Selverajah K: Clinical tests for carpal tunnel syndrome: an evaluation. Br J Rheumatol 25:388, 1986

Hunter JM, Schneider LH, Mackin EJ, Callahan AD: Rehabilitation of the Hand. 3rd Ed. Mosby, St. Louis, 1989

Kaplan SJ, Glickel SZ, Eaton RG: Predictive factors in the nonsurgical treatment of carpal tunnel syndrome. J Hand Surg (Br) 15B:106, 1990

Kelly CP, Pulisetti D, Jamieson AM: Early experience with endoscopic carpal tunnel release. J Hand Surg (Br) 19B:18, 1994

Kulick MI, Gordillo G, Javidi T et al: Long-term analysis of patients having surgical treatment for carpal tunnel syndrome. J Hand Surg IIA:59, 1986

Lamb DW: The Practice of Hand Surgery. 2nd Ed. Blackwell Scientific Publications, Boston, 1989

Lister GD, Bledsole RB, Klein H: The radial tunnel syndrome. J Hand Surg 4:52, 1979

Litchmeen HM, Triedman MH, Silver CM, Simon SD: The carpal tunnel syndrome (a clinical and electrodiagnostic study). Int Surg 50:269, 1968

Lucketti R, Schoenhuber R, Landi A: Assessment of sensory nerve conduction in carpal tunnel syndrome before, during, and after operating. J Hand Surg 13B:386, 1988

Lundborg G, Stanstrom AK, Sollerman C et al: Digital vibrogram: a new diagnostic tool for sensory testing in compression neuropathy. J Hand Surg 11A:693, 1986

Masear VR, Hayes JM, Hyde AG: An industrial cause of carpal tunnel syndrome. J Hand Surg 11A:222, 1986

Mesgarzadeh M, Schenk CD, Bonakdarpour A: Carpal tunnel: MR imaging, part I: normal anatomy. Musculoskel Radiol 171:743, 1989

Mesgarzadeh M, Schenk CD, Bonakdarpour A et al: Carpal tunnel: MR imaging, part II: normal anatomy. Musculoskel Radiol 171:749, 1989

Murphy RX, Jennings JF, Wukich DK: Major neurovascular complications of endoscopic carpal tunnel release. J Hand Surg 19A:114, 1994

Nathan P, Kenistan R: CTS and its relation to general physical condition. Hand Clin 9:253, 1993

Nelson R, Currier D: Clinical Electrotherapy. Appleton & Lange, East Norwalk, CT, 1987

Omer G: Median nerve compression at the wrist. Hand Clin 8:317, 1992

Phalen G: The carpal tunnel syndrome. J Bone Joint Surg 48A:211, 1966

Spinner M: Injuries to the major branches of peripheral nerves in the forearm. WB Saunders, Philadelphia, 1978

Sunderland S: Nerve and Nerve Injuries. 2nd Ed. Churchill Livingstone, New York, 1978

Waylett-Rendall J: Sensibility evaluation and rehabilitation peripheral nerve problems. Orthop Clin North Am 19:43, 1988

Wild E, Geberich SG, Hunt K et al: Analysis of wrist injuries in workers engaged in repetitive tasks. AAOHN J 35:356, 1987

Tendon Transfers for Radial Nerve Palsy

25

Arlynne Pack Brown

Injury to the radial nerve at the humerus results in limited forearm supination, absent wrist extension, metacarpophalangeal (MCP) joint extension, and thumb abduction and extension. These clinical limitations result in the functional limitation of decreased ability to open the hand to grasp.

When it is clear that the muscles are not likely to be reinnervated, tendon transfers are frequently performed. Tendon transfers transmit the muscle power of one muscle to another by moving the tendon insertion from the original muscle to that of the denervated muscle. There are multitudes of muscles available for transfer. The pronator teres muscle is usually the donor of choice to provide wrist extension and the flexor carpi ulnaris muscle is usually used for MCP joint extension. Thumb extension and abduction are commonly provided by the palmaris longus, one-half of the flexor carpi radialis, and the ring finger sublimus muscles. The following rehabilitation guidelines are based on using these muscles as transfers.

The result of tendon transfers can be enhanced in a number of ways. When a transfer crosses several joints, one of which is unstable, the action of the tendon transfer can be improved with an arthrodesis of that joint. The arthrodesis allows the force to be transmitted across the newly stable joint to the joints where the motion is desired. Another consideration is the phase of the original action of the donor muscle with the new desired action. It is typically easier to re-educate muscles transferred within phase. That is, a muscle that is originally a wrist flexor is best transferred to a digital extensor. Recall the tenodesis coordination between these motions during normal hand function: during wrist flexion the extrinsic digital extensors, in phase with the wrist flexors, naturally cause digital extension.

DEFINITION

Schneider[1] defines tendon transfers as "the application of the motor power of one muscle to another weaker or paralyzed muscle by the transfer of its tendinous insertion."

SURGICAL PURPOSE

Loss of extensor muscle function is most commonly associated with radial nerve interruption. It is impossible for the patient with this condition to open the hand to grasp objects; therefore the transfer of normally functioning muscle–tendon units is frequently used to overcome the deficit. The radial nerve supplies all of the wrist extensors and finger extensors including the thumb. Depending on the level of nerve interruption, tendon transfer planning may or may not include wrist extension. Preoperative instruction and splinting may supplement postoperative rehabilitation when the patient is knowledgeable about the function of the transferred units.

Some surgeons perform tendon transfers (internal splints) during the nerve repair recovery phase (i.e., pronator teres to extensor carpi radialis brevis [ECRB]) so that patients do not have to wait for nerve recovery to have a functional hand.

Restoration of lost muscle action by the transfer of available and effective muscle units is the goal of this form of treatment.

TREATMENT GOALS

I. Preoperative goals
   A. Maximize passive range of motion (PROM), particularly the thumb–index web space, and wrist extension.[2–4]
   B. Establish tissue equilibrium.[2,4]
   C. Educate patient about new muscle–joint relationship.
   D. Maximize power of donor muscle.[2,3,5]
   E. Maintain function and grip strength, discourage habit of using tenodesis between wrist and MCP joints for function.[4,5]
   F. Monitor sensation; if median nerve distribution sensation is absent, patient is unlikely to use transfer.[3]
II. Postoperative goals
   A. Protect transferred tendon.[2]
   B. Maintain range of motion (ROM) of uninvolved joints.[2]
   C. Maximize functional ROM of involved joints (i.e., flex wrist to 20 degrees when digits are in composite flexion).
   D. Establish firm scar at juncture site that is able to glide through adjacent structures.[3]
   E. Return to functional use of hand.

POSTOPERATIVE INDICATIONS/ PRECAUTIONS FOR THERAPY

I. Indications
   Surgical tendon transfers
II. Precautions
   A. Neuroma
   B. Overestimation of donor muscle strength
   C. Less than full ROM before surgical transfer[1]

PREOPERATIVE THERAPY

I. Techniques to maximize active ROM (AROM) and PROM[1–4]
II. Techniques to maximize strengthening[2,3]
III. Techniques to maximize scar mobility[2–4]
IV. Monitor sensation[3]
V. Assess strength of and strengthen possible donor muscles[1,5]
VI. Provide splints to promote normal use of hand[6] (Fig. 25-1)

POSTOPERATIVE THERAPY

I. Weeks 0 to 3 or 4: Immobilization of elbow 90 degrees (option of surgeon), forearm pronation 30 degrees to 90 degrees, wrist dorsiflexion 30 degrees to 45 degrees, MCP joints 0 degree, proximal interphalangeal (PIP) joints free or flexed 20 degrees to 45 degrees, thumb full abduction and extension or slightly less than full abduction and extension (Fig. 25-2).

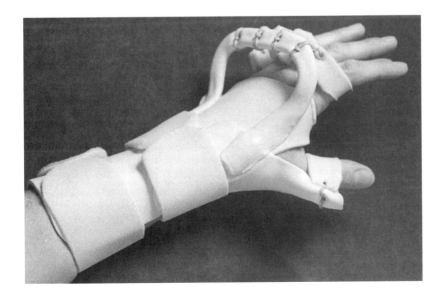

Fig. 25-1. Splints can promote normal use of hand.

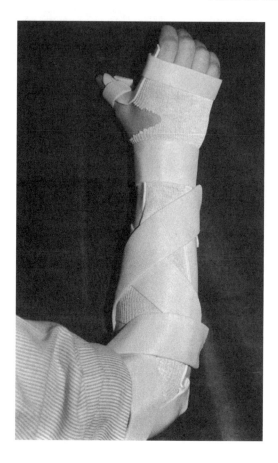

Fig. 25-2. Example of splint used for posoperative positioning.

    A. ROM uninvolved joints of neck, shoulder, distal interphalangeal (DIP) joint
    B. Protective ROM individual joints: elbow, wrist within 10 degrees to 30 degrees of dorsal flexion arc, MCP joints, interphalangeal (IP) joints[5]
    C. Avoid composite flexion
    D. Scar management
    E. Desensitization
 II. Week 3 or 4: Fabricate splint, according to surgeon's guidance, which may or may not include elbow. Position the hand and wrist in same position as that in the original cast.
III. Weeks 5 to 6: Begin brief sessions of muscle contractions and education of transferred muscle and progress to full ROM during light pick up–release activities for digits and twisting activities for thumb (i.e., nut and bolt assembly).[4]
IV. Week 7: Begin dynamic flexion splinting if extrinsic extensor tendon tightness is present.
 V. Week 8: Discontinue protective daytime splinting; introduce resistive exercises.[5]
VI. Week 12: Resume unrestricted activities.

POSTOPERATIVE COMPLICATIONS

   I. Scarring of tendon to surrounding structures, particularly at sites of pulleys
  II. Bowstringing of transferred tendon
 III. Rupture of tendon juncture[1,3]
  IV. Overstretching of transferred tendon[1,2]
   V. Wrist postures in slight radial deviation when flexor carpi ulnaris is used as a donor muscle

EVALUATION TIMELINE

   I. Week 0
      A. ROM of uninvolved joints
      B. Protected ROM of individual involved joints
      C. Sensibility evaluation
  II. Week 5: Composite AROM flexion and extension joints involved in tendon transfer.
 III. Week 7: Composite PROM flexion and extension joints involved in tendon transfer.
  IV. Week 10: Manual muscle testing.

REFERENCES

1. Schneider LH: Tendon transfers in the upper extremity. p. 669. In Hunter JM, Schneider LH, Mackin EJ, Callahan AD (eds): Rehabilitation of the Hand: Surgery and Therapy. Mosby, St. Louis, 1990
2. Reid RF: Radial nerve palsy. Hand Clin 4:179, 1988
3. Riordan RC: Principles of tendon transfers. p. 410. In Hunter JM, Schneider LH, Mackin ER (eds): Tendon Surgery in the Hand. Mosby, St. Louis, 1987
4. Omer GE: Tendon transfers in radial nerve paralysis. p. 425. In Hunter JM, Schneider LH, Mackin EJ (eds): Tendon Surgery in the Hand. Mosby, St. Louis, 1987
5. Reynolds CC: Preoperative and postoperative management of tendon transfers after radial nerve injury. p. 696. In Hunter JM, Schneider LH, Mackin EJ, Callahan AD (eds): Rehabilitation of the Hand. 3rd Ed. Mosby, St. Louis, 1990
6. Colditz JC: Splinting for radial nerve palsy. J Hand Ther 1:18, 1987

Replantation 26

Lauren Valdata Eddington

Experiments on limb replantation were reported in the late 1800s, but it was not until the operating microscope allowed repair of small vessels in the 1960s that microvascular surgery began. More and more reports of successful replantations occurred following improvements in instrumentation, surgical techniques, suture materials, patient selection, and in preoperative and postoperative management. With the success of replantation, greater focus has now been placed on the functional recovery of the replanted digits.

Replantation is defined as "the reattachment of a body part that has been totally severed from the body without any attachments. This term differs from revascularization, which is defined as the reattachment of an incompletely amputated part, in which vessel reconstruction is necessary to assure viability …"[1]

After amputation occurs, recovery of function depends on the preservation of cellular structure, as well as on the restoration of blood flow. Cellular damage may develop as an immediate result of ischemia. Extreme or irreversible ischemic tissue damage before replantation procedures is often seen and can be prevented by proper cooling.[1–3] Two basic methods have been described for care of the amputated part. One method involves wrapping the part in a cloth moistened with lactated Ringer's solution, then placing it in a plastic bag on ice. Another method is to immerse the part in lactated Ringer's solution in a plastic bag and place this bag on ice.[1] A compressive dressing is placed on the stump.

When replanting, the sequence to follow for digital and hand replantation is to shorten and fix bone with repair of the periosteum (especially the volar plate if possible). Extensor tendons are repaired followed by flexor tendons. When possible, both arteries, with or without interpositional vein grafts, are repaired. Finally, nerves and veins are repaired (one and one-half to two veins per arterial repair attempted), and/or vein grafts, if necessary. Lastly, skin is closed without constriction.[1,4,5]

Postoperative care begins with application of the proper bulky dressing and plaster splint. A protocol of no smoking, no caffeine, hourly or more frequent color and warmth checks (to be maintained above 30°C), capillary refill, and elevation of arm to heart level with the patient in as restful an atmosphere as possible is followed. After the first week the patient is referred for hand therapy and evaluation.

DEFINITION

Replantation is the reattachment of a body part that has been totally severed from the body without any attachments[1,4] (Fig. 26-1).

SURGICAL PURPOSE

Under many circumstances, totally amputated parts of the upper limb can be reattached using current surgical techniques. Amputation causes damage to every anatomic structure. Restoration of the critical components such as bone, tendons, arteries, nerves, veins, and skin is essential for the survival of the amputated segment or segments. Not all of these segments will be suitable for replantation, nor will they all survive replantation. The purpose is to restore those parts necessary for good arm and hand function.

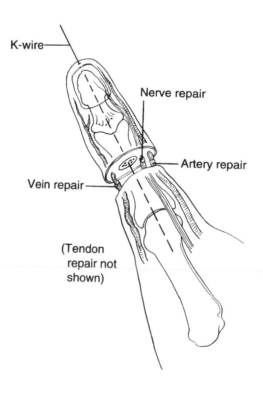

Fig. 26-1. Replantation is the reattachment of a totally severed body part.

TREATMENT GOALS

    I. Protect all repaired structures [i.e., vessels, nerves, tendon(s), fracture(s)].

    II. Promote/monitor wound healing and care.

    III. Maintain range of motion (ROM) of all proximal uninvolved joints of the upper extremity.

    IV. Reduce edema, taking into consideration vein repairs over repaired parts.

    V. Splint hand and fingers in as functional a position as possible.

    VI. Minimize complaints of pain as indicated of proximal joints.

    VII. Educate patient in the care of replanted part and treatment.

    VIII. Promote independence in activities of daily living (ADL) for the patient, with assists as needed.

    IX. Evaluate and give support as needed by hand social work referral.

OPERATIVE INDICATIONS/PRECAUTIONS

    I. Indications

        A. Thumbs and any suitable digits where there have been multiple amputations are replanted, especially at zones III and IV.[1,2]

        B. All digits in children are replanted, if possible.[1,2]

        C. Individual digits are replanted where all fingers may be required for professional or social purposes (e.g., musicians).[2]

        D. Incomplete amputations of individual digits are revascularized, especially where the flexor tendon and/or digital nerves are intact.[2]

        E. Finger replantations distal to flexor digitorum superficialis insertion (zones I, II, III).[2]

        F. Limb severed at or above the wrist if (1) the amputated part is cooled promptly and appropriately, the warm ischemia time is less than 6 hours, and total ischemia time is less than 12 hours; (2) the amputated part and portion of the limb proximal to the amputation has not suffered extensive or other soft tissue injuries; or (3) there are no life-threatening conditions.[2,6,7]

    II. Precautions

        A. Avulsion injuries generally are not advised except for the thumb.[2]

        B. Double level fractures, gross crush, and amputations distal to the middle of the middle phalanx.[2]

        C. Amputations in patients older than 70 years.[2]

        D. Amputations with a warm ischemia time greater than 6 hours are not replanted.[2]

        E. Amputations proximal to the flexor digitorum superficialis insertion (in zones IV and V).

        F. Limb contraindications to replant include (1) avulsion of the brachial plexus, (2) severe mangling injuries of the amputated part, or (3) excessive ischemia time.

IMMEDIATE POSTOPERATIVE COMPLICATIONS

I. Temperature of replant drops below 30°C (86°F); if it cannot be returned to adequate tissue perfusion, surgical re-exploration is necessary.
II. Return to the operating room within 24 to 48 hours after initial replantation can increase the salvage rate to greater than 50 percent. After this time, the result is usually a failure and surgery may not be performed.
III. Infection: daily wound checks are done.

POSTOPERATIVE INDICATIONS/ PRECAUTIONS FOR THERAPY

I. Indications: Replanted digit or part that has been cleared by the surgeon for its viability after initial postoperative dressing is removed and replaced with a lighter dressing by the surgeon.
II. Precautions
   A. Change in temperature of replanted part.
   B. Pressure on replanted part by straps too narrow or splint too small.
   C. Increase in edema of replanted part.
   D. Any changes in the circulation and/or condition of the wounds.

POSTOPERATIVE THERAPY

I. 0 to 5 days: Thermoplastic splinting once referred by physician 0 to 5 days after replantation with wrist in neutral or slightly flexed position with the fingers in metacarpophalangeal (MCP) flexion and the interphalangeals (IP) in a relaxed position of extension. Dorsal splint preferred to better hold the hand in as functional a position as is indicated (Fig. 26-2). Skin and temperature checks continue hourly.
II. 5 to 7 days to 3 weeks.
   A. Gentle, protected passive ROM (PROM) of wrist flexion/extension, then MCP gentle PROM protected flexion/extension and IP protected, gentle PROM flexion/extension, if there is good bony fixation. The tenodesis advantage should be utilized; that is, gentle, passive assisted flexion of wrist with simultaneous MCP and IP joint extension and then extension to neutral or to slightly flexed wrist with subsequent MCP and IP flexion. In addition, gentle, protected IP flexion with the MCPs extended (hook position), as well as IP extension with MCP flexion (tabletop or military salute), can begin passively but no active ROM (AROM) is begun until 3 weeks status postreplantation.

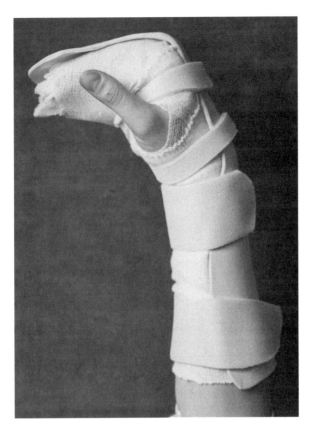

Fig. 26-2. Postoperative splint that may be used upon doctor referral.

    B. Wound care and daily dressing changes that are lighter, using petroleum impregnated fine-mesh gauze or nonadherent porous interface material and gauze;[6] no whirlpool so as not to compromise circulation.

    C. Edema control by positioning of involved extremity at heart level continues; no constrictive dressings or other edema reducing techniques are begun until approximately 3 weeks or if approved by physician.

    D. Skin and temperature checks continue.

    E. AROM, active assisted ROM (AAROM), and PROM to all non-involved joints proximal to finger or wrist so as to avoid joint tightness proximal to the replantation.

III. 3 to 6 weeks: Continuation of passive, protected ROM for fingers and hand with active, protected ROM begun for wrist, MCP, and IPs. Passive and active protected tenodesis exercises can continue with patient instruction in home active, protected flexion and extension exercises in the splint initially. Progression of exercises actively in splint to out of splint continues each week to 6 weeks when patient can be out of the splint at home, but should still wear the splint when sleeping or out in public. Splint may be cut down to hand based after 4 to 6 weeks if for digital replantation. Scar mobilization with fluid flushing edema techniques should continue. Patient should continue to elevate arm to heart level.

At 4 to 6 weeks patient can begin minimal gentle functional activities to pick up light objects or assist in minimal ADL. AROM continues with decreasing the protective positions and including full excursion exercise as the pre-work hardening activities increase.

IV. 6 to 12 weeks: Continue scar mobilizing techniques, as well as, AROM, AAROM, and PROM exercises. After 8 weeks, begin resistive exercises for full excursion and blocked positions. Continue protective splinting in public or when sleeping. Begin dynamic flexion/extension splinting and/or static flexion/extension splinting to increase AROM and PROM for replanted parts. Care and instruction to patient for continued circulation checks with splints on and to gradually increase wear time of the specific splints without any circulation compromise.

During this time, an initial sensory evaluation should be done as a baseline to monitor future nerve growth and regeneration. 30 cps, 256 cps, heavy moving touch, light moving touch, heavy constant touch, and light moving touch tests should be evaluated and recorded. Monofilaments are also used for further sensory evaluations. (See sensory evaluation guidelines, Ch. 7.)

Work hardening will begin to increase use of the involved hand and gradually increase the patient's independence and work tolerance.

V. Greater than 12 weeks: Barring no bone healing problems, the patient can either simulate his or her actual job tasks or return to work after evaluation. All home exercises for ROM and strengthening should continue. Dynamic or static splinting will also continue as needed to further increase active flexion and/or extension. Sensory evaluations should continue every 5 to 8 weeks until indicated to begin patient on early and late phase sensory re-education. (See sensory re-education guidelines, Ch. 7.) Discharge as appropriate.

POSTOPERATIVE COMPLICATIONS

If any changes occur as noted below, contact the patient's physician immediately.

I. Change in temperature of replanted part
II. Change in color of replanted part
III. Replanted part begins to bleed
IV. Increase in necrotic tissue noted over repaired sites
V. Any pus discharge or any other signs of infection
VI. Any sudden increase in edema of the hand and/or replanted part
VII. Any sudden increase in pain of the hand and/or replanted part

EVALUATION TIMELINE

I. 0 to 5 days: Surgeon and nurses monitor for any changes in temperature and/or color of replanted part through observation and Doppler checks. Monitor changes in edema of hand and/or replanted part(s).

II. 5 to 7 days: Protective thermoplastic splint made. Patient and therapist monitor and check temperature, color, and inability of replanted part. No PROM measurements taken at this time. Note in chart the position the fingers are held in the splint.

III. 3 to 4 weeks: Active protected ROM measurements can be recorded. Evaluate and record wound viability, scar adhesions, and techniques used to increase mobility; also, record any painful regions and check for Tinel's sign.

IV. 4 to 6 weeks: Record AROM and PROM measurements in a protected position. Evaluate splint and adjust to increase the functional protect position for hand and replanted parts. Continue with wound evaluation, scar mobilization, and begin more vigorous edema reducing techniques, if approved by physician.

V. 7 to 9 weeks: Record active and gentle PROM measurements. Evaluate joint stiffness and begin, with physician approval, dynamic flexion and/or extension splinting. Continue with edema reduction and scar mobilization techniques.

VI. 9 to 12 weeks: AROM and PROM measurements taken, early grip and pinch measurements (if bone fixation is good). Sensory evaluation and record of progressing Tinel's sign. Prework hardening activities continue with evaluation of patient's ability for return to work activities.

VII. 16 weeks: Active and passive evaluation measurements, grip and pinch measurements. Sensory evaluation and record of progressing Tinel's (or desensitization techniques to begin if patient's hand is overly sensitive to touch).

VIII. Greater than 20 weeks: 1 month follow-ups for ROM, active and passive, grip and pinch, and sensory evaluation with early and late phase sensory re-education beginning when appropriate.

REFERENCES

1. Urbaniak JR: Microsurgery for Major Limb Reconstruction. CV Mosby, St. Louis, 1987, pp. 2–37 and 56–66

2. Morrison WA, O'Brien BMcC, MacLeod AM: Digital replantation and revascularizations. A long term review of one hundred cases. Hand 10:125, 1978

3. Smith AR, van Alphen B, Faithfull NS, Fennema M: Limb preservation in replantation surgery. Plast Reconstr Surg 75:227, 1985

4. Weiland AJ, Villareal-Rios A, Kleinert HE et al: Replantation of digits and hands: analysis of surgical techniques and functional results in 71 patients with 86 replantations. J Hand Surg 2:1, 1977

5. Kader PB: Therapist's management of the replanted hand. Hand Clin 2:179, 1986
6. Silverman P, Mac N, Willette GV: Early protective motion in digital revascularization and replantation. J Hand Ther 2:84, 1989
7. Gelberman RH, Urbaniak JR, Bright DS, Levin LS: Digital sensibility following replantation. J Hand Surg 3:313, 1978

SUGGESTED READINGS

Amadio PC, Lin GT, An KN: Anatomy and pathomechanics of the flexor pulley system. J Hand Ther 2:138, 1989

Axelrod TS, Buchler U: Severe complex injuries to the upper extremity: revascularization and replantation. J Hand Surg 16A:574, 1991

Baker GL, Kleinert JM: Digit replantation in infants and young children: determinants of survival. Plast Reconstr Surg 94:139, 1994

Browne EZ, Ribik CA: Early dynamic splinting for extensor tendon injuries. J Hand Surg 14A:72, 1989

Bunke HJ, Jackson RL, Bunke GM, Chan SW: The surgical and rehabilitative aspects of replantation and revascularization of the hand. p. 1075. In Hunter JM, Mackin EJ, Callahan AD (eds): Rehabilitation of the Hand: Surgery and Therapy. Mosby, St. Louis, 1995

Dellon AL: Sensory recovery in replanted digits and transplanted toes: a review. J Reconstr Microsurg 2:123, 1986

Doyle JR: Anatomy of the flexor tendon sheath and pulley system: a current review. J Hand Surg 14A:349, 1989

Duran RJ, Houser RG: Controlled passive motion following flexor tendon repair in zones 2 & 3. p. 105. In AAOS: Symposium of Tendon Surgery in the Hand. Mosby, St. Louis, 1975

Evans RB: Therapeutic management of extensor tendon injuries. Hand Clin 2:157, 1986

Evans RB, Burkhalter WE: A study of the dynamic anatomy of extensor tendons and implications for treatment. J Hand Surg 11A:774, 1986

Glickman LT, MacKinnon SE: Sensory recovery following digital replantation. Microsurgery 11:236, 1990

Goldner RD, Stevanovic MV, Nunley JA, Urbaniak JR: Digital replantation at the level of the distal interphalangeal joint and distal phalanx. J Hand Surg 14A:214, 1989

Jupiter JB, Pess GM, Bour CJ: Results of flexor tendon tenolysis after replantation in the hand. J Hand Surg 14A:35, 1989

Kleinert HE, Kutz JE, Cohen MJ: Primary repair of zone 2 flexor tendon lacerations. p. 91. In AAOS: Symposium on Tendon Surgery in the Hand. Mosby, St. Louis, 1975

Milford L: The Hand. 2nd Ed. Mosby, St. Louis, 1982

O'Brien B McC: Reconstructive microsurgery of the upper extremity. J Hand Surg 15A:316, 1990

Strickland JW: Biologic rationale, clinical application and results of early motion following flexor tendon repair. J Hand Ther 2:71, 1989

Tark KC, Kim YW, Lee YH, Lew TD: Replantation and revascularization of hands: clinical analysis and functional results of 261 cases. J Hand Surg 14A:17, 1989

Werntz JR, Chester SP, Breidenbach WC et al: A new dynamic splint for postoperative treatment of flexor tendon injury. J Hand Surg 14A:559, 1989

Whitney TM, Lineaweaver WC, Buncke HJ, Nugen K: Clinical results of bony fixation methods in digital replantation. J Hand Surg 15A:328, 1990

Digital Amputation and Ray Resection 27

Linda Coll Ware

Partial digit amputations are the most common type of amputation seen in the upper extremity.[1] Various ways to treat these injuries include: split-thickness skin grafts, bone shortening with primary closure, healing by secondary intention, V–Y flap, volar flap, cross-finger flap, thenar flap, and hypothenar flap.[1-4] Regardless of surgical technique, the goals of surgery are (1) to preserve functional length, (2) to preserve useful sensibility, (3) to prevent symptomatic neuromas, (4) to prevent adjacent joint contractures, (5) to achieve short-duration morbidity, and (6) to return the patient quickly to work or play.[1]

Partial digit amputations can occur at different levels. The level of the amputation can affect the amount of recoverable movement. If the amputation is distal to the sublimis insertion, the middle phalanx segment will be able to participate effectively in grasping activities. If the amputation occurs proximal to the insertion, however, there will be no active flexion of the remaining middle phalanx. Once an amputation has occurred proximal to the proximal interphalangeal (PIP) joint, the remaining proximal segment is controlled by the intrinsic muscles and the extensor digitorum communis. This may only allow 45 degrees of active flexion of the metacarpophalangeal (MCP) joint. If the amputation occurs at the MCP level, the patient is left with a space that makes it difficult to keep small objects in the palm. At this point a ray resection may be considered.[1]

A ray resection or ray resection with digital transposition can be an elective operation decision. Before making this decision, the patient should regain maximum function from the initial injury and live with the altered hand. There is a significant loss of power grip with ray resection because of flexor tendon loss and narrowing of the palm. However, the cosmesis and symmetry of the hand are improved.[5]

Loss of a digit can be devastating for the patient. Emotional support and a referral to social work or psychiatry may be necessary.

DEFINITION

Partial digit amputation is the loss of skin or pulp, or with exposed bone of the finger (Fig. 27-1). A ray resection is an amputation through the metacarpal. Ray resection with a transposition involves an osteotomy of an adjacent metacarpal and its fixation to the remaining metacarpal of the resected digit (Fig. 27-2 and Fig. 27-3).

SURGICAL PURPOSE

Badly damaged fingers may require partial amputations to remove devitalized or infected tissues that are irreparable or irretrievable. In cases of sharp digital injuries, when replantation is not possible, an amputation with soft tissue closure is required. Closure of amputation stumps may require soft tissue advancement flaps, skin grafts, or skeletal shortening. Trimming and protection of nerve ends are frequently required. It is important to maintain the integrity and mobility of the more proximal joints for optimum hand function.

Ray resection, with or without digital transposition, is performed to close the space between fingers when the intervening finger is absent. The digital absence may be due to injury, disease, or birth defect. This form of surgery provides improved hand function and appearance by eliminating the space between fingers.

TREATMENT GOALS

   I. Promote wound closure and optimal scar formation
  II. Maintain full range of motion (ROM) of all uninvolved joints
 III. Maximize ROM of all involved joints
 IV. Desensitization/sensory re-education of injured tip
  V. Return patient to previous level of function

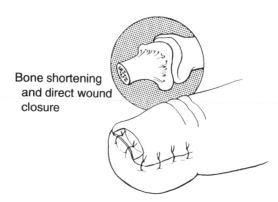

Bone shortening and direct wound closure

Fig. 27-1. Digital amputation.

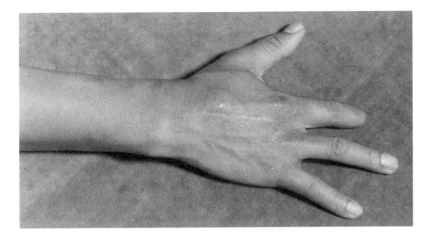

Fig. 27-2. Ray resection with transposition and partial amputation.

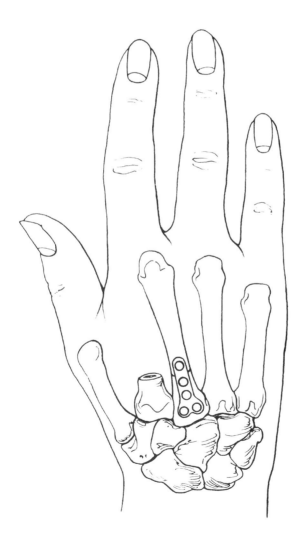

Fig. 27-3. Ray resection with transposition.

NONOPERATIVE INDICATIONS/ PRECAUTIONS FOR THERAPY

    I. Indications: digit amputations allowed to heal by secondary intention.
   II. Precautions
      A. Exposed bone
      B. Associated nail bed injury
      C. Associated fractures
      D. Associated nerve lacerations
      E. Associated tendon lacerations

NONOPERATIVE THERAPY

      I. Wound care (see Ch. 1)
     II. Protective splinting
   III. ROM
   IV. Edema control
    V. Desensitization/sensory re-education
   VI. Scar management once wound is healed
 VII. Strengthening
VIII. Fine motor and functional activities
  IX. Fitting of cosmetic prosthesis

NONOPERATIVE COMPLICATIONS

      I. Infection
     II. Prolonged open wound
   III. Hypersensitivity
   IV. Diminished sensation
    V. Neuroma
   VI. Poorly shaped tip
 VII. Adherent scar
VIII. Limited ROM
  IX. Alienation of digit
   X. Quadrigia syndrome
  XI. Empty space when fisting

POSTOPERATIVE INDICATIONS/ PRECAUTIONS FOR THERAPY

    I. Indications
      A. Partial digit amputations closed by sutures, skin grafts, or flaps.
      B. Ray amputations with or without digital transposition.

II. Precautions
   A. Presence of graft or flap
   B. Associated nail bed injuries
   C. Associated fractures
   D. Associated nerve lacerations
   E. Associated tendon lacerations

POSTOPERATIVE THERAPY

  I. Wound care including donor site
 II. Protective splinting
   A. If the third or fourth ray has been surgically resected, it is important to apply firm circumferential support to the palmar arch to prevent the metacarpals from spreading apart. This can be achieved by a palmar bar splint, which supports the transverse and longitudinal arches of the palm. The splint can be discontinued at 6 to 8 weeks postoperatively.[6]
   B. With a ray resection of the second metacarpal and a transfer of the first dorsal interossei, an index proximal phalanx block should be added to the palmar bar to prevent motion at the MCP joint and stretching of the transfer.[6]
III. Edema control
IV. ROM
   A. Active range of motion (AROM) may begin immediately with partial tip amputations and most ray resections.
   B. When a ray resection of the index finger with a first dorsal interossei transfer has been performed, AROM is started 3 to 4 weeks postoperatively and passive range of motion (PROM) is started 6 weeks postoperatively in the middle finger MCP joint.
   C. The type of fixation determines when to begin AROM of a ray resection with digital transposition. Rigid fixation with plates and screws allows motion early.[5] Consult with the physician.
  V. Desensitization/sensory re-education
 VI. Scar management once wound is closed
VII. Strengthening
   A. Strengthening can begin once amputation wound is healed.
   B. Strengthening can begin 6 to 8 weeks after a ray resection.
   C. Strengthening can begin once osteotomy has healed with a ray resection and digital transposition.
VIII. Fine motor, functional activities, and work hardening
 IX. Fitting of cosmetic prosthesis

POSTOPERATIVE COMPLICATIONS

  I. Graft or flap infection, hematoma, necrosis
 II. Donor site infection

   III. Hypersensitivity in fingertip and/or donor site
   IV. Diminished sensation in fingertip and/or donor site
    V. Neuroma
   VI. Poorly shaped tip
  VII. Adherent scar
 VIII. Limited ROM
   IX. Alienation of digit
    X. Spreading of metacarpals
   XI. Scissoring of digits

EVALUATION TIMELINE

    I. Nonoperative
      A. Immediately
        1. Wound assessment
        2. AROM and PROM measurements of all joints
      B. Once wound is healed
        1. Scar assessment
        2. AROM and PROM measurements of all joints
        3. Strength measurements
        4. Sensory evaluation
        5. Fine motor and functional assessments
   II. Operative
      A. Immediately
        1. Wound assessment including donor site.
        2. AROM and PROM of uninvolved joints.
        3. ROM of involved joints may be delayed until graft or flap, first dorsal interossei transfer or osteotomy has fixation. Consult physician.
      B. Once graft or flap is well established
        1. Scar assessment
        2. AROM and PROM of all joints
          a. AROM at 3 to 4 weeks of the middle finger MCP when first dorsal interosseous is transferred and PROM at 6 weeks.
          b. AROM and PROM for ray resection with digital transposition depends on type of fixation used
        3. Strength measurements: 6 to 8 weeks for ray resection/transposition.
        4. Sensory evaluation.
        5. Fine motor and functional assessments.

REFERENCES

1. Louis DS: Amputations. p. 55. In Green DP (ed): Operative Hand Surgery. Churchill Livingstone, New York, 1982
2. Beasley RW: Surgery of hand and finger amputations. Orthop Clin North Am 12:763, 1981

3. Schenck RR, Cheema TA: Hypothenar skin grafts for fingertip reconstruction. J Hand Surg 9A:750, 1984

4. Tupper J, Miller G: Sensitivity following volar V-Y plasty for fingertip amputations. J Hand Surg 10B:183, 1985

5. Burkhalter WE: Mutilating injuries of the hand. p. 1052. In Hunter JM, Mackin EJ, Callahan AD (eds): Rehabilitation of the Hand: Surgery and Therapy. Mosby, St. Louis, 1995

6. Cannon NM (ed): Diagnosis and Treatment Manual for Physicians and Therapists. The Hand Rehabilitation Center of Indiana, Indianapolis, IN, 1991

SUGGESTED READINGS

Chow SP: Hand function after digital amputation. J Hand Surg 18B:125, 1993

Murray JF et al: Transmetacarpal amputation of the index finger: a clinical assessment of hand strength and complications. J Hand Surg 2:6, 1977

Pillet J, Mackin EJ: Aesthetic hand prosthesis: its psychologic and functional potential. p. 1253. In Hunter JM, Mackin EJ, Callahan AD (eds): Rehabilitation of the Hand: Surgery and Therapy. Mosby, St. Louis, 1995

Preprosthetic Management of Upper Extremity Amputations

28

Lorie Theisen

Complete or partial loss of an upper extremity (UE) is devastating, whether the loss is due to trauma or some advanced disease. A comprehensive treatment program is necessary for the patient with a complete or partial amputation of the hand or limb. Keep in mind that each patient with an amputation has a unique set of circumstances that includes, but is not limited to, level of amputation, condition of residual limb, condition of contralateral limb, and stage of adjustment to the loss.

DEFINITION

The initial phase of rehabilitation begins during the initial hospitalization. Later phases of rehabilitation usually occur in an outpatient setting. As a result of the typically shorter inpatient stay, many initial phase treatment goals are addressed as an outpatient.

Fitting a patient within 1 month of trauma with a UE prosthesis (even a temporary device) increases acceptance of the prosthesis.[1,2]

SURGICAL PURPOSE

To remove useless or nonviable extremity parts that have been severely damaged by disease or trauma. Amputations are commonly performed for life-threatening infections, irreversible vascular compromise, tissue damage beyond hope of repair, and advanced loss of function so that the extremity becomes a biologic parasite for the patient (Fig. 28-1). Rarely, chronic pain is a reason for amputation. The level of amputation is important and must be determined by the surgeon. The more length that can be safely preserved, the better the prognosis for efficient and compliant prosthetic wear and use.

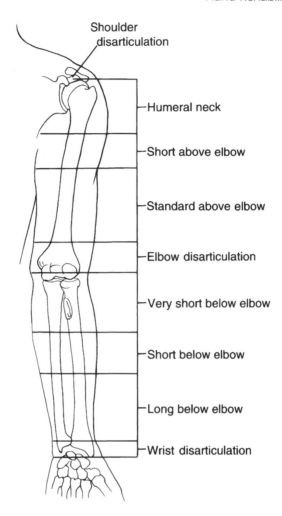

Fig. 28-1. Upper extremity amputations are performed for useless or nonviable parts severely damaged by disease or trauma.

TREATMENT PURPOSE

    I. Promote early mobilization.
   II. Promote proper shaping of the residual stump.
  III. Maximize independence in activities of daily living (ADL).
  IV. Provide orientation to the next rehabilitation phase (i.e., initial phase rehabilitation should orient the patient to follow-up with outpatient treatment).
   V. Introduce options with regard to UE prosthesis, if indicated.

TREATMENT GOALS

I. Promote wound healing.
II. Reduce edema of residual stump.
III. Control or reduce incisional and phantom pain.
IV. Maintain or increase active range of motion (AROM) and passive range of motion (PROM).
V. Promote ADL independence.
VI. Explore patient's and family's feelings about loss of limb.
VII. Explore resources for continuation of preprosthetic training, prosthetic training, and other necessary services.

POSTOPERATIVE INDICATIONS/ PRECAUTIONS FOR THERAPY

I. Indications: any patient with an amputation, complete or partial, who is otherwise medically stable and able to participate in ADL and exercise programs.
II. Precautions
   A. Unstable medical status.
   B. Others as noted by physician.

POSTOPERATIVE THERAPY

I. Evaluation
   A. Database should include age, sex, hand dominance, occupation, avocations, date of injury, date of surgery, level of amputation, mechanism of injury, current medical status, past medical history.
   B. Note skin condition at site of amputation. Note other structures (e.g., tendon or bone) that may have suffered trauma in both upper extremities.
   C. Presence of edema, girth measurements.
   D. Range of motion (ROM) of residual joints and of sound UE. Pay special attention to shoulder girdle and radioulnar joints. In a below elbow amputation, maximizing supination and pronation is an important goal.
   E. Muscle strength of residual musculature and of sound UE. Adhere to precautions with respect to orthopedic condition and other soft tissue injuries.
   F. Presence and quality or description of pain.
   G. Sensibility and hypersensitivity at stump.
   H. ADL status.
   I. Posture and balance.
   J. Note need for additional support from a social worker or psychologist.

II. Treatment plan
   A. Wound care as prescribed by physician. Adhere to special precautions (e.g., skin graft).
   B. Edema control: consider use of compression pump, elevation, and stump wrapping as condition of vascular system and soft tissues allows.
   C. Splinting as necessary for protecting any repaired structures or for decreasing limitations in ROM.
   D. Active, active assistive, or passive range of motion exercise program as indicated, paying special attention to shoulder girdle and radioulnar joints.
   E. Consider transcutaneous electric nerve stimulator (TENS) for pain control.
   F. Desensitization program as condition of wounds allows; include deep pressure when tolerated.
   G. ADL training should include compensatory techniques and adaptive equipment. Consider use of temporary pylon to aid in ADL independence.
   H. Postural exercises, if indicated.
   I. Initiate appropriate intervention from a social worker, psychologist, or psychiatrist.
III. Discharge planning evaluation from inpatient unit
   A. Identify initial problems and any additional problems.
   B. Note progress or lack of progress; include explanation for lack of progress (e.g., complications).
   C. Potential for additional rehabilitation.
   D. Follow-up plan
      1. Location and date of initial visit for further outpatient rehabilitation.
      2. Follow-up with primary surgeon.
      3. Social work, psychologist, or psychiatrist follow-up as indicated.
      4. Follow-up via amputee clinic or physician for prosthetic prescription and other necessary services.

POSTOPERATIVE COMPLICATIONS

   I. Infection
   II. Delayed healing.
   III. Decreased ROM due to immobilization period.
   IV. Neuroma and other scar adherence problems.

EVALUATION TIMELINE

   I. Initial assessment when medically stable.
   II. Re-evaluation every week thereafter during initial phase of rehabilitation.
   III. In late phases or rehabilitation, re-evaluate at least monthly.

REFERENCES

1. Malone J, Fleming L, Roberson J et al: Immediate, early and late postsurgical management of upper-limb amputation. J Rehabil Res Dev 21:33, 1984
2. Fletchall S, Hickerson W: Early upper extermity prosthetic fit in patients with burns. J Burn Care Rehabil 12:234, 1991

SUGGESTED READINGS

Atkins D, Meir III R: Comprehensive Management of the Upper Extremity Amputee. Springer-Verlag, New York, 1989

Helpa M: The Union Memorial Hospital Lower Extremity Amputee Program, Baltimore, 1990

Olivett B: Adult amputee management and conventional prosthetic training. p. 1057. In Hunter J, Schneider L, Mackin E: Rehabilitation of the Hand: Surgery and Therapy, 3rd Ed. Mosby, St. Louis, 1990

Pinzur MS, Angelats J, Light TR et al: Functional outcome following traumatic upper limb amputation and prosthetic limb fitting. J Hand Surg 19A:836, 1994

Upper Limb Prosthetics. 2nd Rev. New York University Post-Graduate Medical School, New York, 1986

Proximal Humeral Fractures

29

Mary Schuler Murphy

Proximal humeral fractures are the most common of all humeral fractures (approximately 45 percent[1-4]) and account for approximately 4 to 5 percent of all fractures.[1,2,5] In 80 percent of all proximal humeral fractures, there is no significant displacement of the fracture, and these can be treated nonsurgically.[1,2,5] The most common mechanism of injury is falling onto outstretched hands from standing height or lower.[1-4,6] Osteoporosis is a major contributing factor in proximal humeral fractures in adults over 40 years old.[1,2] The incidence of proximal humeral fractures after age 40 increases 76 percent, with a 2:1 ratio of women to men.[1-4] Proximal humeral fractures in younger age groups are usually secondary to high velocity injury and typically do not fall into the category of minimally displaced fractures.[1,2] For the purpose of this chapter, a therapeutic treatment protocol has been designed for the treatment of minimally displaced fractures and those fractures stabilized by surgery, permitting early rehabilitation.

Rehabilitation should be initiated early for instruction in control of distal edema and stiffness, as well as increasing mobility of the stabilized fractured shoulder. Bertoft et al.[7] suggest that the greatest improvement in shoulder ROM after proximal humerus fracture occurs in the initial 3 to 8 weeks. Movement of the fractured shoulder depends on the individual's rate of healing and the stability of the fracture. Clinical unity and clinical union play a paramount role in the physician's decision as to how quickly to move the patient through the rehabilitation program.

Clinical unity occurs when the fracture fragments move in unison. This typically occurs in 1 to 4 weeks and is tested by having the patient stand with the affected arm at their side with the elbow flexed. While the physician places one hand on the humeral head, the humerus is gently rotated by the physician's other hand. When the fracture fragments move in unison, clinical unity has been reached. This may be achieved immediately when internal fixation stabilizes the fracture site.[8] When the physician determines clinical unity, the therapy program outlined, initiating movement of the shoulder, can begin.

Clinical union is evidence of cancellous healing as seen radiographically. This can occur as early as 6 weeks.[6] Once clinical union is reached, more aggressive movement can be performed safely.

Close communication with the patient's physician will provide the therapist with the necessary information to advance the patient's program.

DEFINITION

The proximal humerus comprises the humeral head, lesser and greater tuberosities, bicipital groove, and proximal shaft. Proximal humeral fractures may occur between one or all of the four major segments. The anatomic neck of the humerus is at the junction of the humeral head and the tuberosities. With anatomical neck fractures, the blood supply to the humeral head is disrupted, increasing the chance of avascular necrosis. The surgical neck of the humerus is below the tuberosities. Fractures here are more common and have a better prognosis (Fig. 29-1). Types of humeral fractures vary greatly, complicating medical management. Proximal humeral fractures are frequently described by using Neers' four segment classification system.[3] The system provides a guideline for diagnosis and treatment. This system is based on the number of displaced segments and the amount of their displacement and not the number of fracture lines. A one-part fracture has no segments displaced more than 1 cm or angulation greater than 45 degrees. These fractures are typically treated conservatively with a sling. In a two-part fragment, one segment is displaced in relationship to the other three. Depending on the type of two-part fracture, treatment may include either an open or closed reduction. In a three-part fracture, two segments are displaced in relationship to the other segments that are in opposition and in a four-part fracture, all four segments are displaced (Fig. 29-2). In general, three-part fractures are

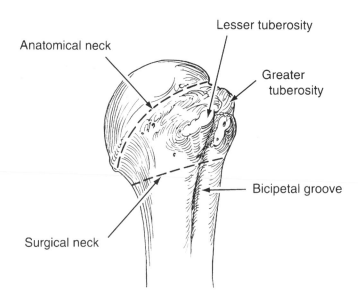

Fig. 29-1. Anatomy of proximal humerus.

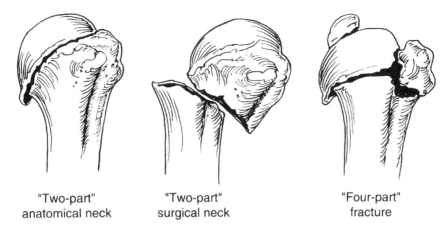

"Two-part"   "Two-part"   "Four-part"
anatomical neck   surgical neck   fracture

Fig. 29-2. Displaced humeral fractures.

treated with open reduction and internal fixation. Humeral head prosthesis is frequently the treatment of choice for four-part fractures.

Another classification system, devised by the American Orthopedic group, emphasizes the vascular supply to the articular segments. In a type A fracture, the articular segment is not isolated from its vascular supply. The type B fracture is partially isolated and a type C fracture is totally separated from its blood supply. Decrease in vascular supply to the articular surface directly correlates with fracture prognosis secondary to the increased possibility of avascular necrosis.[1]

SURGICAL PURPOSE

Fractures of the proximal humerus have varying degrees of severity. Those that have a sufficient degree of displacement or comminution may require open reduction and internal fixation (ORIF). The surgical purpose is to restore joint integrity for optimum function following fracture healing. Ideally, fixation of the bone fragments will be constructed with sufficient strength to allow shoulder joint motion during the bone healing phase. In a small percentage of cases, a humeral head prosthesis may be inserted when the humeral head displacement is severe or the vascular integrity of the joint surface is deemed irreparably damaged. Shoulder joint congruity and availability of early motion are the goals.

TREATMENT GOALS

I. Promote maximal painfree shoulder range of motion (ROM) and function.

II. Promote normal distal ROM and function.

NONOPERATIVE INDICATIONS/ PRECAUTIONS FOR THERAPY

I. Indications
   A. Nondisplaced/minimally displaced humeral fractures that are stable.
II. Precautions
   A. Greater tuberosity fractures require special consideration secondary to the attachment of the rotator cuff muscles and the potential for displacement of the greater tuberosity fragment. Other considerations with a greater tuberosity fracture is the possibility of a rotator cuff tear, as well as the potential for impingement of the greater tuberosity against the acromion and posterior glenoid.
   B. Associated soft tissue injury (i.e., ligaments, tendons).

NONOPERATIVE THERAPY

I. Day 1
   A. Use of sling for proximal stabilization.
   B. Decrease shoulder pain through the use of modalities.
   C. Wrist and hand ROM exercise and edema reduction techniques.
II. Day 3 to 7
   A. Initiate weaning from sling: when sitting support arm on pillow on a supporting surface.
   B. Initiate pendulum exercises.
   C. Incorporate elbow and forearm ROM into distal ROM exercises and continue edema control.
III. Day 7 to 3 weeks
   A. Passive range of motion (PROM), active assistive range of motion (AAROM) in supine; assisted elevation in the frontal plane and the plane of the scapula and external rotation.
   B. Initiate pulleys for forward elevation.
   C. Progression from gravity eliminated position to PROM, AAROM while sitting with arm supported on a tabletop (Fig. 29-3).
   D. Sling discontinued.
IV. 3 1/2 weeks: PROM, AAROM in extension and internal rotation
V. 3 to 4 weeks: isometric strengthening
VI. 4 to 6 weeks
   A. Initiate place and hold active range of motion (AROM) in supine.
   B. Progress to tabletop activities with the arm supported on a table while performing active reaching activities (placing pegs in a pegboard, dusting) (Fig. 29-4).
VII. 6 to 8 weeks
   A. Initiate light functional strengthening activities (e.g., copper tooling on an incline board, sanding, etc.).
   B. Continue with PROM, AAROM exercises to increase shoulder mobility/function.

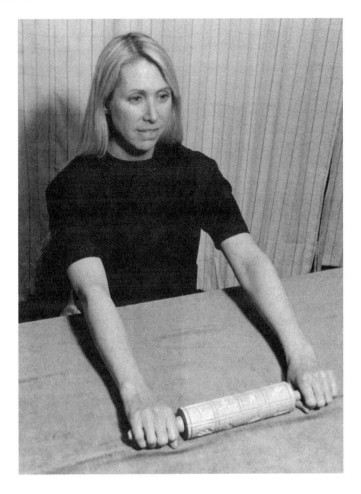

Fig. 29-3. Tabletop activity provides support during exercise.

    C. Initiate Baltimore Therapeutic Equipment (BTE) Work Simulator and use of theraband.
VIII. 8 to 12 weeks
    A. Continue with stretching ROM exercises to regain end ROM.
    B. Continue and progress strengthening exercise; initiate use of free weights (start with 1 lb weight and progress to maximum of 5 lbs).

NONOPERATIVE COMPLICATIONS

    I. Stiff and painful shoulder
   II. Distal edema and stiffness
  III. Delayed union
  IV. Nonunion
   V. Degenerative arthritis
  VI. Frozen shoulder

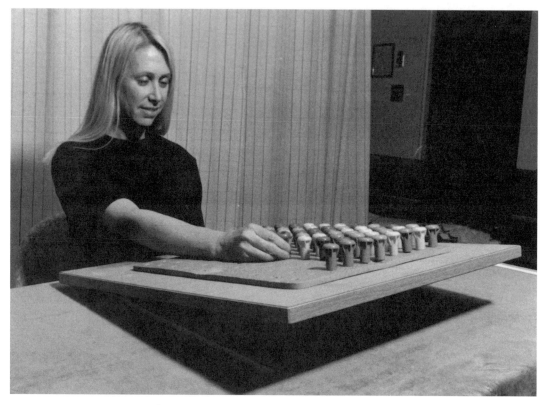

Fig. 29-4. Active reaching exercises on tabletop.

VII.   Avascular necrosis
VIII. Myositis ossificans
IX.   Neurovascular injuries
X.   Reflex sympathetic dystrophy (RSD)

POSTOPERATIVE INDICATIONS/ PRECAUTIONS FOR THERAPY

I. Indications: Humeral fractures stabilized through surgical reduction.
II. Precautions
   A. Infection
   B. Associated soft tissue injuries and/or repairs.

POSTOPERATIVE THERAPY

The progression of postsurgical repairs (i.e., internal fixation, open reduction internal fixation [ORIF]) of proximal humeral fractures follow the same treatment guidelines as nonoperative treatment but may progress at a faster rate secondary to the stabilization of the fracture provided by the surgery. An example of this would be the tension band wiring supplemented by lag-screw fixation used in two- and three-part fractures as reported by Cornell. He advocates early aggressive therapy with PROM initiated on day 1 and AROM and strengthening after the fourth postoperative week.[8] Hawkins et al.[9] also describe early AAROM 5 to 7 days postfixation of a three-part fracture with the wire band principle. On the contrary, poor fracture stabilization may delay the progression of treatment. If significant pain or crepitation accompanies early motion, they describe delaying ROM 3 to 4 weeks.[9] Secondary to the soft osteogenic bone found frequently in patients with osteoporosis, many ORIFs may be minimally stable. In such cases, patients are frequently treated cautiously with a delayed rehabilitation program. Significant injury and repair of the rotator cuff may also delay the progression of therapy. Communication with the surgeon is of paramount importance. Thus the therapist must consult with the surgeon about fracture stabilization and any soft tissue repairs before proceeding with the rehabilitation program.

POSTOPERATIVE COMPLICATIONS/ CONSIDERATIONS

   I. Infection
  II. Hardware failure
 III. Failure to stabilize the fracture
 IV. Soft tissue repairs
  V. All nonoperative complications

EVALUATION TIMELINE

   I. Nonoperative
    A. Day 1
      1. Wrist and hand ROM (active and passive)
      2. Distal edema
      3. Sensory screening
      4. Pain assessment
      5. Activity of daily living assessment
    B. Day 3 to 7: Elbow and forearm ROM (active and passive).
    C. Week 1: Passive shoulder flexion and external rotation.
    D. Week 3: Passive shoulder extension and internal rotation.
    E. Week 4 to 6: Active shoulder ROM and distal grasp and pinch strength.
    F. Week 12: Proximal strength.
  II. Operative as per above but will vary according to the type of surgical procedure (e.g., soft tissue repair) performed.

REFERENCES

1. Bigliani LU, Craig EV, Butters KP: Fractures of the proximal humerus. p. 871. In Rockwood CA Jr, Green DP (ed): Fractures in Adults. 3rd Ed. Vol. I. Lippincott-Raven, Philadelphia, 1990
2. Bigliani LU: Fractures of the proximal humerus. p. 278. In Rockwood CA, Matsen FA (eds): The Shoulder. Vol. 1. W.B. Saunders, Philadelphia, 1990
3. Basti JJ, Dionysian E, Sherman PW, Bigliani LU: Management of proximal humeral fractures. J Hand Ther 7:111, 1994
4. Basti JJ, Dionysian E, Sherman PW, Bigliani LU: Management of proximal humeral fractures and fracture dislocations. J Bone Joint Surg 72B:1050, 1990
5. Neer CS: Fractures. p. 363. In Neer CS (ed): Shoulder Reconstruction. W.B. Saunders, Philadelphia, 1990
6. Loder RT, Mayhew HE: Common fractures from a fall on an outstretched hand. Am Fam Physician 37:327, 1988
7. Bertoft ES, Lundh I, Ringqvist I: Physiotherapy after fracture of the proximal end of the humerus: comparison between two methods. Scand J Rehabil Med 16:11, 1984
8. Cornell CN: Tension-band wiring supplemented by lag-screw fixation of proximal humerus fractures: a modified technique. Orthop Rev Aspects of Trauma, May, Suppl:19–23, 1994
9. Hawkins RJ, Angelo RL: Displaced proximal humeral fractures. Orthop Clin North Am 18:421, 1987

SUGGESTED READINGS

DeLee JC, Drez D: Orthopaedic Sports Medicine: Principles and Practice. Vol. I. W.B. Saunders, Philadelphia, 1994

Kristiansen B, Kofoed H: Transcutaneous reduction and external fixation of displaced fractures of the proximal humerus, a controlled clinical trial. J Bone Joint Surg 70B:821, 1988

Moda SK, Chadia NS, Sangwan SS et al: Open reduction and fixation of proximal humeral fractures and fracture dislocation. J Bone Joint Surg 72B:1050, 1990

Young TB, Wallace WA: Conservative treatment of fractures and fracture-dislocations of the upper end of the humerus. J Bone Joint Surg 67B:373, 1985

Zych GA: Complex upper-extremity fractures. Instructional Course Lectures 39:259–63, 1990

Shoulder Arthroplasty **30**

Anne Edmonds

Shoulder arthroplasty is used to provide a painless range of motion (ROM) by replacing or resurfacing the articulating surface of the humeral head and the glenoid. Patients who present with a history of rheumatoid arthritis, osteoarthritis, avascular necrosis, sickle cell infarction, irradiation necrosis, ochronosis, and gout may benefit from this procedure[1] (Fig. 30-1).

Hemiarthroplasty is used for severely displaced and comminuted humeral fractures or dislocations with an interrupted vascular supply.

With a properly supervised rehabilitation program, following either of these procedures, patients can obtain a functional outcome.

DEFINITION

I. *Total shoulder arthroplasty* (TSA): replacement of the humeral head and the glenoid articulating surface with components made of polyethylene or titanium.
   A. Three types of replacement components are used:
      1. Unconstrained: humeral component that articulates with a scapular component. If musculotendinous units are intact or able to be reconstructed, this implant has the potential for good results.[2] This is the most widely used component (Figs. 30-2 and 30-3).
      2. Constrained: designed for patients who have severe deterioration without a reconstructible rotator cuff but with a functioning deltoid muscle.[1] The glenoid and humeral components are coupled and fixed to bone. The forces acting across the point of coupling cause increasing rates of breakage and loosening.[3]

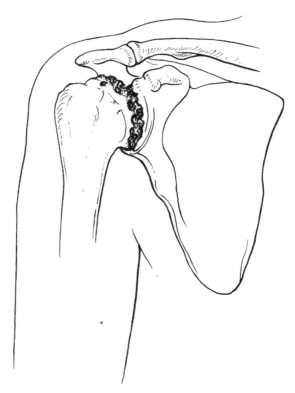

Fig. 30-1. Arthritis of a glenohumeral joint of a shoulder.

Arthritic shoulder joint

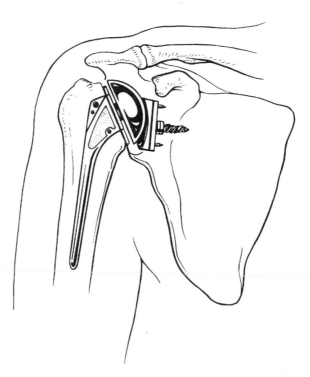

Fig. 30-2. Unconstrained prosthesis of a shoulder.

Shoulder replacement

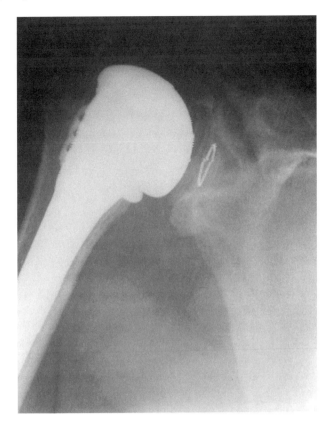

Fig. 30-3. X-ray of unconstrained shoulder prosthesis.

3. Semiconstrained: monospherical. The humeral head is smaller and spherical with a head–neck angle of 60 degrees and reportedly permits increased ROM. The glenoid component is matched to the humeral head prosthesis to allow constant surface contact.[1]

II. *Hemiarthroplasty*: replacement of the humeral head with a stemmed intramedullary implant that articulates with the glenoid, acromion, and distal clavicle[2] (Figs. 30-4 and 30-5).

SURGICAL PURPOSE

To remove painful, irregular, and deformed glenohumeral joint surfaces and replace them with metal or plastic. Restoration approximating normal skeletal alignment and joint stability with an effective pain-free ROM is derived.

The hemishoulder arthroplasty is used to replace a humeral head damaged from a fracture, an avascular necrosis of known or unknown cause, or destructive tumor. These conditions do not involve the glenoid fossa. Hemiarthroplasty does not disturb the glenoid and is a lesser procedure. It

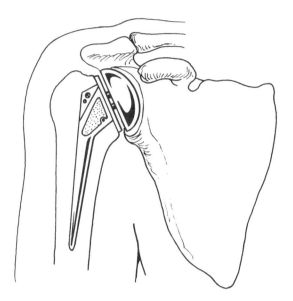

Fig. 30-4. Hemiarthroplasty prosthesis.

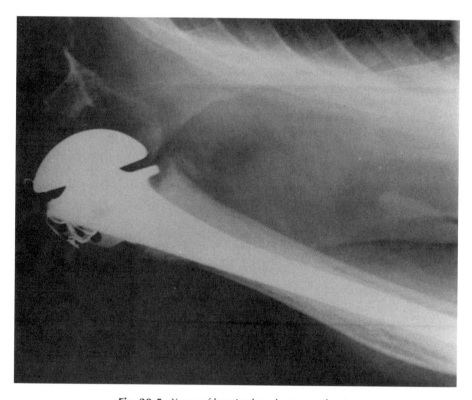

Fig. 30-5. X-ray of hemiarthroplasty prosthesis.

reduces postoperative wound complications, and there are fewer risks of joint component failure compared with a total replacement. This facilitates rehabilitation and improved potential for good shoulder function.

TREATMENT GOALS FOR TOTAL SHOULDER ARTHROPLASTY

I. To concentrate on the rehabilitation of the soft tissues encompassing the implant and to be aware of and monitor the reconstructed structures.
II. To restore maximum pain-free ROM
III. To increase function
IV. To maximize strength

POSTOPERATIVE INDICATIONS/ PRECAUTIONS FOR THERAPY FOR TOTAL SHOULDER ARTHROPLASTY

I. Indications
   A. Decreased ROM and function
   B. Decreased strength
II. Precautions
   A. Infection
   B. Integrity of muscle tissue surrounding the implant
   C. Stability of the implant

POSTOPERATIVE THERAPY FOR TOTAL SHOULDER ARTHROPLASTY

I. Unconstrained prosthesis
   A. ROM
      1. Phase I: 0 to 8 days
         a. Local heat and passive range of motion (PROM) or active assistive range of motion (AAROM) exercises within first 2 days: assess PROM.
         b. Pendulum exercises with the body in a forward flexed position. Forearm pronated and then supinated while doing circular motion.
         c. External rotation and flexion initiated while in supine. Support is given by towels or pillow under humerus.
         d. Assisted overhead pulley.
         e. Assisted abduction.[4]

2. Phase II
   a. 8 to 10 days: exercises initiated in standing position.
   b. 10 to 14 days: internal rotation exercises begun. Assess PROM/AAROM.
   c. Continue external rotation exercises in standing position until 40 to 60 degrees is obtained.[4]
   d. 17 to 21 days: isometric exercises begin with elbow flexed to 90 degrees and held close to body. Opposite hand, wall or door jamb provides resistance.
3. Phase III
   a. 3 to 6 weeks: assisted shoulder elevation to obtain last 20 degrees of motion.[4] Assess active ROM (AROM) and PROM.
   b. Assisted external rotation in standing position leaning against wall and stretching axilla.
   c. Assisted internal rotation: standing with arm behind back with hand resting supine on table.
B. Strengthening
   1. Phase I: 6 to 8 weeks: assess strength-gross manual muscle testing (MMT) upper arm
      a. Exercises done supine without gravity.
      b. Primarily supraspinatus and anterior deltoid.
   2. Phase II: 8 to 10 weeks
      a. Targets deltoid and rotator cuff.
      b. Exercises performed against gravity in standing or sitting position.
   3. Phase III: 10 to 12 weeks
      a. Isolates anterior, middle, and posterior deltoid and individual rotator cuff muscles.
      b. Theraband used for resistance.[4]

POSTOPERATIVE COMPLICATIONS FOR TOTAL SHOULDER ARTHROPLASTY

I. Infection
II. Nerve palsy
III. Subluxation/dislocation
IV. Intraoperative fracture
V. Pulmonary embolus
VI. Pneumonia[3]

TREATMENT GOALS FOR HEMIARTHROPLASTY

I. To achieve full PROM gradually rather than quickly.
II. To increase function.
III. To regain strength.

POSTOPERATIVE INDICATIONS/
PRECAUTIONS FOR THERAPY FOR
HEMIARTHROPLASTY

I. Indications
  A. Decreased ROM and function.
  B. Decreased strength.
II. Precautions
  A. Stability of implant.
  B. Strength of repaired tendons and soft tissue to avoid anterior instability.
  C. Infection.

POSTOPERATIVE THERAPY FOR
HEMIARTHROPLASTY

I. Phase I
  A. 1 to 7 days: Codman exercises, passive flexion within pain-free range.
  B. Day 3: passive external rotation to limits defined at surgery.[5]
  C. Overhead pulleys and wooden dowel passively.
  D. 1 week: isometrics begin if good tuberosity fixation at surgery.[5]
II. Phase II
  A. 2 to 3 weeks: gentle active assistive exercises.
  B. 4 to 6 weeks: more aggressive passive stretching; AROM to begin.
  C. 6 weeks: resistive exercises with rubber tubing.
  D. 2 months: should achieve 90 degree active forward flexion.[5]
III. Phase III
  A. 4 months: increased resistance using light hand weights.
  B. Strengthening to continue 1 year or more with improvements.

POSTOPERATIVE COMPLICATIONS FOR
HEMIARTHROPLASTY

I. Improper positioning of tuberosities, which could cause impingement, anterior or posterior subluxation.
II. Detachment of subscapularis tendon causing anterior instability.[5]
III. Disassociation of humeral head component.

EVALUATION TIMELINE FOR TOTAL
SHOULDER ARTHROPLASTY

I. Stretching
  A. 0 to 8 days: assess PROM and active assistive ROM while supine.
  B. 10 to 14 days: assess AROM against gravity.
  C. 3 to 6 weeks: assess AROM.
II. Strengthening

A. 6 to 8 weeks: gross MMT upper extremity.

B. 8 to 10 weeks: MMT.

C. 10 to 12 weeks: MMT.

EVALUATION TIMELINE FOR HEMIARTHROPLASTY

I. 1 day to 1 week: PROM assessment and initiation of exercises; supine progressing to sitting or standing.

II. 2 to 3 weeks: AAROM exercises against gravity.

III. 4 to 6 weeks

A. MMT upper extremity.

B. AROM exercises.

IV. 6 weeks: continue exercises; resistance initiated.

V. 8 to 10 weeks: AROM evaluation: MMT evaluation.

VI. 4 months to 1 year: continue strenthening with re-evaluation every 3 to 4 weeks.

REFERENCES

1. Sisk TD, Wright PE: Arthroplasty of shoulder and elbow. p. 1503. In Crenshaw AH (ed): Campbells Operative Orthopaedics. Vol. II, Mosby, St. Louis, 1987

2. Swanson AB, Cerdo RD, Hynes D et al: Bipolar implant shoulder arthroplasty long term results. Clin Orthop 249:227, 1989

3. Johnson RL: Total shoulder arthroplasty. Orthop Nurs 12:1, 1993

4. Brems JJ: Rehabilitation following total shoulder arthroplasty. Clin Orthop 307:70, 1994

5. Dines DM, Warren RF: Modular shoulder hemiarthroplasty for acute fractures. Clin Orthop 307:18, 1994

SUGGESTED READINGS

Clayton ML, Ferlic DC, Jeffers PD: Prosthetic arthroplasties of the shoulder. Clin Orthop 164:184, 1982

Neer CS, Kirby RM: Revision of humeral head and total shoulder arthroplasties. Clin Orthop 170:189, 1982

Neer CS, Watson KL, Stanton FJ: Recent experience in total shoulder replacement. J Bone Joint Surg 64A:319, 1982

Weiland A, Weiss AP, Adams M, Moore R: Unconstrained shoulder arthroplasty: a five year average follow-up study. Clin Orthop 257:86, 1990

Elbow Fractures and Dislocations **31**

Jane Imle Schmidt

The elbow joint provides an essential link to the forearm, wrist, and hand, which allows the hand to be moved into position for activities of daily living (ADLs), as well as transmit heavy loads.[1] The elbow joint allows the motions of flexion, extension, and forearm rotation. Injury to this joint complex can lead to loss of these motions and subsequent loss of upper extremity function.[2] The elbow joint has three articulations. The ulnohumeral joint resembles a hinge joint and allows flexion and extension, and the radiohumeral and proximal radioulnar joint (trochoid joint) allow forearm rotation.[3] Normal range of motion (ROM) into flexion is 140 degrees and into extension is 0 degrees, with 75 degrees of supination and 70 degrees of pronation available. Most ADLs can be performed with a ROM from 30 to 130 degrees of flexion, and 50 degrees each of pronation and supination[4] (Fig. 31-1).

Post-traumatic stiffness is a common result after both operative and nonoperative treatment to fractures and dislocations of the elbow.[5] Soft tissue structures including the medial and lateral collateral ligaments, the flexor pronator muscle groups, the extensor supinator muscle groups, and the brachialis are all subject to damage in these injuries. The brachial artery, as well as the median, radial, and ulnar nerve, are also vulnerable in elbow fractures and dislocations.[6] To restore functional ROM through rehabilitation, good communication is required between the physician and therapist. The therapist must know which structures were injured, how they were reduced or repaired, and how stable the reduction or fixation is in order to be able to treat safely and effectively elbow fractures and dislocations. To prevent the adverse effects of immobilization, early active motion to noninjured areas and early protective exercise for injured areas are advocated as soon as the inflammatory process allows.[7]

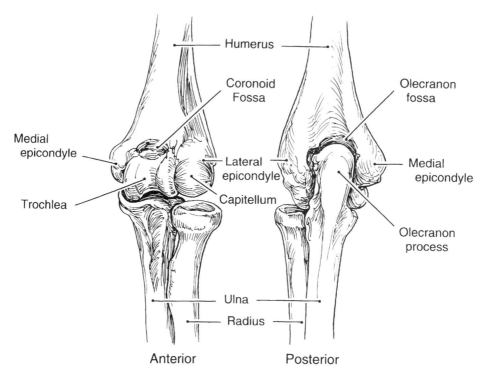

Fig. 31-1. Normal elbow anatomy (left).

DEFINITION

I. Fractures of the distal humerus: One-third of all elbow fractures involve the distal humerus. The mechanism of injury is a fall on an outstretched hand or a direct blow in the case of the epicondylar fracture. Distal humeral fractures may be classified as extra-articular: supracondylar, transcondylar or epicondylar, or intra-articular: T and Y condylar, lateral condylar, medial condylar or articular (capitellum, trochlea). Depending on their severity, these fractures are treated by closed manipulation or surgical stabilization.[8] Those fractures extending into the joint generally involve open reduction and internal fixation[12] (Fig. 31-2).

II. Fractures of the proximal ulna and olecranon: These fractures account for one-fifth of all elbow injuries in adults and generally occur indirectly in a fall on the outstretched hand with the elbow in some flexion, or via a direct blow to the olecranon.[9] These fractures are classified as undisplaced, displaced, transverse or oblique, or comminuted. Undisplaced fractures are managed with short immobilization while the other types require surgical intervention[10] (Fig. 31-2).

III. Fractures of the proximal radius: These fractures of the radial head and neck account for nearly half of all fractures about the elbow in

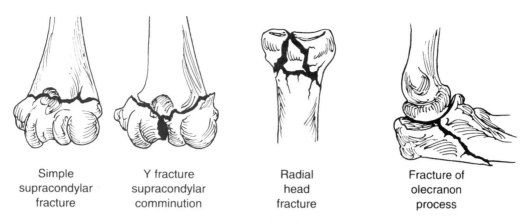

| Simple supracondylar fracture | Y fracture supracondylar comminution | Radial head fracture | Fracture of olecranon process |

Fig. 31-2. Elbow fractures.

the adult.[9] These fractures occur when there is an axial load placed when the forearm is in pronation, as in a fall on an outstretched hand. They may be classified as undisplaced, displaced, and comminuted. Undisplaced fractures are treated with early active motion. Displaced fractures may be treated nonoperatively, or they may require operative treatment including excision of the fracture or entire radial head, or open reduction with internal fixation. Comminuted fractures of the radial head that are not accompanied by other instabilities are generally treated by complete excision[11] (Fig. 31-2).

IV. Dislocations of the radius and/or ulna: The elbow joint is the second most commonly dislocated joint in the body.[12,13] The mechanism of this injury is a fall on an outstretched hand.[3,13–15] The most common pattern of elbow instability is posterolateral rotatory instability and this instability varies in degree of displacement from subluxation to full dislocation with the coronoid resting behind the humerus.[15] Reduction of these injuries is typically closed unless they have been neglected or fail with closed manipulation, thus requiring open reduction.[12] Frequently these dislocations are accompanied by a shear fracture of the coronoid.[15]

V. Fractures associated with dislocations: *Monteggia lesions* include all ulnar fractures associated with dislocations of the radiocapitellar articulation. They are divided into four types, with type I (anterior angulation and anterior dislocation of the radial head) being the most common and only type discussed here.[16] These lesions are relatively uncommon, but can present with serious problems. The mechanism of injury may be a direct blow to the ulnar aspect of the forearm or a fall with hyperpronation or hyperextension.[10] Closed methods may be used to treat children, but open reduction with internal fixation of the ulna and either closed or open reduction of the radial head is required in adults.[10,17] The *Essex-Lopresti* fracture includes a fracture of the radial head and instability of the distal radioulnar joint (DRUJ), in combination with a partial or complete disruption of the inter-osseous membrane. In this injury the brachialis muscle can be torn from its insertion and the brachial artery and the median nerve can also be damaged. The mechanism of injury is a forceful fall onto an outstretched hand and surgical management is required.[18] A *sideswipe fracture* occurs when the elbow is protruding from a car window and is struck by an oncoming car or a fixed object. Many different combinations of fractures and soft tissue injuries may be produced, but the most common is an open fracture of the olecra-non, anterior dislocation of the head of the radius and the distal fragment of the ulna, and a comminuted fracture of the humerus.

SURGICAL PURPOSE

Fractures and dislocations that interrupt the normal elbow anatomy may interfere with effective joint motion and have the potential to cause pain. This joint is complex and not only allows for flexion and extension, but also forearm pronation and supination through the radial head capitellar articulation. Unless normal anatomic relationships are restored after injury, severe limitations of elbow movement will occur. This will impair an individual's ability to carry out ADLs as well as to hold productive jobs in the workforce.

TREATMENT GOALS

I. Nonoperative
   A. Control edema.
   B. Maintain ROM of uninvolved joints.
   C. Initiate early protective exercise for the injured joints.
   D. Avoidance of positions of instability.
   E. Return to previous level of function.
II. Operative
   A. Control edema.
   B. Promote wound healing.
   C. Control scar formation.
   D. Maintain ROM of uninvolved joints.
   E. Initiate early protective exercise for the injured joints.
   F. Avoidance of positions of instability.
   G. Return to previous level of function.

NONOPERATIVE INDICATIONS/ PRECAUTIONS FOR THERAPY

I. Indications
   Elbow fractures and/or dislocations that have achieved stability through closed techniques.

II. Precautions
  A. Associated muscle and/or ligamentous injury.
  B. Associated nerve or blood vessel injury.
  C. Unresolved hematoma and/or edema.
  D. Unstable reduction or history of recurrent dislocations.

NONOPERATIVE THERAPY

Vigorous stretching, whether active or passive, is never permitted in the rehabilitation of elbow fractures and dislocations. These techniques can result in increased periarticular hemorrhage and fibrosis, causing decreased ROM, and can lead to complications of myositis ossificans and the formation of heterotopic bone.[7,17] Communication with the surgeon is necessary to determine when fractures are stable enough to withstand active motion and what ranges of motion are the "safe zone" (the range of motion that creates no displacement of the fracture or subluxation). Continuous passive motion (CPM) machines and hinged elbow splints (commercial and custom fabricated) allow protected motion while preventing medial and lateral instability. These devices can be valuable adjuncts to a therapy program. Timelines for strengthening need to be determined by the physician based on radiographic union.

  I. Therapy following distal humeral fractures treated with closed manipulation
    A. Extra-articular supracondylar and transcondylar fractures are immobilized in a posterior splint with the elbow flexed to approximately 90 degrees and the forearm neutral for a period of 2 to 6 weeks depending on the stability of the fracture. Gentle active motion into flexion can be started at 2 to 3 weeks with a gradual increase into extension. Strengthening can begin when cleared by the physician.
    B. Medial epicondylar fractures are immobilized in a posterior splint with the elbow flexed to 90 degrees, the forearm in pronation, and the wrist in slight flexion to relax the flexor pronator muscle group. These fractures are immobilized for 1 to 2 weeks followed by gentle active motion, progressing to strengthening activities as directed by the physician.
    C. Lateral epicondylar fractures are rare in the adult, and treatment consists of immobilization of the elbow in 90 degrees of flexion, the forearm in supination and the wrist extended to relax the muscles that originate from the fracture surface. Immobilization is for 1 to 2 weeks followed by gentle active motion.
    D. Intra-articular T and Y condylar fractures are treated by 3 weeks of immobilization with the elbow in 90 degrees of flexion followed by splinting with intermittent gentle active mobilization for another 2 to 3 weeks, progressing to strengthening activities as directed by the physician. Displaced fractures of these types require surgical intervention, and their postoperative therapy is described below. In the elderly patient, who is not a candidate

for surgical intervention with a severe comminution, the "bag-of-bones" technique may be used. This technique uses compressive manipulation of the distal articular fragments. The elbow is immobilized in as much flexion as possible without compromising circulation for 2 weeks with active motion into flexion starting at the end of this period. The hand and wrist are mobilized from the day of injury and the shoulder within 2 weeks. At 4 weeks, the elbow should have from 90 degrees to full flexion. The patient progresses to a sling, which is adjusted to allow more elbow extension as tolerated, with the sling being discontinued by 6 weeks.

E. Medial and lateral condylar fractures that are undisplaced are splinted or casted for 4 to 5 weeks with the elbow in flexion. These fractures may become displaced, resulting in limitations in motion and arthritis; therefore, communication is needed with the physician to proceed safely with rehabilitation.

F. Capitellar fractures with large fragments that are anteriorly displaced are treated with closed reduction and immobilization with the elbow in 90 degrees of flexion and the forearm supinated for approximately 3 weeks.

II. Therapy following fractures of the proximal ulna and olecranon.

A. Undisplaced fractures are immobilized in a posterior splint in midflexion and begin gentle ROM after 7 to 10 days. Full flexion is avoided for 4 to 6 weeks until bony union is complete. When union is evident, the patient may progress to gentle resistive activities.

III. Therapy following fractures of the proximal radius.

A. Undisplaced and minimally displaced radial head fractures are managed with immediate active range of motion (AROM) or are immobilized in flexion for a period of 2 to 3 weeks followed by AROM and progression to strengthening activities as directed by the physician. A loss of full elbow extension can be expected and displacement can sometimes occur with early motion.

IV. Therapy following dislocations of the radius and/or ulna.

A. These dislocations are immobilized in a posterior plaster splint in 90 degrees of elbow flexion and neutral forearm rotation. The circulatory and neurologic status is closely monitored during the first 24 hours for sign of ischemia and compartment syndrome. Motion in the uninvolved joints is begun the day after reduction and gentle active flexion from the splint may start the first week. The physician may be able to indicate a "safe zone" (ROM not producing subluxation) for AROM so that a thermoplastic splint blocking extension at the end of the "safe zone" can be fabricated. If no subluxation is evident with extension at week 3, unprotected flexion and extension exercises can be initiated, progressing to strengthening exercises, particularly of the triceps. At 10 to 12 weeks if an extension loss is still apparent, static progressive splinting may be initiated.

V. Therapy following fractures associated with dislocation (see Postoperative Therapy).

NONOPERATIVE COMPLICATIONS

  I. Loss of motion
  II. Nerve injury
  III. Malunion
  IV. Instability of the fracture and/or recurrent dislocation
  V. Vascular injuries and compartment syndrome
  VI. Myositis ossificans
  VII. Heterotopic ossification
  VIII. Nonunion
  IX. Residual pain
  X. Post-traumatic arthritis
  XI. Reflex sympathetic dystrophy

POSTOPERATIVE INDICATIONS/ PRECAUTIONS FOR THERAPY

  I. Indications
     Elbow fractures and/or dislocations that have achieved stability through surgical techniques.
  II. Precautions
     A. Associated muscle and/or ligamentous injury.
     B. Associated nerve or blood vessel injury.
     C. Unresolved hematoma and/or edema.
     D. Unstable reduction or history of recurrent dislocations.

POSTOPERATIVE THERAPY

Vigorous stretching, whether active or passive, is never permitted in the rehabilitation of elbow fractures and dislocations. These techniques can result in increased periarticular hemorrhage and fibrosis, causing decreased ROM, and can lead to complications of myositis ossificans and the formation of heterotopic bone.[7,17] Communication with the surgeon is necessary to determine when fractures are stable enough to withstand active motion and what ranges of motion are the "safe zone" (the range of motion that creates no displacement of the fracture or subluxation). CPM machines and hinged elbow splints (commercial and custom fabricated) allow protected motion while preventing medial and lateral instability. These devices can be valuable adjuncts to a therapy program (Fig. 31-3). Timelines for strengthening need to be determined by the physician based on radiographic union.

  I. Therapy following distal humeral fractures treated with surgical stabilization.
     A. Extra-articular supracondylar and transcondylar fractures that require limited open reduction or percutaneous pinning are immobilized in less elbow flexion than if closed methods are used. The ulnar nerve is sometimes transposed in these frac-

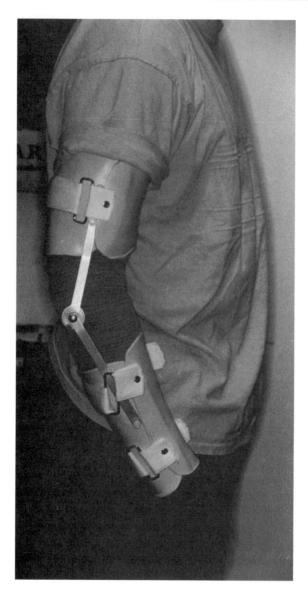

Fig. 31-3. Hinged elbow splint.

tures. Gentle AROM into flexion may begin at 2 to 3 weeks with a gradual increase into elbow extension. Some surgeons prefer earlier active motion or CPM when fixation is stable. Strengthening may begin when cleared by the surgeon.

B. Medial epicondylar fracture (see Nonoperative Therapy).

C. Lateral epicondylar fracture (see Nonoperative Therapy).

D. Intra-articular T and Y condylar fractures that require fixation with screws and Kirschner wires or full exposure with plating of the fracture are splinted in 45 to 90 degrees of elbow flexion postoperatively and are kept elevated. Those fractures requiring full exposure may involve osteotomy of the proximal ulna or release or reflection of the triceps and transposition of the ulnar nerve. Depending on bone quality and stability of the hardware as indicated by the surgeon, gentle AROM may begin in 3 to 5 days. The patient is encouraged to use the extremity in light ADLs with protective splinting continued between exercise sessions. Strengthening is begun at 6 weeks or at the time the fracture demonstrates healing on radiograph.

E. Medial and lateral condylar fractures stabilized with screws and/or Kirschner wires will begin AROM 5 to 10 days postoperatively, with the extremity splinted in flexion between exercise sessions for 3 to 5 weeks. If a medial condylar fracture requires plating, the ulnar nerve may have been transposed anteriorly; this possibility should be considered in the rehabilitation.

F. Capitellar fractures treated with either surgical excision or surgical reduction and secure fixation with either screws or threaded Kirschner wires may begin gentle AROM in 2 to 3 days progressing to strengthening as directed by the surgeon.

II. Therapy following fracture of the proximal ulna and olecranon.

A. These fractures that are fixated with Kirschner wires, intramedullary fixation, bicortical screws, plates or excision of the fracture fragments may begin gentle AROM between 3 to 7 days postoperatively. Extremes of motion, specifically flexion, are avoided during the first 4 weeks. The elbow may be supported in a protective splint in between exercise sessions during this time. Strengthening exercises may be started when the union is firm or at least 8 weeks postoperatively when excision has been performed.

III. Therapy after fracture of the proximal radius

A. Displaced radial head fractures may be treated with open reduction and internal fixation, or if the fragment cannot be fixed, surgical excision of the radial head is the treatment of choice. Postoperatively the patients are immobilized in 90 degrees of elbow flexion and neutral forearm rotation. Gentle AROM is begun at 5 to 10 days, and the patient may be moved from a splint to a sling. At 3 weeks the sling is removed. Strengthening may begin as directed by the physician.

IV. Therapy following dislocation of the radius and/or ulna (see Nonoperative Therapy).

V. Therapy following fractures associated with dislocations.

A. Monteggia fractures can be reduced surgically in a variety of ways: (1) internal fixation of the ulna with closed reduction of the radial head, (2) open reduction of the radial head and internal fixation of the ulna, and occasionally (3) internal fixation of the ulna with excision of the radial head. Radial neuropathy, particularly the posterior interosseous branch, is frequently seen in these fractures. Postoperatively these patients with type I fractures are immobilized in 90 to 120 degrees of elbow flexion with moderate forearm supination for 4 weeks. AROM is begun at 4 weeks, and gentle pronation and supination are permitted. The patient may need to be supported in a sling or protective splint between exercise sessions. Extension of the elbow beyond 90 degrees is not permitted until 4 to 6 weeks after surgery.

B. Essex-Lopresti fractures can be managed with open reduction internal fixation (ORIF) of the radial head in conjunction with reduction of the DRUJ and repair of the triangular fibrocartilage complex (TFCC) and pinning of the DRUJ. If there has been severe comminution of the radial head, a prosthetic replacement may be used with repair and pinning of the DRUJ. Immobilization is in a Muenster cast, which allows gentle elbow flexion and extension while preventing forearm rotation. At 6 weeks the pin is removed from the DRUJ and gentle forearm rotation may begin. These patients may develop chronic problems necessitating future reconstructions.

C. Sideswipe fractures are frequently stabilized with an external fixator. Initial treatment may include management of an open wound. Therapeutic treatment depends on each individual injury and the surgical stabilization performed. Nonunion, infection, and residual disability are often complications in these injuries.

POSTOPERATIVE COMPLICATIONS

See Nonoperative Complications

EVALUATION TIMELINE

I. Edema measurements: taken on initial evaluation and checked weekly thereafter until resolved or within normal limits (WNL).

II. Pain levels: taken on initial evaluation and checked at each visit during the first 2 weeks and weekly thereafter until resolved or WNL.

III. Sensory status: taken on initial evaluation and checked every 4 to 6 weeks or earlier if the patient is indicating a change of status.

IV. Circulatory status: taken on initial evaluation and checked each visit during the first week.

V. AROM to the uninvolved joints: started on initial evaluation and checked weekly until WNL.

VI. AROM to the involved joints: started as described specifically for each injury in the nonoperative and postoperative therapy sections, and checked weekly thereafter.

VII. Strengthening: started as described specifically for each injury in the nonoperative and postoperative therapy sections, and checked every 3 to 4 weeks thereafter.

VIII. CPM: may be initiated after approval by the physician; generally CPM is indicated early with AROM in the "safe zone" ranges.

IX. Static progressive splinting and dynamic splinting: may be initiated after approval by the physician; generally when radiographic union is firm.

REFERENCES

1. Werner FW, Kai-Nan A: Biomechanics of the elbow and forearm. Hand Clin 10:357, 1994
2. Bass RL, Stern PJ: Elbow and forearm anatomy and surgical approaches. Hand Clin 10:343, 1994
3. Morrey BF: Anatomy of the elbow joint. p. 7. In Morrey BF (ed): The Elbow and Its Disorders. W.B. Saunders, Philadelphia, 1985
4. Morrey BF, Askew LJ, An KN et al: A biomechanical study of normal functional elbow motion. J Bone J Surg 63:872, 1981
5. Weiss AC, Sachar K: Soft tissue contracture about the elbow. Hand Clin 10:439, 1994
6. Conwell HE: Injuries to the elbow. Clin Symp 21: 1969
7. Nirschl RP, Morrey BF: Rehabilitation. p. 147. In Morrey BF (ed): The Elbow and Its Disorders. W.B. Saunders, Philadelphia, 1985
8. Bryan RS, Morrey BF: Fractures of the distal humerus. p. 302. In Morrey BF (ed): The Elbow and Its Disorders. W.B. Saunders, Philadelphia, 1985
9. Nicholson DA, Driscoll PA: The elbow. Br Med J 307:1058, 1993
10. Cabanela ME: Fractures of the proximal ulna. p. 382. In Morrey BF (ed): The Elbow and Its Disorders. W.B. Saunders, Philadelphia, 1985
11. Morrey BF: Radial Head Fracture. p. 355. In Morrey BF (ed): The Elbow and Its Disorders. W.B. Saunders, Philadelphia, 1985
12. Linscheid RL: Elbow Dislocations. p. 414. In Morrey BF (ed): The Elbow and Its Disorders. W.B. Saunders, Philadelphia, 1985
13. Royle SG: Posterior dislocation of the elbow. Clin Orthop 269:201, 1991
14. O'Driscoll SW, Morrey BF, Korinek S: Elbow subluxation and dislocation: a spectrum of instability. Clin Orthop 280:186, 1992
15. O'Driscoll SW: Elbow instability. Hand Clin 10:405, 1994
16. Bado JL: The Monteggia lesion. Clin Orthop 50:71, 1967
17. Crenshaw AH: Cambell's Operative Orthopedics. 8th Ed. Mosby, St. Louis, 1992
18. Morgan WJ, Breen TF: Complex fractures of the forearm. Hand Clin 10:375, 1994

SUGGESTED READINGS

Aitken GK: Distal humeral fractures in the adult. Clin Orthop 207:191, 1986

Bell SN, Morrey BF: Chronic posterior subluxation and dislocation of the radial head. J Bone J Surg 73:392, 1991

Inglis AE: The rehabilitation of the elbow after injury. Instr Course Lect 40:45, 1991

Jupiter JB: Heterotopic ossification about the elbow. Instr Course Lect 40:41, 1991

McKee MD, Jupiter JB: A contemporary approach to the management of complex fractures of the distal humerus and their sequelae. Hand Clin 10:479, 1994

Rockwood CA, Green DP, Bucholz RW: Rockwood and Green's Fractures in Adults. 3rd Ed. J.B. Lippincott, Philadelphia, 1991

Sponseller PD: Problem elbow fractures in children. Hand Clin 10:495, 1994

Elbow Arthroplasty 32

Anne Edmonds

In the early 1970s, total elbow arthroplasty came into vogue as a new procedure to eliminate pain primarily for patients with rheumatoid arthritis (Fig. 32-1). Secondarily, the total elbow arthroplasty restored stability and improved active range of motion (AROM).

DEFINITION

Prostheses that attempt to duplicate the normal surface anatomy of the distal humerus and proximal ulna.

I. Constrained: constructed with either metal-to-metal or metal-to-high density polyethylene, through a bushing or a separate polyethylene piece.[1] This type of prosthesis is rarely used.

II. Semiconstrained: also a hinge, with stemmed humeral and ulnar components, but allows a few degrees of lateral motion. These may tolerate insufficient soft tissue or loss of metaphyseal bone stock, more than the resurfacing implants[2] (Figs. 32-2 to 32-4).

III. Unconstrained: not hinged and there is no attachment between the humeral and ulnar components. Sufficient bone stock and soft tissue support is a prerequisite for this type[3] (Figs. 32-5 and 32-6).

SURGICAL PURPOSE

To remove the irregular and painful ulna–humeral joint and replace these surfaces with new, usually metal or plastic, surfaces. The radial head is excised and often not replaced to improve pronation and supination. Joint stability is restored and a painless but effective range of motion (ROM) is derived.

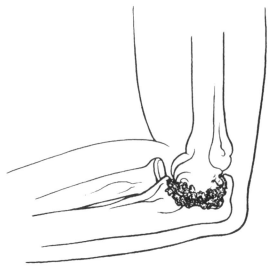

Fig. 32-1. Arthritis of elbow joint.

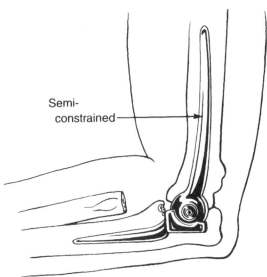

Semi-constrained

Fig. 32-2. Semiconstrained elbow prosthesis.

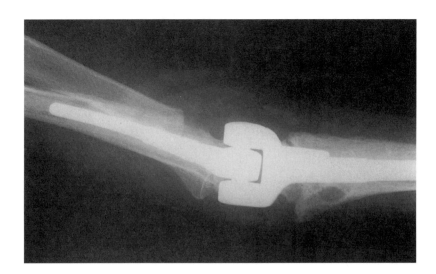

Fig. 32-3. Anterior/posterior radiograph of semiconstrained prosthesis.

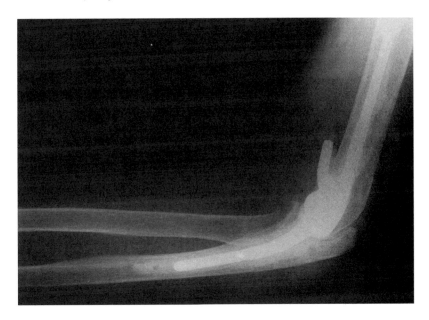

Fig. 32-4. Lateral radiograph of same semiconstrained prosthesis.

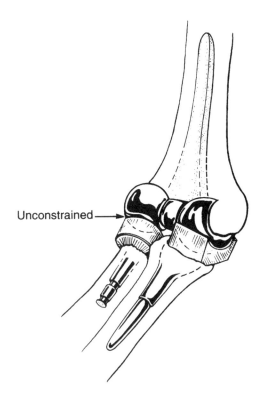

Unconstrained

Fig. 32-5. Unconstrained elbow prosthesis.

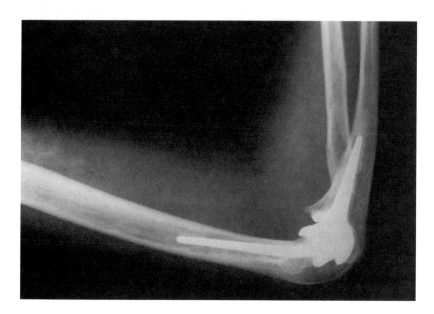

Fig. 32-6. Radiograph of unconstrained capito–condylar elbow prosthesis.

TREATMENT GOALS

I. Regain maximum elbow ROM to within the limits of the prosthesis.
II. Regain maximum strength.
III. Assist the patient's proficiency of self-care skills.
IV. Assess the patient's home environment for proper discharge.

POSTOPERATIVE INDICATIONS/ PRECAUTIONS FOR THERAPY

I. Indications
   A. Immobilization of nonconstrained arthroplasty at 90 degrees of flexion for 2 to 3 weeks may be necessary if instability is a problem. If implant is stable, then immobilization for 1 week. Usually protected motion is initiated at 3 to 5 days if ligament repair is stable. Bulky dressing is removed after first week and a long arm splint (LAS) is applied.
   B. Elbow motion in the rheumatoid patient is generally better following arthroplasty than a patient with traumatic open reduction internal fixation.[1]
II. Precautions
   A. Stability of ligamentous repair.
   B. Clinical manifestations and selected surgical repair.
   C. Avoidance of angular stress or torque on elbow, especially abduction and external rotation.
   D. Eliminating stress on triceps repair.
   E. Signs or symptoms of ulnar neuropathy.
   F. Infection.
   G. Neurovascular status.

POSTOPERATIVE THERAPY

    I. Immediate AROM to hand and wrist only.

   II. Compressive gloves as needed for edema.

  III. At 1 week when bulky dressing is removed, LAS applied for support. This should be worn at all times when not exercising.

  IV. At 3 to 5 days: begin protected active assisted elbow flexion/extension.

   V. At 5 to 8 days: begin gentle passive extension and active assisted supination/pronation.

  VI. At 5 to 8 days: begin simple activities of daily living (ADL), keep arm adducted, can move shoulder gently. Use LAS up to 6 weeks.

 VII. At 12 to 14 days: eat with fingers, buttoning, some grooming.

VIII. At 14 to 15 days: if little or no pain, begin graded resistive exercise to fingers if no pain.

  IX. At 3.5 to 4 weeks: maintain adducted position while exercising. May discontinue day splint at 4 weeks, continue at night to 6 weeks.

   X. At 5 to 6 weeks: begin resistive activities in pure planar motions.

  XI. At 6 to 7 weeks: isometrics.

 XII. 6 to 8 weeks: begin continuous passive motion (CPM) (Fig. 32-7).

XIII. Up to 6 months: no lifting, jarring, pounding, pushing, or weight bearing.

XIV. Restrictions

    A. No racquet sports.

    B. No golf or bowling.

    C. No competitive sport activities.

    D. No heavy labor.

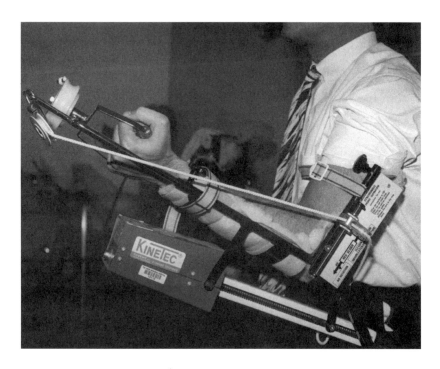

Fig. 32-7. Continuous passive motion may be used in postoperative treatment.

POSTOPERATIVE COMPLICATIONS

   I. Infection
  II. Triceps weakness
 III. Ulnar neuropathy
 IV. Prosthesis loosening

EVALUATION TIMELINE

     I. Active ROM of hand and wrist can be measured immediately.
    II. Active assisted ROM of elbow measured at 3 to 5 days.
   III. 5 to 8 days: passive extension should be measured. ROM should be measured thereafter every 2 to 3 weeks.
   IV. 14 to 15 days: resistive exercises to fingers.
    V. 3.5 to 4 weeks: assess grip and pinch strength and thereafter every 2 to 3 weeks.
   VI. 5 to 6 weeks: resistive exercises in pure planar motion.
  VII. 6 to 7 weeks: isometrics. Assess grip and pinch.
 VIII. 6 to 8 weeks: initiate CPM.
   IX. Up to 6 months: no lifting, pounding, pushing, or weight bearing.

REFERENCE

1. Ferlic DC: Rheumatoid arthritis in the elbow. p. 1767. In Green DP (ed): Operative Hand Surgery. 2nd Ed. Vol. 3. Churchill Livingstone, New York, 1988
2. Goldberg VM, Figgie HE, Inglis AE, Figgie MP: Current concepts review. Total elbow arthroplasty. J Bone Joint Surg 70:778, 1988
3. Dale KG, Orr PM, Harrell PB: Total elbow replacement. Orthop Nurs 2:23, 1992

SUGGESTED READINGS

Ewald FC: Operative Techniques for the Capitello-Condylar Total Elbow Prosthesis. Brigham and Women's Hospital and Harvard University Medical School, Boston
Ewald FC, Jacobs MA: Total elbow arthroplasty. Clin Orthop 182:137, 1984
Kudo H, Iwaro K: Total elbow arthroplasty with a nonconstrained surface—replacement prosthesis in patients who have rheumatoid arthritis. J Bone Joint Surg 72:355, 1990
Occupational Therapy Section, Good Samaritan Hospital, Baltimore, MD. Capitella-Condylar Total Elbow Replacement Protocol
Weiland AJ, Weiss AP, Wills RP, Moore JR: Capitellar-condylar total elbow replacement: long term follow-up. Department of Orthopaedic Surgery. The Johns Hopkins University School of Medicine, Baltimore, J Bone Joint Surg 71A:217, 1989

Proximal Row Carpectomy 33

Bonnie Aiello

Injury to the proximal carpal row can lead to long-standing pain and disability. Wrist fusion is often offered to these patients, but proximal row carpectomy is a valid option that can decrease pain and still maintain motion.

The triquetrum, lunate, and all or a piece of the scaphoid are removed. The distal carpus then articulates with the radius, not the ulna.

The success of the surgery depends on the distal pole of the capitate and the lunate fossa being in good shape. This will be the major articulation of the wrist.

Postoperative therapy calls for approximately 1 month in a cast to provide stability and allow for healing. This is then followed by progressive motion and strengthening.

DEFINITION

Removal of the proximal row of carpal bones allowing the capitate to articulate with the lunate fossa (Fig. 33-1). Usually done in severe perilunate dissociation and Kienböck's disease to decrease pain and retain wrist motion.

SURGICAL PURPOSE

To relieve wrist pain, retain some wrist motion, and achieve joint stability. The proximal row includes the scaphoid, the lunate, and the triquetrum. The success of the procedure is dependent on good to excellent articular surfaces of the face of the capitate and the lunate fossa of the radius into which the capitate nestles.

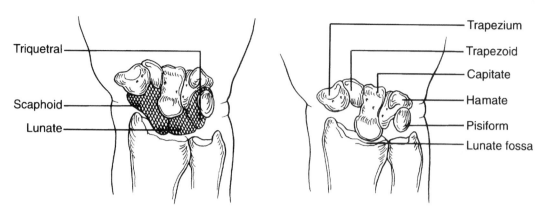

Fig. 33-1. Removal of the proximal row of carpal bones allowing the capitate to articulate with the lunate fossa.

TREATMENT GOALS

I. Decrease wrist pain
II. Maintain wrist motion 50 to 70 percent
III. Maintain 50 to 80 percent grip strength

POSTOPERATIVE INDICATIONS/ PRECAUTIONS FOR THERAPY

I. Indications
   A. Long-standing perilunate dislocation
   B. Scaphoid malunion/nonunion
   C. Unsuccessful Silastic implant
   D. Advanced Kienböck's disease
   E. Radiocarpal arthrosis
   F. Rheumatoid arthritis
   G. Spastic wrist contractures
II. Precautions
   Poor articular surface of proximal pole of capitate or lunate fossa.

POSTOPERATIVE THERAPY

Bulky dressing with volar forearm plaster cast for 5 days. Cast for 4 weeks with range of motion (ROM) of fingers and thumb. May use cockup for support for 2 to 4 weeks. Cast removed week 4 and active ROM (AROM) started, progress to resistance as tolerated.

POSTOPERATIVE COMPLICATIONS

   I. Pain
  II. Weakness
 III. Limited ROM

EVALUATION TIMELINE: POSTOPERATIVE

   I. Digital ROM day 1
  II. Wrist AROM week 4
 III. Wrist passive ROM (PROM) week 6
  IV. Strength week 6

SUGGESTED READINGS

Culp RW, McGuigan FX, Turner MA et al: Proximal row carpectomy: a multi-center study. J Hand Surg (Am) 18:19, 1993

Ferlic DC, Clayton ML, Mills MF: Proximal row carpectomy: a review of rheumatoid and non-rheumatoid wrists. J Hand Surg (Am) 16:420, 1991

Green D: Management of wrist problems. Hand Clin 3:163, 1987

Green D: Operative Hand Surgery. p. 198. 2nd Ed. Vol. 1. Churchill Livingstone, New York, 1988

Green D: Operative Hand Surgery. p. 927. 2nd Ed. Vol. 2. Churchill Livingstone, New York, 1988

Inglis A, Jones E: Proximal row carpectomy for diseases of the proximal row. J Bone Joint Surg 59A:45, 1977

Jorgenson E: Proximal row carpectomy. J Bone Joint Surg 51A:1104, 1969

Lin HH, Stern PJ: "Salvage" procedures in the treatment of Keinbock's disease. Proximal row carpectomy and total wrist arthrodesis. Hand Clin 9:521, 1993

Nevaiser R: Proximal row carpectomy for posttraumatic disorders of the carpus. J Hand Surg 8:301, 1983

Tsuge K: Comprehensive Atlas of Hand Surgery. p. 207. Year Book Medical Publishers, New York, 1990

Ulnar Head Resection 34

Frank DiGiovannantonio

The distal radioulnar joint (DRUJ) is an important and integral part of wrist and hand function. The radius and hand move in relation to and function about the distal ulna.[1] Even the most minor modifications to the relationship among the distal radius, ulna, and ulnar carpus can lead to significant load changes at the distal ulnar and triangular fibrocartilage (TFC).[1]

The current literature describes many variations and modifications to the widely used ulnar head resection. This chapter describes four of the following procedures and their appropriate treatment: (1) Darrach procedure, (2) Bowers: hemiresection-interposition technique (HIT), (3) matched ulna resection, and (4) the Sauve–Kapandji procedure. Communication between therapist and physician is critical because of the variations in surgical technique and purpose for each patient.

Indications for the appropriate surgical procedure to be used during ulnar head resection vary greatly within the literature, as well as among physicians. A review of the literature, however, reveals several diagnoses that are commonly referred for some form of ulnar head resection. They include but are not limited to degenerative arthritis,[2–9] unreconstructable fractures of the ulnar head,[3,4] ulnocarpal impingement,[3,4,6,8–10] chronic painful TFC tears,[3,6,9,11] malunion of a distal radius fracture,[2–6,8,10–12] Madelung's deformity,[3–5,8,10,12] and rheumatoid arthritis.[3,5–11]

DEFINITION

I. Darrach procedure: Resection of the distal end of the ulna just proximal to the sigmoid notch of the radius[11] (Fig. 34-1).

II. Hemiresection-interposition technique: Resection of only the ulnar articular head, leaving the shaft/styloid relationship intact. An interposition "anchovy" of tendon, capsule, or muscle is placed in the

297

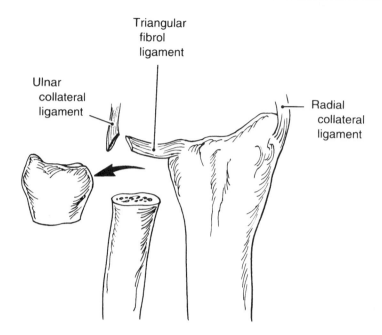

Fig. 34-1. Darrach procedure.

vacant distal radioulnar joint cavity to limit contact of the radial and ulnar shafts. It is important to remember that this procedure presupposes an intact or reconstructible triangular fibrocartilage complex (TFCC).[10]

III. Matched procedure: The resection of the distal ulna in a smooth, curved, convex fashion to match the contour of the radius throughout forearm rotation.[4]

IV. Sauve–Kapandji procedure: A distal radioulnar arthrodesis with the surgical creation of a pseudoarthrosis in the distal ulna[7] (Fig. 34-2).

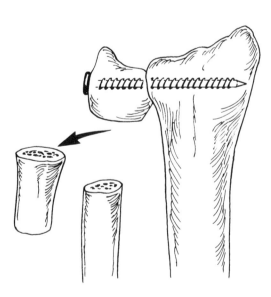

Fig. 34-2. Sauve–Kapandji procedure.

SURGICAL PURPOSE

Pain at the DRUJ may be caused by a variety of reasons. It is often due to arthritis between the radius and ulna at that level. This arthritis often can be caused by a malalignment of the joint after distal radial fracture, by dislocation, by systemic arthritis, or by other conditions causing malalignment that brings on cartilage surface changes. The most frequent type of surgery is the resection or reshaping of the distal ulna as it articulates with the radius. These procedures eliminate the joint surfaces and prevents them from rubbing together, thereby decreasing the symptoms of pain.

TREATMENT GOALS

I. Maintain/increase range of motion (ROM) of uninvolved joints.
II. Protective healing through proper immobilization.
III. Control edema.
IV. Decrease pain.
V. Restore active ROM at wrist and forearm.
VI. Prevent infection at surgical site.
VII. Restore patient to maximum functional capacity.

OPERATIVE INDICATIONS/PRECAUTIONS

I. Indications
   A. Rheumatoid arthritis.
   B. Degenerative arthritis.
   C. Malunited distal radius fracture.
   D. TFCC tears.
   E. Madelung's deformity.
   F. Ulnar head fractures.
   G. Ulnocarpal impingement.
   H. Chronic dislocation of the DRUJ.
II. Precautions
   A. Associated tendon injuries.
   B. Associated bony injury.
   C. Associated nerve injury.
   D. Associated vascular injury.

POSTOPERATIVE INDICATIONS/ PRECAUTIONS FOR THERAPY

I. Indications
   A. Distal ulnar resection.
   B. Arthrodesis with pseudoarthrosis.
   C. Painful ROM.
   D. Edema.
   E. Splinting.

II. Precautions
  A. Ulnar stump instability.
  B. Combined tendon interposition or transfer.
  C. Painful or nonpainful clicking or popping of the wrist during the early stages of active ROM.
  D. Disproportionate pain.

POSTOPERATIVE THERAPY

  I. Therapy following the Darrach procedure, HIT, and the Matched procedure:
  A. Immediately after surgery the patient is immobilized in a long arm cast at neutral forearm rotation for 7 to 10 days.
  B. At 7 to 10 days postoperatively, the cast is removed by the treating physician and stability is assessed.
    1. If the patient is *stable*, he or she is placed in a short arm wrist splint.
      a. The patient can move safely within 45 to 60 degrees of wrist flexion and extension, as well as forearm supination and pronation within the first 2 to 4 weeks postoperatively. If the patient is relatively pain free after that 2 to 4 week period, the wrist splint is discontinued and normal ROM may be attempted.
      b. Strengthening may begin at 4 to 6 weeks as tolerated by the patient. However, power grasp should be avoided until 8 to 12 weeks.
    2. If after removal of cast the patient is assessed to be *unstable*, the patient is placed in a long arm splint in neutral forearm rotation or as directed by the physician until 4 weeks postoperatively.
      a. Active ROM to within 45 to 60 degrees of wrist flexion and extension and supination and pronation may begin at 7 to 10 days postoperatively. AROM should be performed within pain-free limits and only in the presence of the therapist. The patient is to continue to wear their splint at all other times. Consult with the physician with regard to motion that may promote instability.
      b. At 4 to 6 weeks postoperatively the long arm splint may be discontinued and gradual strengthening may begin.
      c. Avoid power grasp until 8 to 12 weeks postoperatively.
          If in either of the preceding cases the patient presents with any clicking or popping of the wrist during the early phases of ROM, the physician should be contacted, and consideration should be given to immobilizing the patient in a long arm splint until 6 weeks postoperatively.
  II. Therapy following Sauve–Kapandji procedure.
  A. The patient is immobilized in a long arm cast for 7 to 10 days postoperatively.

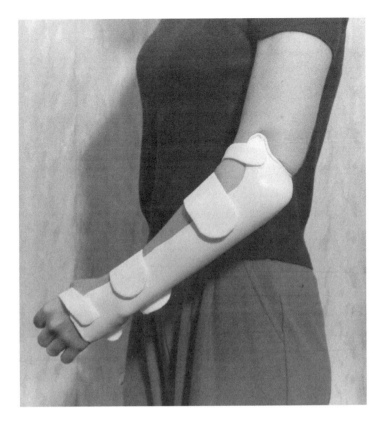

Fig. 34-3. Munster-type splint.

B. If internal fixation was attained using Kirschner (K) *wires*, the patient is placed in a long arm or Munster type splint (Fig. 34-3) at neutral forearm rotation until 3 to 4 weeks postoperatively.[8]
   1. The patient may remove the long arm splint to perform active supination and pronation exercises, within 45 to 60 degrees, again avoiding end range of motion.
C. If internal fixation is attained through the use of a *screw*, the patient can be placed in a wrist splint at 7 to 10 days postoperatively, and active forearm supination and pronation within 45 to 60 degrees can begin.
D. In patients with either K-wire or screw fixation, ROM of the wrist may begin at 4 weeks postoperatively.
E. The wrist splint should be worn between exercise for approximately 6 weeks postoperatively or until fusion between the radius and ulna is achieved. At this point, strengthening may begin.

POSTOPERATIVE COMPLICATIONS

   I. Stylocarpal impingement.[3]
  II. Radioulnar impingement.[4]
 III. Regeneration of the distal ulna.[5]

IV. Radial deviation of the wrist.[5]
V. Wrist instability.[5,6,8,9,11,12]
VI. Tendon rupture.[6,11]
VII. Nerve impairment.
VIII. Reflex sympathetic dystrophy.
IX. Wrist synovitis.[7]
X. Instability of the distal ulna.
XI. Inadequate bony resection.

EVALUATION TIMELINE

I. Therapy following Darrach procedure, HIT, or Matched procedure.
  A. Stable wrist
    1. Week 1
      a. Wrist splint fabricated with wrist at neutral to 30 degrees of extension.
      b. Active ROM of all uninvolved joints.
    2. Weeks 2 to 4
      a. Active ROM wrist and forearm, within pain-free limits, to 45 to 60 degrees from neutral.
      b. Light activities of daily living (ADL) may also be performed at this time as tolerated by the patient.
    3. Weeks 4 to 6
      a. If the patient is relatively pain free, the wrist splint may be discontinued and full ROM may be attempted.
      b. Gradual strengthening of the hand, wrist, and forearm.
    4. Weeks 6 to 10
      a. More progressive strengthening and return to normal function.
      b. Power grasp may be attempted at week 8 if relatively pain free.
  B. Unstable wrist
    1. Weeks 1 to 4
      a. Long arm splint is fabricated.
      b. Active ROM wrist and forearm to 45 to 60 degrees from neutral only in the presence of the therapist and avoiding any motions promoting instability as per physician.
      c. Active ROM of all uninvolved joints.
    2. Weeks 4 to 6
      a. If the patient is relatively pain free and the physician has been consulted, the long arm splint may be discontinued.
      b. Gradual strengthening may begin at this time, as well as attempts at normal ROM.
    3. Weeks 6 to 12
      a. Progressive strengthening and return to normal function. However, power grasp should be avoided until at least week 8.

II. Therapy following Sauve–Kapandji procedure.
  A. Internal fixation via K wires
    1. Weeks 1–4
      a. Fabrication of a long arm or Munster type splint.
      b. Active ROM of all uninvolved joints.
      c. Long arm splint is removed to perform active forearm supination and pronation to 45 to 60 degrees from neutral avoiding end range.
    2. Weeks 4 to 6
      a. Long arm splint discontinued and a wrist splint fabricated to be worn between exercises.
      b. Active ROM wrist as tolerated.
    3. Week 6
      a. Wrist splint may be discontinued as long as the treating physician confirms fusion between radius and ulna.
      b. Gentle strengthening.
    4. Weeks 8 to 12: progressive strengthening and return to normal function. Avoid power grasp activities until week 8.
  B. Internal fixation via screw
    1. Weeks 1 to 4
      a. Fabrication of wrist splint.
      b. Active forearm supination and pronation within 45 to 60 degrees from neutral avoiding end range.
    2. Weeks 4 to 12: Follow protocol for K-wire fixation.

REFERENCES

1. Palmer AK, Werner FW: Biomechanics of the distal radioulnar joint. p. 26. In Leach RE (ed): Clinical Orthopedics and Related Research, Lippincott-Raven, Philadelphia, 1984
2. Bowers WH: Instability of the distal radioulnar articulation. p. 311. In Cramer LE, Schneider LH (eds): Hand Clinics. Vol. 7. W.B. Saunders, Philadelphia, 1991
3. Bowers WH: Distal radioulnar joint arthroplasty: the hemiresection-interposition technique. J Hand Surg 10A:169, 1985
4. Gabuzda GM, Watson HK: Matched distal ulnar resection for posttraumatic disorders of the distal radioulnar joint. J Hand Surg 17A:724, 1992
5. Dingman PVC: Resection of the distal end of the ulna (Darrach operation). J Bone Joint Surg 34A:893, 1952
6. Eaton RG, Nolan WB: A Darrach procedure for distal ulnar pathology derangements. p. 85. In Urist MR: Clinical Orthopedics and Related Research. J.B. Lippincott, Philadelphia, 1992
7. Agee JM, Szabo RM, Vincent KA: The Sauve-Kapandji procedure for reconstruction of the rheumatoid distal radioulnar joint. J Hand Surg 18:1125, 1991
8. Taleisnik J: The Sauve-Kapandji procedure. p. 110. In Urist MR: Clinical Orthopedics and Related Research. Lippincott-Raven, Philadelphia, 1992
9. Frederick HA, Hontas RB, Saunders RA: The Sauve-Kapandji procedure: a salvage operation for distal radioulnar joint. J Hand Surg 16A:1125, 1991

10. Bowers WH: The distal radioulnar joint. p. 973. In Green DP (ed): Operative Hand Surgery. 3rd Ed. Churchill Livingstone, New York, 1993

11. Eaton RG, Eberhart RE, Tulipan DJ: The Darrach procedure defended: technique redefined and long-term follow-up. J Hand Surg 16:438, 1991

12. Gordon L, Levinsohn DG, Moore SV, et al: The Sauve-Kapandji procedure for the treatment of posttraumatic distal radioulnar joint problems. p. 397. In Cramer LE, Schneider LH (eds): Hand Clinics. Vol. 7. W.B. Saunders, Philadelphia, 1991

SUGGESTED READINGS

Bieber EJ, Linscheid RL, Dobyns JH, Beckenbaugh RD: Failed distal ulna resection. J Hand Surg 13A:193, 1988

Darrach W: Anterior dislocation of the head of the ulna. Ann Surg 56:802, 1912

Darrow JC, Linscheid RL, Dobyns JH et al: Distal ulnar recession for disorders of the distal radioulnar joint. J Hand Surg 10:482, 1985

Hartz CR, Beckenbaugh RD: Long-term results of resection of the distal ulna for post-traumatic conditions. J Trauma 19:219, 1979

Jackson IT, Milward TM, Lee P et al: Ulnar head resection in rheumatoid arthritis. J Hand Surg 6:172, 1974

Noble J, Arafa M: Stabilization of the distal radioulnar joint: anatomy and clues to prompt diagnosis. Clin Orthop Relat Res 144:154, 1979

Wrist Arthrodesis 35

Beth Farrell Kozera

Total and intercarpal wrist arthrodesis surgery is a very successful reconstructive procedure for stabilizing the wrist.[1] Intercarpal arthrodesis is useful in treating carpal instability resulting from destruction of the carpus as seen in arthritis and advanced Kienböck's disease.[2] This is the surgery of choice when the patient's job requires some wrist mobility and the radiocarpal joint is "relatively free of arthritis involvement."[1]

Total wrist arthrodesis compromises motion for stability and, in most cases, pain relief. It is often performed as salvage surgery for other failed procedures and for heavy laborers with advanced radiocarpal instability.[1] The nondominant wrist is usually fused in the neutral position and the dominant hand is positioned in 10 degrees of extension and 5 degrees of ulnar deviation.[2]

The immobilization phase following surgery can lead to stiff uninvolved joints of the upper extremity. Therefore, one of the primary goals of therapy is to maintain full range of motion (ROM) of all uninvolved joints. This phase also contributes to upper extremity weakness and decreased endurance. Thus, once fusion is complete, it is important to begin general conditioning, strengthening, and instruction in compensatory techniques. These will enhance the patient's level of functioning for return to work and normal activities.

The therapist plays an important role in the success of wrist arthrodesis. Communication between the doctor and therapist in regard to the healing process is important in determining appropriate timing to initiate various phases of treatment. It should be emphasized that this protocol offers only guidelines, which may vary with each patient's particular condition.

DEFINITION

I. Total wrist arthrodesis: the surgical immobilization of the wrist joint. An iliac or distal radius bone graft is inserted with internal fixation to stabilize the wrist in the desired position (Fig. 35-1).

II. Intercarpal arthrodesis: the surgical partial immobilization of the wrist joint for treatment of carpal instability. An iliac or distal radius bone graft is used to replace the subchondral bone and articular cartilage is removed[3] (Fig. 35-2).

SURGICAL PURPOSE

To eliminate wrist pain, to correct joint instability with deformity and concurrent pain. It is done at the expense of wrist joint motion.

The limited wrist fusion applies to fusing two or more carpal bones together. The most common fusions involve the trapezium, scaphoid,

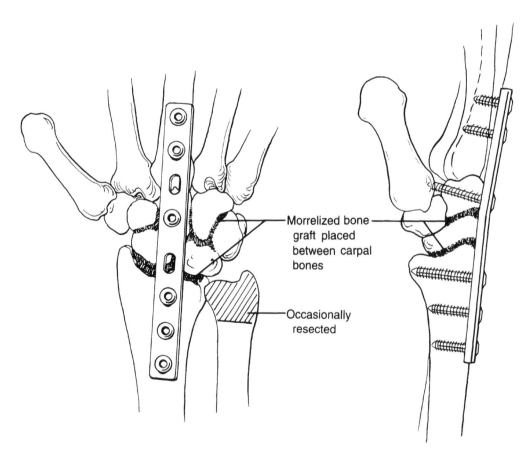

Morrelized bone graft placed between carpal bones

Occasionally resected

Fig. 35-1. Total wrist arthrodesis.

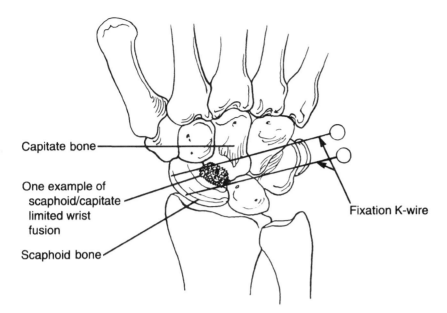

Capitate bone

One example of
scaphoid/capitate
limited wrist
fusion

Scaphoid bone

Fixation K-wire

Fig. 35-2. Intercarpal arthrodesis.

and trapezoid; the scaphoid and capitate; the lunate triquetrum, hamate, and capitate; and the triquetrum and lunate. Other combinations are possible. If a carpal bone is damaged, such as the scaphoid or lunate, these fusions may be performed to allow for replacement. The vacated abnormal bone is substituted with a tendon or fascial "anchovy," but stability is achieved.

The total wrist fusion is performed to stop wrist pain, increase strength along with endurance, and create joint stability. The techniques vary to accomplish this fusion that binds the radius to the carpus and metacarpals. Internal fixation is frequently used in the form of plates and screws or pins. The distal ulna may or may not be excised depending on the circumstances. Bone grafting from the iliac crest or another source is required. The average length of time for bony fusion is approximately 12 weeks. Another 12 weeks is usually necessary to reach maximum benefit.

TREATMENT GOALS

    I. Improve stability of the wrist
    II. Maximize ROM of wrist (if intercarpal arthrodesis)
    III. Protect fusion
    IV. Control edema
    V. Minimize pain
    VI. Minimize adhesions
    VII. Maintain ROM of uninvolved joints
    VIII. Return patient to maximum level of functioning

INDICATIONS/PRECAUTIONS FOR SURGERY

I. Indications
   A. Intercarpal wrist arthrodesis[2]
      1. Localized arthritis of carpus
      2. Carpal instability
      3. Advanced Kienböck's disease
      4. As salvage surgery for partial carpal bone loss.
      5. Sparing of midcarpal joints with destruction limited to radio-carpal area.
   B. Total wrist arthrodesis
      1. Wrist pain and/or instability resulting from degenerative changes.
      2. Heavy laborer with advanced radiocarpal joint destruction.[1]
      3. As salvage surgery for failed procedures[1] (e.g., arthroplasties, partial wrist fusion).
      4. Paralysis of wrist with the potential for tendon reconstruction.[1]
      5. Reconstruction following tumor resection.
      6. Adolescent spastic hemiplegia with wrist flexion deformity.[1]
      7. Wrist extensors are ruptured or nonfunctioning.[2]
II. Precautions for therapy
   Partial arthrodesis: vigorous wrist exercise may exacerbate wrist pain.[2]

POSTOPERATIVE THERAPY

The timetable below is only a guideline. It is important to consult with the patient's physician regarding surgical procedure performed, treatment goals, and healing status of the fused wrist.

I. Partial wrist arthrodesis
   A. Postoperative day 1 through entire rehabilitation program.
      1. Maintain ROM of uninvolved joints.
      2. Edema control.
      3. Pain control as needed.
   B. Cast immobilization for 8 to 10 weeks or until pins are removed (with delayed union or nonunion, immobilization time is increased).[4]
   C. Short arm splint or thumb spica splint (depending on procedure) is applied for 2 to 3 weeks following cast removal[4] (Fig. 35-3).
      1. 8 to 10 weeks: initiate gentle active ROM (AROM) of wrist.[5] Avoid forced wrist motion.[2]
      2. Initiate scar management and edema control of wrist and digits.
   D. Once the fusion is complete and with the physician's consent, begin graded strengthening of the wrist and work hardening.[2]

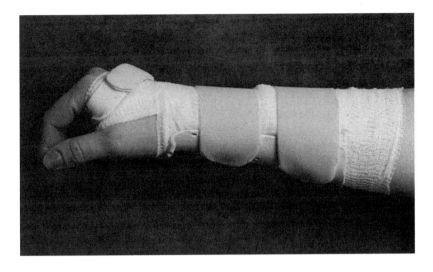

Fig. 35-3. Splint is applied after cast and/or pin removal.

II. Total wrist arthrodesis

Postoperative therapy is essentially the same as intercarpal wrist arthrodesis; however, a total wrist arthrodesis is generally immobilized in a plaster cast for a longer period (e.g., 12 weeks).[1]

POSTOPERATIVE COMPLICATIONS

   I. Pseudoarthrosis
  II. Fracture of healed fusion
 III. Nonunion
 IV. Deep wound infection
  V. Superficial skin necrosis
 VI. Vascular insufficiency/gangrene
VII. Hematoma
VIII. Edema
 IX. Pain
  X. Transient median nerve or superficial radial nerve compression.
 XI. Scar adhesions limiting tendon excursion.

EVALUATION TIMELINE

 I. ROM
   A. Intercarpal wrist fusion
     1. 1 week postoperatively measure uninvolved upper extremity joints.
     2. AROM of wrist once pins are removed.
     3. Passive ROM (PROM): measured once fusion is complete.

    B. Total wrist arthrodesis

       1 week postoperatively measure AROM and PROM of uninvolved upper extremity joints.

  II. Sensory: evaluate 1 week postoperatively. If deficits, evaluate at 1-month intervals following initial evaluation.

  III. Pain: evaluate 1 week postoperatively and at every visit thereafter.

  IV. Edema: evaluate 1 week postoperatively and at every visit thereafter.

  V. Scar formation: same as III and IV.

  VI. Strength: evaluate all upper extremity joints for strength once the fusion is complete.

REFERENCES

1. Dick HM: Wrist and intercarpal arthrodesis. p. 127. In Green DP (ed): Operative Hand Surgery. Vol. 1. Churchill Livingstone, New York, 1982
2. Nalebuff EA, Fatti JF, Weil CE: Arthrodesis of the rheumatoid wrist: indications and surgical technique. p. 365. In Lichtman DM: The Wrist and Its Disorders. WB Saunders, Philadelphia, 1988
3. Green DP: Carpal dislocations and instabilities. p. 925. In Green DP (ed): Operative Hand Surgery. 2nd Ed. Vol. 2. Churchill Livingstone, New York, 1988
4. Feldon P: Wrist fusions: intercarpal and radiocarpal. p. 446. In Lichtman DM (ed): The Wrist and Its Disorders. WB Saunders, Philadelphia, 1988
5. Watson HK, Black DM: Instabilities of the wrist. p. 103. In Taleisnick J (ed): Hand Clinics. Vol. 3. WB Saunders, Philadelphia, 1987

SUGGESTED READINGS

Clendenin MB, Green DP: Arthrodesis of the wrist—complications and their management. J Hand Surg 6:253, 1981

Dick HM: Wrist arthrodesis. p. 131. In Green DP (ed): Operative Hand Surgery. 3rd. Ed. Vol. 1. Churchill Livingstone, New York, 1993

Fisk GR: The wrist: review article. J Bone Joint Surg 66B:401, 1984

Nalebuff EA, Fatti JF, Weil CE: Arthrodesis of the rheumatoid wrist: indications and surgical technique. p. 365. In Lichtman DM: The Wrist and Its Disorders. WB Saunders, Philadelphia, 1988

Watson HK, Dhillon HS: Intercarpal arthrodesis. p. 113. In Green DP (ed): Operative Hand Surgery. 3rd. Ed. Vol. 1. Churchill Livingstone, New York, 1993

Internal/External Fixation of Wrist and Distal Forearm Fractures

36

Linda Coll Ware

Joint congruency is essential to ensure a good functional wrist. The fundamental goal of treating a wrist fracture is an accurate and stable reduction.[1] There are many techniques for fracture fixation outlined in the literature: percutaneous pin fixation, pins and plaster, closed reduction and external fixation, open reduction and internal fixation,[1] and arthroscopic reduction and percutaneous external fixation.[2] Which technique a physician chooses depends on many variables, including type of fracture, associated injuries, loss of bone substance, age and occupation of patient, and physician's surgical expertise.

Rehabilitation of wrist fractures begins immediately after fracture reduction and stabilization.[3] Internal fixation and dynamic external fixation may enable active motion of the wrist as early as week 1. External fixation does not allow wrist motion until as early as 6 weeks.

Open communication between physician and therapist is critical. Radiographic changes must be communicated to the therapist. Progressive therapy and strengthening should be started only after consulting the physician between 6 and 12 weeks.

Over a period of several months, the patient progresses from active exercises to increasingly resistive activities. Steady improvement is expected for 8 to 12 months until full functional ability is achieved.[3]

DEFINITION

I. External fixation: a method of holding together the fragments of a fractured bone by using transfixing metal pins through the fragments and a compression device attached to the pins outside the skin surface. The pins are removed at a later procedure when the fracture is healed[4] (Figs. 36-1 and 36-2).

311

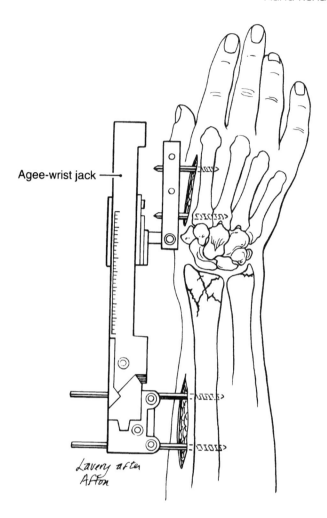

Fig. 36-1. External fixation of fracture.

II. Internal fixation: any method of holding together the fragments of a fractured bone without the use of appliances external to the skin. After open reduction of the fracture, smooth or threaded pins, Kirschner wires (K-wire), screws, plates attached by screws, or medullary nails may be used to stabilize the fragments. In some instances, the device is removed at a later operation, but sometimes it may remain in the body permanently[4] (Figs. 36-3 and 36-4).

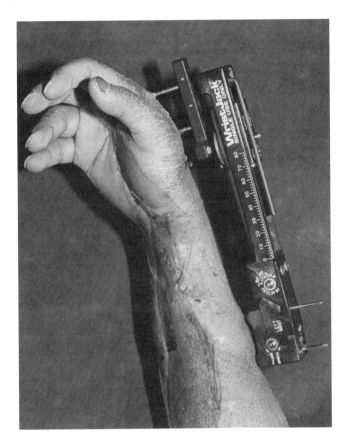

Fig. 36-2. External fixation of a distal forearm fracture.

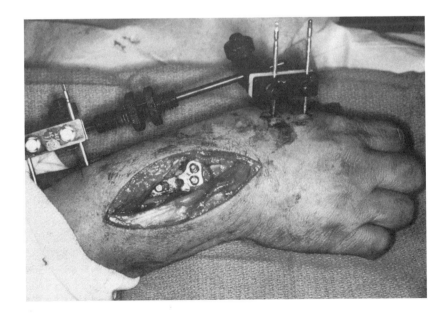

Fig. 36-3. Internal fixation may be used in combination with external device.

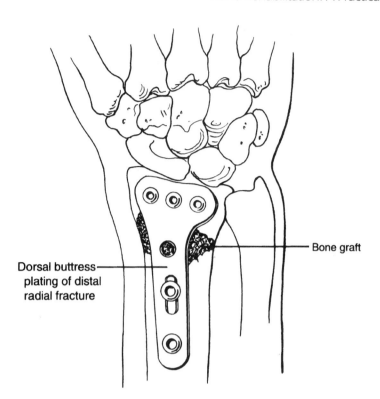

Fig. 36-4. Internal fixation of fracture.

TREATMENT AND SURGICAL PURPOSE

Many fractures of the distal radius and ulnar are unstable. Because the structure of the radius at this level is mostly cancelous, it will not easily stay reduced and may require some form of stabilization. The principal forms of stabilization are pins, bone plates, and external fixation devices. These may be used singly or in combination to achieve and maintain an acceptable reduction of the fracture. On occasion bone grafting to the radius may be necessary when these techniques are used so that sufficient bone stock is present for strong healing. Combinations of fractures and dislocation of the carpal bones, as well as the radius and ulnar, occur and require accurate reduction and stabilization.

TREATMENT GOALS

    I. Maintain full range of motion (ROM) of all uninvolved joints.
   II. Prevent wound or pin tract infection.
  III. Provide mobilization or immobilization of fixated joint as per fixation device.
  IV. Prevent scar adhesions on extensor surface.
   V. Return to previous level of function.

POSTOPERATIVE INDICATIONS/ PRECAUTIONS FOR THERAPY

I. Indications: wrist fractures requiring internal or external fixation.
II. Precautions
    A. Associated soft tissue loss.
    B. Associated tendon injuries.
    C. Associated nerve injuries.

POSTOPERATIVE THERAPY

I. Therapy following internal fixation of wrist.
    A. Week 1
        1. Thermoplastic splint to immobilize fixated fracture for amount of time directed by physician.
            a. Thermoplastic splints are easy to remove for bathing or dressing changes if there is associated soft tissue loss.
            b. If physician prefers a plaster cast, make sure uninvolved joints are not restricted.
        2. Begin active ROM (AROM) of all uninvolved joints. Uninjured joint ROM can be enhanced by static and dynamic splinting.[3]
        3. Begin edema control.
    B. Week 2
        1. Begin gentle mobilization of wrist. Patient continues to wear splint when not exercising.
        2. Begin scar control procedures to prevent extensor adhesions.
    C. Weeks 6 to 12: When physician communicates radiographic union is clearly demonstrated, the splint may be discontinued and aggressive mobilization and strengthening can be started.
    D. Post 6 months: Internal fixators may be removed 6 months after surgery or may remain in the body permanently.
II. Therapy following static external fixation of wrist
    A. Week 1
        1. Thermoplastic splint to immobilize fixated fracture for amount of time directed by physician. Splint may or may not be requested by physician.
            a. Splints are easy to remove for bathing or dressing changes if there is associated soft tissue loss.
            b. If physician prefers a plaster cast, make sure uninjured joints are not restricted.
        2. Begin AROM of all uninvolved joints.[5] Uninjured joint ROM can be enhanced by static and dynamic splinting.[3]
        3. Begin edema control.
        4. Instruct patient on pin site care.
    B. Weeks 6 to 12: Physician removes external fixator when radiographic union is demonstrated.

1. A protective splint is applied to wrist.
2. Begin scar control.
3. Mobilization progressing to strengthening can be started to regain full ROM and power.

III. Therapy following dynamic external fixation of the wrist[6]
   A. Week 1
      1. Begin active and active assisted wrist flexion from the neutral position.
      2. Begin scar control.
      3. Begin AROM of all uninvolved joints.
      4. Begin edema control.
      5. Instruct patient on pin site care.
   B. Week 4: Begin wrist extension and ulnar deviation.
   C. Weeks 8 to 10
      1. External fixation removed by physician.
      2. Begin scar control.
      3. Progressive mobilization and strengthening of wrist started.

POSTOPERATIVE COMPLICATIONS

I. Pin tract infection
II. Pin site fracture
III. Pin loosening
IV. Osteoarthritis/osteoporosis
V. Reflex sympathetic dystrophy
VI. Tendons adhering to internal fixation devices and scars.
VII. Nerve compression
VIII. Malunion and poor articular congruency.
IX. Refracture

EVALUATION TIMELINE

I. Week 1
   A. AROM and passive ROM (PROM) measurements of all uninjured upper extremity joints.
   B. Edema measurements.
   C. Active and active assisted wrist flexion measurements if dynamic external fixation is used.
II. Week 2: AROM measurements of the internally fixated wrist.
III. Week 4: ROM measurements of wrist extension and ulnar deviation if dynamic external fixation is used.
IV. Weeks 6 to 12
   A. AROM measurements.
   B. Grip strength measurements.
   C. Pinch strength measurements.
   D. Sensory screening.

REFERENCES

1. Axelrod TS, McMurtry RY: Open reduction and internal fixation of comminuted, intra-articular fractures of the distal radius. J Hand Surg 15A:1, 1990
2. Cooney WP, Berger RA: Treatment of complex fractures of the distal radius. Hand Clin 9:603, 1993
3. Melone Jr CP: Unstable fractures of the distal radius. p. 160. In Lichtmen DM (ed): The Wrist and Its Disorders. WB Saunders, Philadelphia, 1988
4. Glanze W (ed): Mosby's Medical, Nursing and Allied Health Dictionary. p. 454, 601. Mosby, St. Louis, 1989
5. Reiss B: Therapist's management of distal fractures. p. 348. In Hunter JM, Mackin EJ, Callahan AD (eds): Rehabilitation of the Hand: Surgery and Therapy. Mosby, St. Louis, 1995
6. Clyburn TA: Dynamic external fixation for comminuted intra-articular fractures of the distal end of the radius. J Bone Joint Surg 69:1110, 1987

SUGGESTED READINGS

Foster D, Kopta J: Update on external fixators in the treatment of wrist fractures. Clin Orthop 204:177, 1986

Freeland A, Jabaley M: Stabilization of fractures in the hand and wrist with traumatic soft tissue and bone loss. Hand Clin 4:425, 1988

Frykman G et al: Comparison of eleven external fixators for treatment of unstable wrist fractures. J Hand Surg 14A:247, 1989

Frykman GK, Kropp WE: Fractures and traumatic conditions of the wrist. p. 315. In Hunter JM, Mackin EJ, Callahan AD (eds): Rehabilitation of the Hand: Surgery and Therapy. Mosby, St. Louis, 1995

Leung KS et al (ed): An effective treatment of comminuted fractures of the distal radius. J Hand Surg 15A:11, 1990

McQueen MM et al: Hand and wrist function after external fixation of unstable distal radial fractures. Clin Orthop 285:200, 1992

Penning DW: Dynamic external fixation of distal radius fractures. Hand Clin 9:587, 1993

Riggs Jr SA, Cooney III WP: External fixation of complex hand and wrist fractures. J Trauma 23:332, 1983

Seitz WH: Complications and problems in the management of distal radius fractures. Hand Clin 10:117, 1994

Seitz WH: External fixation of distal radius fractures. Orthop Clin North Am 24:255, 1993

Appendix 36-1

Wrist Fractures and Types of Fixation

Type of Fracture	Type of Fixation	Healing Rate

A. Scaphoid fracture	Cast immobilization
	Closed internal fixation
	Open internal fixation
		Tubercle of
		  scaphoid 8–10 wk
		3 months or more need
		  union on radiography

B. Triquetrum fracture	Cast immobilization	6 weeks
C. Lunate fracture	Cast immobilization Closed internal fixation Open internal fixation	6–8 weeks
D. Hamate body fracture	Cast immobilization Closed internal fixation Open internal fixation	4–6 weeks
E. Trapezium fracture	Surgical reduction with internal fixation	4–6 weeks
F. Colle's fracture (distal radius and ulna styloid)	Closed reduction with cast Closed reduction with internal fixation Open reduction internal fixation	Undisplaced 4 weeks Displaced 4–6 weeks

G. Barton's fracture
  (distal radius)
	Open reduction internal
	  fixation with cast immobilization
		4–6 weeks

H. Smith's fracture (distal radius)	Closed reduction with cast Closed reduction with internal fixation Open reduction internal fixation	6 weeks
I. Comminuted intra-articular fractures of distal radius	Dynamic external fixation External fixation Open reduction internal fixation	8–10 weeks 6–8 weeks
J. Combinations of distal forearm and carpal bone fractures	Combination of internal and external fixation Closed and/or open reduction	6–8 weeks

Finger Fracture Rehabilitation

37

Gregory Hritcko

Hand fractures are a common problem, and the literature indicates secondary complications frequently develop when these injuries are viewed and treated as minor.[1] Foresight and prevention are the guiding principles during the initial stages of management. Range of motion (ROM) of adjacent, noninvolved joints should be initiated as early as possible in the acute injury phase. Splint immobilization generally requires the intrinsic plus position of wrist extension to 30 degrees, metacarpophalangeal (MCP) joints flexed to 70 degrees to 90 degrees, and interphalangeal (IP) joints in neutral 0 degrees to avoid joint contractures as a result of ligament shortening. General goals of hand therapy of preserving and maximizing function apply in the initial stage, as well as after fracture consolidation has been achieved.

An understanding of the anatomy, fracture healing process, and the technique selected by the surgeon will set the fundamental guidelines for the rehabilitation course. Review of the history and mechanism of the injury will offer insight to the complexity of the problems and may point to potential difficulties before they arise; for example, comminuted fractures are associated with soft tissue compromise leading to an increased potential for stiffness.[2] To optimize the end result, specific goals and interventions will be dictated by the type of fracture, location, degree of disruption, and management technique selected by the surgeon.

Fractures of the distal phalanx are reported as the most frequent of all hand fractures at a rate of 40 to 50 percent.[3] They most often involve the thumb and middle finger.[3] Common deformities include a tendon component (e.g., mallet finger with terminal extensor tendon avulsions and the flexor digitorum profundus avulsion fracture in the football jersey injury).

Middle phalanx fractures comprise 8 to 12 percent of hand fractures.[3] The muscle tendon units influence angulation patterns with the middle phalanx fracture. A fracture of the distal one-quarter will angulate apex volar secondary to the pull of the flexor digitorum superficialis. Proximal one-quarter fractures will commonly displace into a configuration with the apex dorsal because of the pull of the central slip of the extensor tendon. The midshaft fracture can angulate in either direction.[4,5]

Fifteen to 20 percent of hand fractures occur at the proximal phalanx level with the thumb and index finger frequently involved.[3] Midshaft proximal phalanx fractures are often spiral or oblique in configuration, which may shorten or rotate because of instability. The flexor tendon or the MCP joints may be compromised with the proximal base fracture and the proximal interphalangeal (PIP) joint may be involved with the distal neck or head fracture.[3–5]

It is beyond the scope of this book to address intra-articular fractures and the rehabilitation management of these injuries. Specific surgical interventions (e.g., Schenck dynamic traction or the Agee force couple) require specific therapy interventions. Refer to the current body of literature or discuss follow-up with the surgeon.

DEFINITION

Structural break in the continuity of a bone, epiphyseal plate, or cartilaginous joint surface (Fig. 37-1).

TREATMENT PURPOSE

Fractured phalanges need to be reduced in as near normal a position as possible. Many times this can be accomplished without open reduction. If this is so, then appropriate cast or splint immobilization is required, leaving free for movement as many of the unaffected joints as possible. Open reduction is used to stabilize a fracture with pins or plates so that realignment of the fragments is accomplished. The potential for early

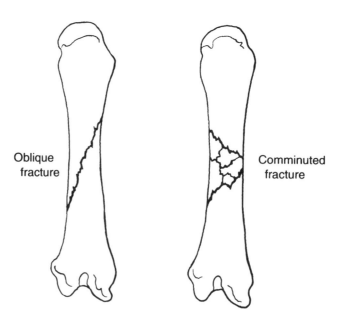

Oblique fracture

Comminuted fracture

Fig. 37-1. Common finger fractures are oblique and comminuted fractures.

mobilization exists in these cases; however, the surgery used to accomplish the task disrupts surrounding soft tissues. These soft tissues must be considered during the healing phase. Percutaneous pinning often can achieve satisfactory fracture alignment and stabilization with minimal interference to the soft tissues. This method is often used when possible.

TREATMENT GOALS

Preventive measures should be taken to preserve and maximize the function of the involved extremity. These measures should include all general goals of all hand therapy management. Specific goals will be dictated by the type of fracture, location, degree of disruption, reduction technique used by the surgeon, and stability of the reduction.

    I. Promote healing through maintaining/protecting reduction (i.e., immobilization splint).
    II. Maintain/increase ROM of noninvolved joints.
    III. Pain control.
    IV. Edema control.
    V. Restore and maximize the functional return of the involved extremity and joint.

NONOPERATIVE INDICATIONS/ PRECAUTIONS FOR THERAPY

    I. Indications: nondisplaced fractures requiring
      A. Splinting
      B. Edema control
      C. Limited passive/active range of motion (PROM or AROM) of noninvolved joints.
      D. Pain control
      E. Limited PROM or AROM of involved joints.
      F. Dynamic splinting
      G. Decreased strength/endurance.
    II. Precautions
      A. Associated concomitant soft tissue injury (neurovascular, tendon).
      B. Fracture stability, influenced by type of fracture, rate of healing, and pain level.
      C. Nonunion or delayed union of fracture site.

NONOPERATIVE THERAPY

    I. Distal phalanx fractures
      A. Tuft fractures
        1. Protective splint to prevent reinjury, worn for 2 to 4 weeks until fracture site is nontender (Fig. 37-2).
        2. Wound care as indicated by injury mechanism.
        3. AROM begins at 2 to 4 weeks, week 0 to 1 week if fracture is stable enough.[3,4]

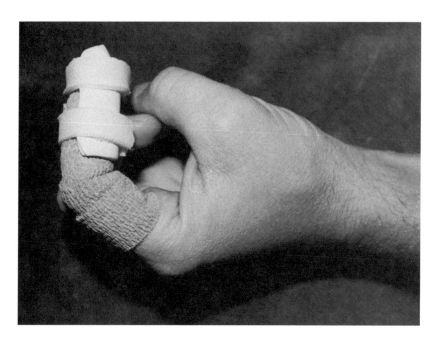

Fig. 37-2. Protective splint for a tuft fracture.

    4. PROM begins at 5 to 6 weeks.
    5. Strength/endurance building begins at 7 to 8 weeks.[3,4]
  B. Shaft fractures
    1. Protective/immobilization splint worn for 3 to 4 weeks.
    2. Wound care as indicated.
    3. AROM begins at 3 to 4 weeks.
    4. PROM begins at 5 to 7 weeks.
    5. Strength/endurance building at 8 weeks.[3,4]
 II. Middle phalanx fractures: nondisplaced
  A. Splinted in intrinsic plus position (Fig. 37-3). Immobilization should not exceed 3 weeks, avoiding PIP stiffness.[6] Buddy splinting may be a splint option requested by surgeon (Fig. 37-4).

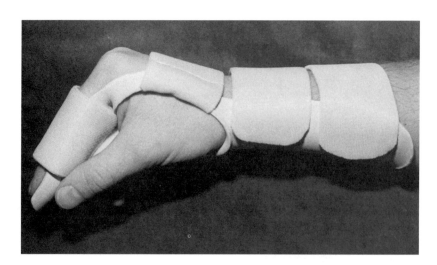

Fig. 37-3. Nondisplaced fractures may be splinted in an intrinsic plus position.

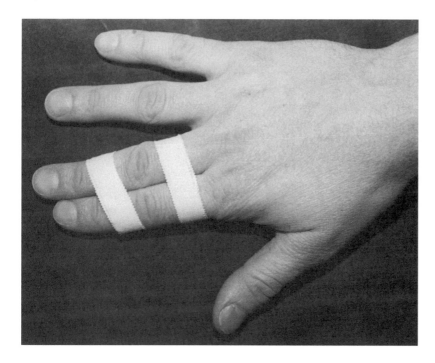

Fig. 37-4. Buddy splinting may be an option for nondisplaced fractures.

   B. AROM initiated when pain/edema subsides.
   C. 3 to 5 days for stable fracture.[4]
   D. 3 weeks for oblique or other unstable fracture.[4]
   E. PROM begins at 4 to 6 weeks.
   F. Strength/endurance building begins at 6 to 8 weeks.
III. Proximal phalanx fractures
   A. Nondisplaced extra-articular
      1. Splinted with buddy tape and AROM initiated immediately.[5]
      2. PROM begins at 5 to 7 weeks.[5]
      3. Strength/endurance building begins at 6 to 8 weeks.
   B. Nondisplaced intra-articular
      1. Splinted in "intrinsic plus" position for 2 to 3 weeks.
      2. AROM begins at 2 to 3 weeks.
      3. PROM begins at 4 to 8 weeks.
      4. Strength/endurance building begins at clinical union, 8 to 12 weeks.[5]

NONOPERATIVE COMPLICATIONS

  I. Distal phalanx fracture
     A. Infection
     B. Nailbed deformities
     C. Hypersensitivity
 II. Middle phalanx fracture
     A. Tendon adhesions and decreased excursion.
     B. Decreased joint mobility and stiffness.[4,5]

   III. Proximal phalanx fracture: decreased joint mobility and stiffness.[4,5]
   IV. General complications
      A. Infection
      B. Delayed union
      C. Malunion

POSTOPERATIVE INDICATIONS/ PRECAUTIONS FOR THERAPY

    I. Indications: displaced fractures requiring
      A. Splinting
      B. Edema control
      C. Limited AROM/PROM of noninvolved joints
      D. Pain
      E. Limited AROM/PROM of involved joints
      F. Dynamic splinting
      G. Decreased strength/endurance
   II. Precautions
      A. Concomitant soft tissue trauma
      B. Fracture stability
      C. Nonunion or delayed union of fracture site

POSTOPERATIVE THERAPY

    I. Distal phalanx fractures
      A. Shaft fractures surgically treated with percutaneous Kirschner wire (K-wire) stabilization (Fig. 37-5).
      B. Wound/pin care.
      C. AROM PIP joint begins at 3 to 5 days.
      D. AROM of distal interphalangeal (DIP) joint begins upon removal of K-wire at 3 to 6 weeks.[3,4,7]
      E. Protective extension splinting continues for 2 to 6 additional weeks.
      F. PROM initiated at 8 weeks.[3,4,7]
      G. Strength/endurance building initiated at 6 to 8 weeks.
   II. Displaced middle phalanx fractures: (Surgeon may select stabilizing or rigid fixation, which will guide therapy intervention.).
      A. Splinted in "intrinsic plus" position to support/protect reduction.
      B. Wound/pin care.
      C. AROM begins at 5 to 15 days at surgeon's recommendation; begin with gentle supported blocking exercise.[5]
      D. Strength/endurance building begins at 7 to 9 weeks.
   III. Displaced proximal phalanx fractures
      A. Splinted in "intrinsic plus" position.
      B. Wound/pin care

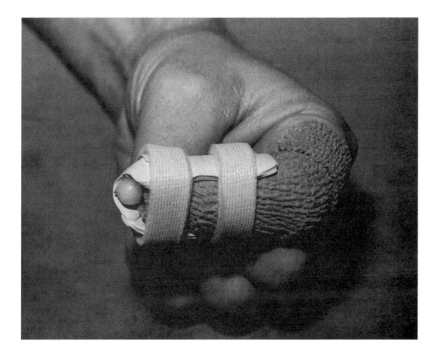

Fig. 37-5. Protective splinting for distal phalanx fracture stabilized with K-wire.

C. AROM initiated at 5 to 15 days at surgeon's recommendation and dependent upon rigid versus stabilizing fixation.[5]
D. PROM begins at 6 to 8 weeks.
E. Strength/endurance building begins at 8 to 10 weeks.

POSTOPERATIVE COMPLICATIONS

I. Distal phalanx fractures
   A. Infection
   B. Nailbed deformities
   C. Hypersensitivity
II. Middle phalanx fractures
   A. Decreased tendon excursion and adhesions.
   B. Decreased joint mobility and stiffness.[4,5]
III. Proximal phalanx fractures
   A. Associated soft tissue injuries
   B. Decreased joint mobility and stiffness.[4,5]
IV. General complications
   A. Infection
   B. Delayed union
   C. Malunion

EVALUATION TIMELINE

Appropriate baseline measures should be taken at initiation of specific exercises and repeated at 4- to 6-week intervals for documentation of progress:

I. Nonoperative

	AROM	PROM	Strength/Endurance
Distal phalanx			
Tuft fracture	2–4 weeks	5–6 weeks	7–8 weeks
Shaft fracture	3–4 weeks	5–7 weeks	8 weeks
Middle phalanx (nondisplaced)			
Stable	3–5 days	4–5 weeks	6–8 weeks
Oblique	3 weeks		
Proximal phalanx (nondisplaced)			
Extra-articular	Immediate	4–7 weeks	6–8 weeks
Intra-articular	2–3 weeks	4–5 weeks	8–12 weeks

II. Operative

	AROM	PROM	Strength/Endurance
Distal phalanx			
Shaft fracture PIP	3–5 days (postoperative)		
(With K-wire fixation) DIP	3–6 weeks (at time of K-wire removal)	8 weeks	8 weeks
Middle phalanx [displaced, open reduction, internal fixation (ORIF)]	5–15 days (postoperative)	6–8 weeks	7–9 weeks
Proximal phalanx (displaced, ORIF)	5–15 days (postoperative)	6–8 weeks	8–10 weeks

REFERENCES

1. Strickland JW, Stiechen JB, Klienman WB, Flynn M: Factors influencing digital performance after phalangeal fracture. p. 126. In Strickland JW, Stiechen JB (eds): Difficult Problems in Hand Surgery. Mosby, St. Louis, 1983
2. Meyer FN, Wilson RL: Management of non-articular fractures of the hand. p. 353. In Hunter JM, Mackin EJ, Callahan AD (eds): Rehabilitation of the Hand: Surgery and Rehabilitation. 4th Ed. Mosby, New York, 1995

3. Kasch MC, Taylor-Mullins PA, Fullenwider L (eds). Hand Therapy Review Course Study Guide. Garnor, NC, 1990

4. Beasley RW: Hand Injuries. WB Saunders, Philadelphia, 1987

5. Sorenson MK: Fractures of the wrist and hand. p. 191. In Moran G (ed): Hand Rehabilitation—Clinics in Physical Therapy. Vol. 9. Churchill Livingstone, New York, 1986

6. Flynn JE: Hand Surgery. Williams & Wilkins, Baltimore, 1982

7. Connolly JF (ed): Depalma's The Management of Fractures and Dislocations. 3rd Ed. WB Saunders, Philadelphia, 1987

SUGGESTED READINGS

Creighton JJ, Stiechen JB: Complications in phalangeal and metacarpal fracture management. In Mitchell MM (ed): Hand Clinics. Vol. 10. WB Saunders, Philadelphia, 1994

Jabaley ME, Freeland AE: Rigid internal fixation in the hand 104 cases. Plast Reconstr Surg 77:288, 1986

Melone CP: Rigid fixation of phalangeal and metacarpal fractures. Orthop Clin North Am 17:421, 1986

Packer JW, Colditz JC: Bone injuries: treatment and rehabilitation. p. 81. In Seyfor AE, Hueston JT (eds): Hand Clinics: Difficult Hand Fractures. WB Saunders, Philadelphia, 1986

Proximal Interphalangeal Joint Fracture Dislocation

38

Arlynne Pack Brown

Proximal interphalangeal (PIP) joint fracture dislocations are produced through axial compression on semiflexed or hyperextended digits. These forces usually result in dorsal dislocations and less commonly in volar dislocations.

PIP joint dislocations are described by two separate classification systems described by Eaton and Bowers.[1] Regardless of which classification system is used, fragments less than 30 percent of the articular surface are usually stable and managed with closed reduction techniques. Those joints with greater than 30 percent of the articular surface involved are usually unstable and require management with open reduction internal fixation techniques.

Stable joints are either secured with buddy tape to the appropriate adjacent digit or protected with an extension block splint or with a combination of both techniques. Active exercises are begun 3 weeks after injury and 1 week later progressed to passive exercises and dynamic splinting. Protective buddy splinting continues as indicated. Strengthening is progressed from approximately 4 weeks after injury while monitoring stability, edema, and pain.

Unstable joints can be managed using a variety of techniques ranging in complexity from closed reduction and volar plate arthroplasty to force couple splints and progressive dynamic traction splinting. The postoperative therapy for each technique is distinct and detailed later.

Possible complications for all PIP joint dislocations are the same for all methods of treatment: recurrent subluxations, infections, limited range of motion (ROM), traumatic arthritis, and adherence of extensor tendons.

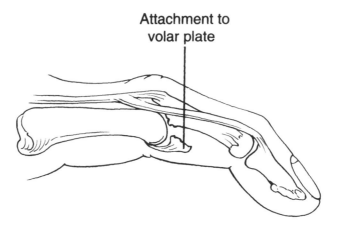

Fig. 38-1. Dorsal dislocation of PIP joint.

DEFINITION

    I. Dorsal dislocation: Middle phalanx moves dorsal in relation to proximal phalanx[1-3] (Fig. 38-1).
    II. Volar dislocation: Middle phalanx moves volar in relation to proximal phalanx. This is an uncommon injury that can present clinically as a boutonniere deformity (Fig. 38-2).

TREATMENT AND SURGICAL PURPOSE

The treatment and surgical purpose of managing a PIP joint fracture dislocation are to restore maximum active ROM (AROM) to the involved joint. The surgical techniques used to achieve the reduction of the fracture with dislocation vary with the surgeon's preferences and skills. The goal is to restore the joint surfaces as accurately as possible. This may require bone grafting using the distal radius as a donor site. The type of fixation may or may not allow joint motion. Several forms of traction (or distraction) devices are used. It is extremely important for the therapist to discuss with the surgeon the operative technique

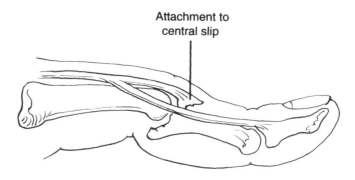

Fig. 38-2. Volar dislocation of PIP joint.

and plans for therapy. Close monitoring of each patient's individual care is mandatory for a good final result.

TREATMENT GOALS

   I. Promote maximum ROM.
   II. Minimize scarring.
   III. Prevent PIP joint flexion contracture.
   IV. Prevent recurrence of dislocation.

NONOPERATIVE INDICATIONS/ PRECAUTIONS FOR THERAPY

   I. Indications
      A. PIP joint fracture dislocation treated with closed reduction, buddy taping, and/or extension block splinting.
   II. Precautions
      A. Unstable reduction.

NONOPERATIVE THERAPY

Stable closed reduction (excluding volar plate arthroplasty).
   I. *Weeks 0 to 3:*
      A. Splints
         1. Buddy tape to appropriate adjacent digit (e.g., to radial digit if radial collateral ligament tear) (Fig. 38-3).
         2. Dorsal extension block splint (Fig. 38-4).
            a. Extension block splint options.[1]
               i. Tape Alumifoam to proximal phalanx and limit extension to 25 to 30 degrees.
               ii. Hand-based splint with extension block incorporated.
               iii. Depending on patient reliability and compliance, include block in a plaster cast/splint positioning wrist 30 to 40 degrees extension, metacarpophalangeal (MCP) joints 90 degrees flexion, PIP joint 25 degrees. Remember to tape to proximal phalanx to avoid rupture of central slip.[1, 3–5]
               iv. If required greater than 30 degrees PIP joint flexion to maintain stability initially, then decrease flexion by 25 percent each week.[6]
         3. Combination buddy tape and dorsal extension block splint.
      B. AROM into full flexion and to limits of extension block splint.[1]
   II. Week 3: Remove extension block splint.[4] Continue buddy taping and AROM.
   III. Week 4: Begin dynamic extension splint.[1]

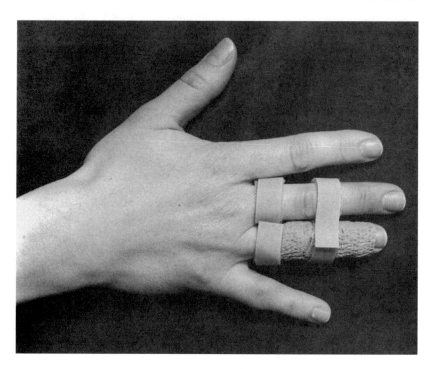

Fig. 38-3. Buddy tape to appropriate digit.

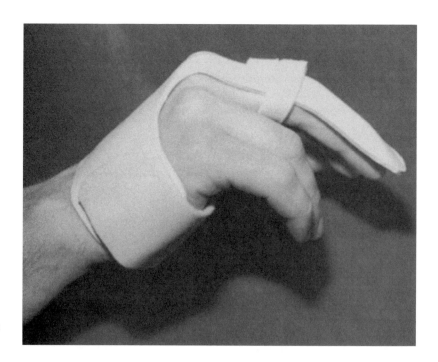

Fig. 38-4. Dorsal extension block splint.

NONOPERATIVE COMPLICATIONS

I. Progress to subluxation.
II. Loss of PIP joint ROM.
III. Permanent joint stiffness.

POSTOPERATIVE INDICATIONS/ PRECAUTIONS FOR THERAPY

I. Indications
   A. PIP joint fracture dislocation treated with open reduction internal fixation, Eaton volar plate arthroplasty, or Agee force couple traction splint.
II. Precautions
   A. Unstable reduction.
   B. Epiphyseal plate fractures.
   C. Internal or external fixation.

POSTOPERATIVE THERAPY

I. Unstable closed reduction or volar plate arthroplasty.
   A. Weeks 0 to 2: Immobilize with Kirschner wire (K-wire).
   B. Weeks 2 or 3: K-wire removal by surgeon.
      1. Begin extension block splint 25 degrees.
      2. Begin active simultaneous extension of the MCP, PIP, and distal interphalangeal (DIP) joints to limit of splint. Begin active blocked extension of the MCP, PIP, and DIP individual joints to patient tolerance.
   C. Week 3: pull out wire removed by surgeon. Begin active extension.
   D. Week 4: Begin progressive extension splinting with surgeon's approval. Begin light work with buddy taping.
II. Unstable acute fracture dislocations managed with Agee force couple splint (Fig. 38-5).
   A. Day 0 to 2: soft dressing.
   B. Day 2: discontinue dressing. Begin antibiotic ointment to pin sites. Begin AROM exercises. Follow "unstable closed reduction or volar plate arthroplasty" guidelines after force couple splint removed by surgeon.
III. Dynamic traction splinting and early passive ROM[7] (PROM) (Fig. 38-6).
   A. Weeks 0 to 3: Wear splint continuously. Move through complete arc of ROM five times, then leave in position of extreme flexion for 2 hours alternating with extreme extension for 2 hours. Perform blocked DIP joint AROM.
   B. Week 3: Remove splint, begin AROM wrist. Replace splint and continue with ROM described for weeks 0 to 3.

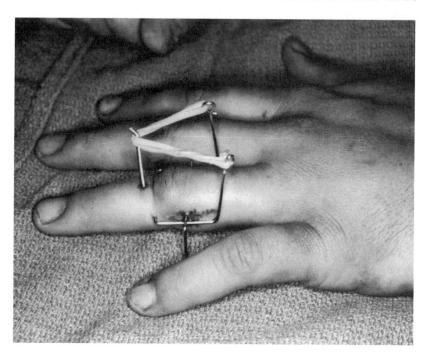

Fig. 38-5. Unstable acute fracture dislocations managed by Agee force couple splint.

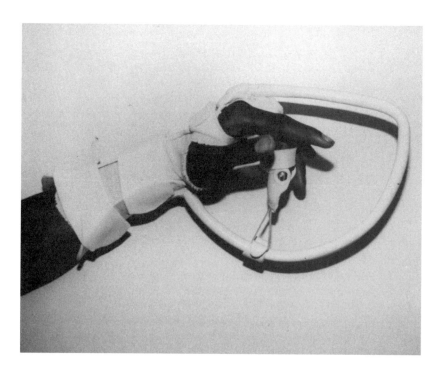

Fig. 38-6. Dynamic traction splinting allows for early PROM.

C. Week 4: Begin active, blocked ROM PIP and DIP.

D. Weeks 4.5 to 8: Remove arc splint. Fabricate protective hand-based splint. Begin composite AROM.

E. Splint: basic features

1. Molded splint extending dorsally from proximal forearm to PIP joint with wrist and MCP joints in "functional position."

2. Modified arc with axis in line with that of PIP joint.

3. Mold a "Dutch-girl's hat" to the shape of the arc of Dowing for full arc of motion. Rubberbands attach to this arc for traction. See Schenck's 1986[7] article for more details.

4. Amount of traction is estimated based on patient comfort and physical principles and then checked on radiograph by surgeon.

POSTOPERATIVE COMPLICATIONS

I. Recurrent subluxations.[2,4]

II. Infections.[2]

III. Loss of DIP joint flexion secondary to flexor tendon adhesions.[2]

IV. Permanent joint stiffness.[2]

V. Traumatic arthritis.[2]

VI. Adherence of extensor tendon.[4]

EVALUATION TIMELINE FOR NONOPERATIVE THERAPY

I. Week 0 to 3

A. Measure and begin active composite ROM to limits of extension block splint and/or buddy tape.

B. Active blocked flexion PIP and DIP.

C. Passive composite and blocked flexion PIP and DIP.

II. Week 3: Measure and begin active composite ROM without splint.

III. Week 4: Measure and begin passive composite and blocked extension ROM.

IV. Weeks 6 to 8: Measure and begin grip strength.

REFERENCES

1. Lubahn JD: Dorsal fracture dislocations of the proximal interphalangeal joint. Hand Clin 4:15, 1988

2. Agee JM: Unstable fracture dislocations of the proximal interphalangeal joint. Clin Orthop Relat Res 214:101, 1987

3. Isani A: Small joint injuries requiring surgical treatment. Orthop Clin North Am 17:407, 1986

4. Eaton RG, Malerich MM: Volar plate arthroplasty of the proximal interphalangeal joint: a review of ten years' experience. J Hand Surg 5:250, 1980

5. Wilson RL, Carter MS: Joint injuries in the hand: preservation of proximal interphalangeal joint function. p. 171. In Hunter JM (ed): Rehabilitation of the Hand. 3rd. Ed. Mosby, Philadelphia, 1978

6. McElfresh EC, Dobyns JH, O'Brien ET: Management of fracture-dislocation of the proximal interphalangeal joints by extension block splinting. J Bone Joint Surg 54:1705, 1972

7. Schenck RR: Dynamic traction and early passive movement for fractures of the proximal interphalangeal joint. J Hand Surg 1A:850, 1986

Metacarpal and Proximal Interphalangeal Joint Capsulectomy

39

Rebecca J. Saunders

Capsulectomies of the metacarpophalangeal (MCP) and proximal interphalangeal (PIP) joints are performed to improve motion and functional use of stiff joints with normal articular surfaces. These procedures are necessary when stiff joints fail to respond to a conservative treatment program including splinting and exercise.

Many anatomic structures within the finger may limit joint motion. These structures are listed below.

I. Limited flexion (extension contracture).
   A. Scar contracture of skin over the dorsum of the finger
   B. Contracted long extensor muscle or adherent extensor tendon.
   C. Contracted interosseus muscle or adherent interosseus tendon.
   D. Contracted capsular ligament, particularly the collateral ligaments.
   E. Bony block or exostosis.
   F. Flexor tendon adherence.
II. Limited extension
   A. Scar of skin on the volar surface of the finger.
   B. Contraction of the superficial fascia in the finger, as in Dupuytren's contracture.
   C. Contraction of the flexor–tendon sheath within the finger.
   D. Contracted flexor muscle or adherent flexor tendon.
   E. Contraction of the volar plate of the capsular ligament.
   F. Adherence of the collateral ligaments with the finger in the flexed position.
   G. Bony block or exostosis.[1]

These multiple factors need to be evaluated clinically and at the time of surgery. Capsulectomies are frequently performed concurrently with other surgical procedures (e.g., intrinsic releases, flexor, and/or extensor tenolysis). To facilitate effective postoperative management the therapist should obtain a copy of the operative report. Curtis has stated that "the results seem to indicate that the more anatomical structures are involved in the limitation of motion, the poorer is the end result."[1]

The therapist's role in postoperative management of capsulectomies begins before surgery. Patient education should emphasize what will be expected of the patient postoperatively and why their postoperative performance is critical in obtaining the maximum functional benefit from the surgery.[2] As Curtis has stated, "one should not expect to restore function completely by this procedure, but one can expect to improve it."[1]

Successful management of the postcapsulectomy patient requires skillful observation, constant reassessment, and adaptation on the part of the therapist as well as a motivated and compliant patient. Maximum gains in range of motion (ROM) are usually obtained 3 to 5 months postoperatively. Patients requiring fewer surgical maneuvers, however, may continue to gain ROM for up to 6 to 8 months.[3]

DEFINITION

I. MCP capsulectomy: surgical release of dorsal and/or volar joint capsule and collateral ligaments.
II. PIP capsulectomy: surgical release of the dorsal and/or volar joint capsule and collateral ligaments.

SURGICAL PURPOSE

I. MCP capsulectomy: to restore metacarpal phalangeal joint motion where either a flexion or extension contracture exists. The capsular structures have contracted or are locally adherent to other surrounding elements (Fig. 39-1). These structures are surgically released and partially excised. Joint stability must be maintained and passive ROM (PROM) obtained at the time of surgery is approximately the active range that can be expected with postoperative wound healing.
II. PIP capsulectomy: to restore motion to the joint that has less than a 45 degree range. The tissues surrounding the PIP joint must be considered as contributing to the contracture (e.g., skin, tendons, joint capsule, and joint surfaces) (Fig. 39-2). Tissue equilibrium (scar maturity) must be present before surgery. Offending scar and capsule are released or excised, but joint stability is maintained. PROM achieved at the time of surgery approximates the expected active ROM (AROM) with healing.

TREATMENT GOALS

I. MCP capsulectomy: increase PROM and AROM of the MCPs to approximately 60 degrees to 70 degrees flexion and to increase functional use of the hand.

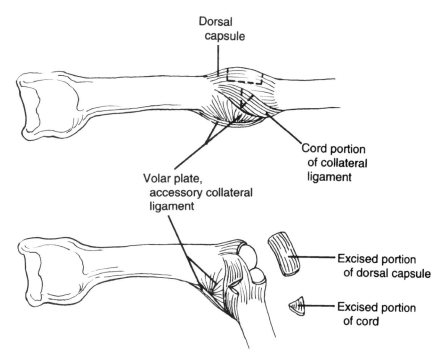

Fig. 39-1. Anatomy of MCP joint structures.

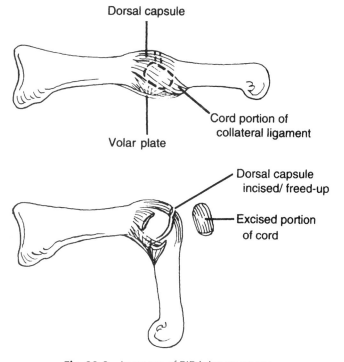

Fig. 39-2. Anatomy of PIP joint structures.

II. PIP capsulectomy: restore AROM and PROM of PIP joint flexion and extension.

III. Functional goal postoperatively for both procedures: achieve AROM equal to the PROM present after the surgical release.

POSTOPERATIVE INDICATIONS/ PRECAUTIONS FOR THERAPY

I. MCP capsulectomy: if tendons are adherent and also limiting flexion, a concurrent tenolysis may have been performed. (See the operative note.)

II. PIP capsulectomy: this procedure is often performed in combination with other surgical procedures (e.g., tenotomy of contracted interossei, flexor, and/or extensor tenolysis). The operative report should be reviewed to ensure adequate protection and treatment of the involved anatomic structures.

   A. Precautions
      1. Intrinsic releases
         Splinting should include an intrinsic stretch splint and instruction in stretching exercises.
      2. Extensor tenolysis with volar capsulectomy secondary to flexion contracture requires dynamic extension splinting to protect the weakened and frequently stretched extensor tendon while promoting active flexion; static extension splinting is required at night.

POSTOPERATIVE THERAPY

I. General treatment principles for capsulectomies secondary to limitations of flexion and/or extension

   A. Edema control

   B. Pain management

   C. Initiation of AROM as per doctor's orders (usually within 24 to 48 hours of surgery).

   D. PROM, instruction in gentle, passive stretching.

   E. Scar management

   F. Splinting

      1. An appointment for postoperative therapy should be made when the surgery is scheduled.

      2. Dynamic splints are used during the day as an adjunct to the patient's active exercise program (and to protect weakened structures).

      3. Static progressive splints are used at night to maintain gains in ROM and provide a prolonged gentle stretch to the involved soft tissues.

4. All splints need to be monitored and adjusted frequently, as the soft tissues respond to the stresses applied through active and passive exercise. The patient should be provided with detailed wearing instructions and precautions.

5. Splinting is continued until the patient is able to maintain the ROM present postoperatively with AROM and PROM (approximately 3 to 5 months).

6. When passive motion exceeds active motion the emphasis on active exercise should be increased to overcome tendon weakness or adherence.

G. Functional activities and light use of the hand should be incorporated early to promote use of available ROM and to increase strength.

H. Grip strengthening can be initiated at 6 weeks postoperatively; however, if a concurrent tenolysis was performed, it is deferred until 8 to 10 weeks postoperatively.

II. Postoperative management of MCP capsulectomy

A. Begin AROM 1 to 3 days postoperatively as per doctor's orders. Active exercises should include blocked and full excursion flexion and extension.

B. PROM: instruction in *gentle* passive stretching.

C. Splinting

1. Instruction in skin care and routine checking for pressure areas to prevent skin breakdown.

2. Static splint MCPs placed near the limit of obtainable flexion with the wrist in extension to be used at night; this needs to be monitored closely and adjusted frequently as flexion increases; continue night splinting until ROM goals are met and maintained for a few weeks (Fig. 39-3).

3. Dynamic splinting to increase MCP flexion should be used intermittently during the day. Splint use should be followed by active exercise to help maintain gains in PROM achieved by splinting (Fig. 39-4).

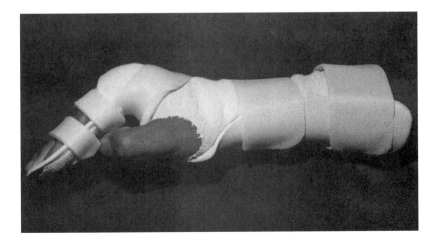

Fig. 39-3. Postoperative night positioning for MCP capsulectomy.

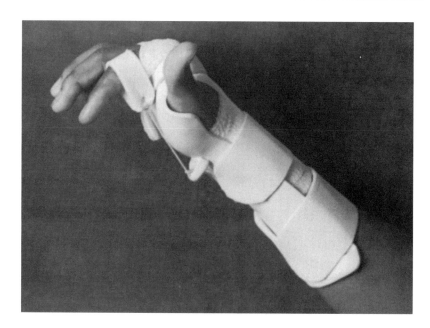

Fig. 39-4. Dynamic MCP flexion splint used intermittently during day.

    4. If an extension lag is present, dynamic flexion splinting should be alternated with dynamic extension splinting (Fig. 39-5).

D. Functional activities should be promoted to utilize gains in ROM and to increase strength.

E. Muscle re-education of wrist extensors may be necessary, as patients may have been substituting their digital extensors for wrist extension, and this pattern can contribute to stiffness in extension of MCPs and also interfere with grip strength.[2]

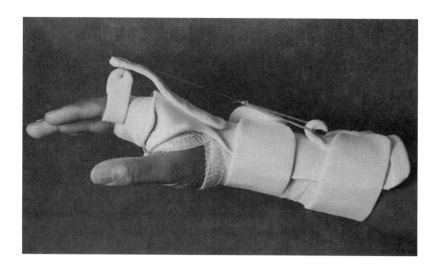

Fig. 39-5. Dynamic extension splint should be used during day if an extension lag is present.

F. Continuous passive motion (CPM) can be a useful adjunct to help decrease postoperative pain and edema while increasing PROM.

III. Postoperative management of PIP capsulectomy
   A. PIP capsulectomy secondary to extension contracture.
      1. Dynamic flexion and extension splinting are alternated during the day (ratio of flexion vs. extension splinting is determined by the available ROM).
      2. AROM should emphasize blocked active flexion and extension exercises.
      3. Static night splint position is determined by available range and anatomic structures involved.
   B. PIP capsulectomy secondary to flexion contracture.
      1. Depending on the severity of the contracture and the surgeon's preferred method, the PIP joint may be pinned in extension postoperatively with initiation of exercise and splinting deferred until pin removal at 1 to 2 weeks postoperatively.
      2. The static splint maintains PIP joint extension at night and in between active exercise sessions (Fig. 39-6).
      3. Alternate dynamic extension and flexion splinting can be used during the day (as indicated by ROM) (Figs. 39-7 and 39-8).

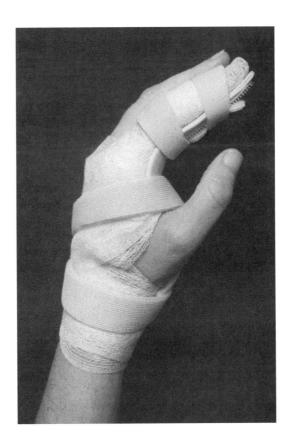

Fig. 39-6. Static PIP extension splint used at night and between active exercises.

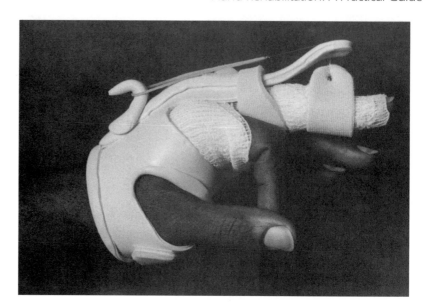

Fig. 39-7. Dynamic extension splint can be used during day for increasing extension.

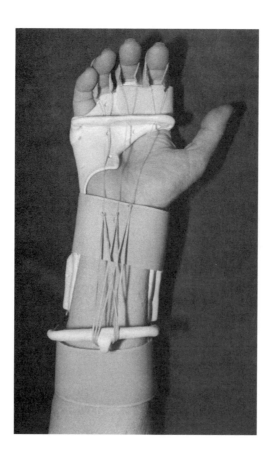

Fig. 39-8. Dynamic flexion splint can be used during day for increasing flexion.

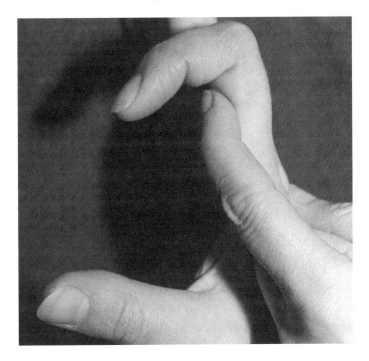

Fig. 39-9. Blocked ROM exercises should be included in exercise program.

4. An active exercise program should include blocked PIP flexion and extension (Fig. 39–9). If an extension lag is present it is important to protect it, via splinting, and prevent further loss of extension as ROM into flexion improves. Failure to monitor PIP joint extension closely can result in recurrence of the flexion contracture.

5. The oblique retinacular ligament may have become tight secondary to the flexion contracture, and stretching exercises should be initiated (Fig. 39–10).

POSTOPERATIVE COMPLICATIONS

   I. Infection
  II. Limitations in ROM secondary to edema and/or pain.
 III. Weakness of previously adherent tendons.
 IV. Joint subluxation secondary to excessive ligament excision.
  V. Reflex sympathetic dystrophy.

EVALUATION TIMELINE

   I. Preoperative evaluation 1 to 2 weeks before surgery to include
      A. AROM/PROM
      B. Grip and pinch strength.
      C. Sensation

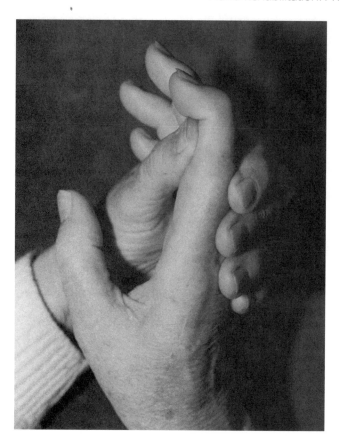

Fig. 39-10. Stretching exercise for oblique retinacular ligament.

      D. Functional assessment of activities of daily living, vocational and avocational activities.

II. Postoperative evaluation

    A. Initial AROM postoperatively.

    B. Weekly re-evaluation of AROM/PROM.

    C. At 6 to 8 weeks: evaluation of ROM, sensation, and strength. If a concurrent tenolysis was performed, evaluation of strength is deferred until 8 to 10 weeks postoperatively.

REFERENCES

1. Curtis RM: Capsulectomy of the interphalangeal joints of the fingers. J Bone Joint Surg (Am) 36:1219, 1954
2. Laseter G: Postoperative management of capsulectomies. p. 364. In Hunter JM, Schneider LH, Mackin EJ, Callahan AD (eds): Rehabilitation of the Hand. 3rd Ed. Mosby, St. Louis, 1990
3. Gould JS, Nicholson BG: Capsulectomy of the metacarpophalangeal and proximal interphalangeal joints. J Hand Surg 4:482, 1979

SUGGESTED READINGS

Campbell's Operative Orthopaedics. 7th Ed. Mosby, St. Louis, 1987

Cannon N: Postoperative management of metacarpophalangeal joint capsulectomies. p. 1173. In Hunter JM, Mackin EJ, Callahan AD (eds): Rehabilitation of the Hand: Surgery and Therapy. 4th Ed. Mosby, St. Louis, 1995

Diao E, Eaton G: Total collateral ligament excision for contractures of the proximal interphalangeal joint. J Hand Surg 18A:395, 1993

Flowers KR: Edema: differential management based on stages of wound healing. p. 87. In Hunter JM, Mackin EJ, Callahan AD (eds): Rehabilitation of the Hand: Surgery and Therapy. 4th Ed. Mosby, St. Louis, 1995

Flynn MD: Hand Surgery. 3rd Ed. Williams & Wilkins, Baltimore, 1982

Green DP (ed): Operative Hand Surgery. 2nd Ed. Churchill Livingstone, New York, 1988

Innis PC, Clark GL, Curtis RM: Management of the stiff hand. p. 1129. In Hunter JM, Mackin EJ, Callahan AD (eds): Rehabilitation of the Hand: Surgery and Therapy. 4th Ed. Mosby, St. Louis, 1995

McEntee P: Therapists management of the stiff hand. p. 328. In Hunter JM, Schneider LH, Mackin EJ, Callahan AD (eds): Rehabilitation of the Hand. 3rd Ed. Mosby, St. Louis, 1990

Young VL, Wray RC, Jr, Weeks PM: The surgical management of stiff joints in the hand. Plast Reconstr Surg 62:835, 1978

Metacarpophalangeal Joint Arthroplasty

40

Lorie Theisen

Metacarpophalangeal (MCP) joint flexible implant arthroplasty is frequently indicated for patients with rheumatoid arthritis. Pain, joint instability, and deformities are common problems. Typically, in rheumatoid arthritis, ulnar drift of the fingers and subluxation of the MCP joint occur. Radial deviation of the metacarpals secondary to wrist malalignment is thought to cause the ulnar drift deformity. Other causes include posture, gravitational forces, and dynamic flexion forces.[1-3]

In flexible implant arthroplasty the term *implant* refers to a flexible Silastic spacer rather than a joint. One of the main functions of the spacer is to maintain alignment and spacing during the early stages of healing and rehabilitation. Early motion is important in promoting the development of a fibrous joint capsule. The process whereby the implant acts as a spacer to support the newly forming fibrous capsule is the encapsulation process.[4-7] Early protected motion ensures a greater range of motion, assists in decreasing edema, promotes an organized arrangement of collagen fibers, and prevents malalignment.

DEFINITION

A surgical formation or reformation of the MCP joints, typically a flexible implant, is used (Fig. 40-1).

SURGICAL PURPOSE

To restore skeletal alignment and tendon repositioning for more effective and efficient finger function. Flexible implant arthroplasty is most commonly used for patients with rheumatoid arthritis. The surgery is also

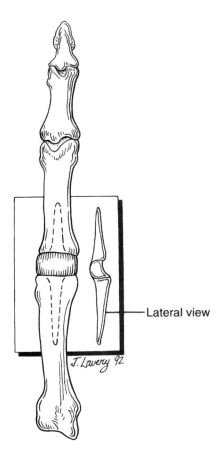

Lateral view

J. Lowery 92

Fig. 40-1. Views of implant.

performed in cases of other types of arthritic conditions resulting from trauma, infection, or systemic diseases. The silicone implant acts primarily as a bone spacer. Soft tissue reconstruction around the joint may include collateral ligament repair and extensor tendon realignment. Postoperative therapy and monitoring are integral parts of the treatment to ensure a satisfactory result. Greatly improved appearance of the hand is also achieved.

TREATMENT GOALS

    I. Monitor wound healing.
    II. Decrease edema.
    III. Prevent scar adherence.
    IV. Active MCP flexion to 70 degrees and extension to neutral.
    V. Neutral alignment of each digit with the corresponding metacarpal.
    VI. Prevent rotational deformities.

POSTOPERATIVE INDICATIONS/ PRECAUTIONS FOR THERAPY

I. Indications: MCP arthroplasty with flexible implant.
II. Precautions
   A. Extensive reconstruction of soft tissues, limited bone stock, or arthrodesis of adjacent joints may require a delay in initiating postoperative rehabilitation and may require additional protective splinting during the postoperative rehabilitation.
   B. Delay in wound healing that may be due to medical conditions and/or nonsteroidal anti-inflammatory drug or steroid use.
   C. Presence of osteoporosis.
   D. Greater than expected postoperative pain may indicate a flare-up of rheumatoid arthritis or infection.

POSTOPERATIVE THERAPY

I. 2 to 6 days postoperatively: the bulky dressing is removed and a dynamic MCP extension splint is applied over a lightly padded dressing (Fig. 40-2). The surgeon should be consulted if there is any question about the timing of the first visit. The pull of the slings is full MCP extension when at rest and appropriate tension to allow active MCP flexion. Keep in mind that the final goal is 70 degrees

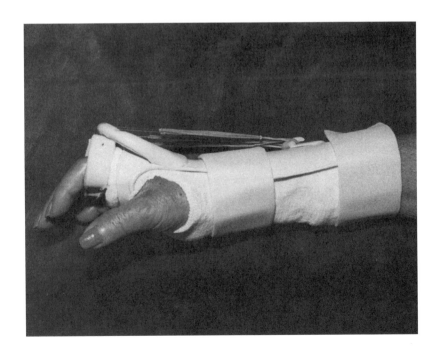

Fig. 40-2. Dynamic extension splint for postoperative treatment.

MCP flexion. The slings should also pull in approximately 15 degrees of radial direction to prevent ulnar forces. Interphalangeal (IP) extension blocks or troughs to prevent proximal interphalangeal (PIP) flexion during active MCP flexion exercises may be applied. If the troughs are applied volarly, care should be taken so that the digits are not positioned in an ulnar direction. Dorsally applied troughs may be easier to apply correctly. The dynamic splint is worn continuously (a static splint may be fabricated for night use) (Fig. 40-3) and active MCP flexion exercises performed intermittently throughout the waking hours.

II. 2 to 3 weeks postoperatively: MCP flexion assists (e.g., dynamic flexion splinting) may be initiated for intermittent use throughout the day. The MCP flexion splint should not pull the fingers in an ulnar direction. It is important to work diligently to obtain MCP extension and flexion goals in the first 3 weeks.[8,9]

III. 6 weeks postoperatively: dynamic MCP extension splinting is gradually tapered to night splinting only, with the following exceptions:
A. Presence of MCP extension lag.
B. Presence of MCP flexion contracture. In these cases continue splinting for the existing deformities. Initiate appropriate activities of daily living (ADL) and education on joint protection techniques.

IV. 8 to 10 weeks: mild isometric resistive exercises may be initiated, if ulnar forces are avoided. Isometric exercises may be useful in preventing ulnar forces.

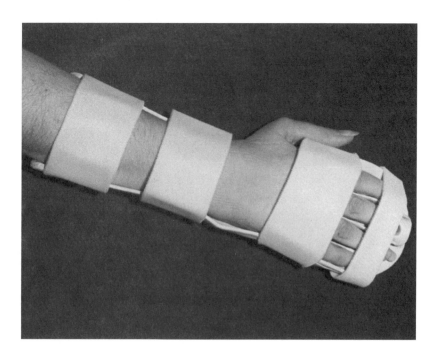

Fig. 40-3. Static positioning splint.

POSTOPERATIVE COMPLICATIONS

I. Pronation deformity or medial rotation may occur. To resolve this deformity, additional outriggers to provide a rotational force at the MCP joint may be necessary. The combined pull of a force couple (force couple is two equal and opposite forces that act along parallel lines)[9] may be necessary. The force couple is obtained by applying another outrigger to the digit with a pronation tendency. The combined forces produce a force in supination direction of the digit and allow MCP extension and flexion.[10]

II. Extension contracture at the fifth digit may occur. Therefore, the dynamic splinting and range of motion (ROM) programs should be carefully monitored. Tension on the dynamic MCP portion may need to be reduced for the fifth digit.

III. Dislocation or fracture of implant may occur.

IV. Slow healing with steroid medication (wound care precautions).

EVALUATION TIMELINE

I. 2 to 7 days postoperatively: initial assessment including active ROM measurement of the MCP joints.

II. Reassessment of ROM every week thereafter.

III. 8 to 10 weeks: grip strength using a modified blood pressure cuff may be initiated.[11]

REFERENCES

1. Flatt A: Care of the Rheumatoid Hand. 4th Ed. Mosby, St. Louis, 1983
2. Smith RR, Kaplan E: Rheumatoid deformities at the MCP joints. J Bone Joint Surg 49A:31, 1967
3. Hakstan R, Tubiana R: Ulnar deviation of the fingers: the role of joint structure and function. J Bone Joint Surg 49A:299, 1967
4. Flatt AS: Restoration of rheumatoid finger joint function. J Bone Joint Surg 45A:753, 1961
5. Swanson A: Flexible implant arthroplasty for arthritis finger joints. J Bone Joint Surg 54A:435, 1972
6. Swanson A, Swanson G, Leonard J: Postoperative rehabilitation programs in flexible implant arthroplasty of the digits. p. 912. In Hunter J (ed): Rehabilitation of the Hand. 3rd Ed. Mosby, St. Louis, 1990
7. Leonard J, Swanson A, Swanson G: Post-operative care for patients with silastic finger joint implants. 4th Ed. Dow Corning Corporation, Midland, MI, 1985
8. Madden J, Devore G, Arem A: A rational post-operative management program for metacarpophalangeal joint implant arthroplasty. J Hand Surg 2:358, 1977
9. Swanson A, Swanson G, Leonard J: Postoperative rehabilitation programs in flexible implant arthroplasty of the digits. p. 912. In Hunter J (ed): Rehabilitation of the Hand. 3rd Ed. Mosby, St. Louis, 1990

10. Devore G, Muhleman C, Sasarita S: Management of pronation deformity in metacarpophalangeal joint implant arthroplasty. J Hand Surg 11A:859, 1986
11. Melvin J: Evaluation of muscle strength. p. 291. In: Rheumatic Disease Occupational Therapy and Rehabilitation. 2nd Ed. FA Davis, Philadelphia, 1982

SUGGESTED READINGS

Aren A, Madden J: Effects of stress on healing wounds: intermittent noncyclical tension. J Surg Res 20:93, 1976

Beckenbaugh R, Dobyns J, Linscheid R: Review and analysis of silicone—rubber metacarpophalangeal implants. J Bone Joint Surg 58A:483, 1976

Bieber E, Weiland A, Volence Dowling S: Silicone rubber implant arthroplasty of the metacarpophalangeal joints for rheumatoid arthritis. J Bone Joint Surg 68A:206, 1986

Bryant M: Wound healing. Clin Symp 29:2, 1977

Ehrlich G: Rehabilitation Management of Rheumatic Conditions. 2nd Ed. Williams & Wilkins, Baltimore, 1986

El-Gammal TA, Blair W: Motion after metacarpophalangeal joint reconstruction in rheumatoid disease. J Hand Surg 18:504, 1993

Gardner R, Mowat A: Wound healing after operations on patients with rheumatoid arthritis. J Bone Joint Surg 55B:134, 1973

Kirschenbaum D, Schneider LH, Adams DC, Cody RP: Arthroplasty of the metacarpophalangeal joints with use of silicone-rubber implants in patients who have rheumatoid arthritis. J Bone Joint Surg Am 75:3, 1993

Kloth L, McCulloch J, Feedar J: Wound Healing: Alternatives in Management. FA Davis, Philadelphia, 1990

Lundborg G, Branemark PI, Carlsson I: Metacarpophalangeal joint arthroplasty based on the osseointegration concept. J Hand Surg 18:693, 1993

Melvin J: Rheumatic Disease in the Adult and Child. 3rd Ed. FA Davis, Philadelphia, 1982

Peimer CA, Medige J, Eckert BS et al: Reactive synovitis after silicone arthroplasty. J Hand Surg II:624, 1986

Stephens J, Pratt N, Parks B: The reliability and validity of the Tekdyne hand dynamometer: part I. J Hand Therapy 9:10, 1996

Stephens J, Pratt N, Michlovitz S: The reliability and validity of the Tekdyne hand dynamometer: part II. J Hand Therapy 9:18, 1996

Stothard J, Thompson AE, Sherris D: Correction of ulnar drift during silastic metacarpophalangeal joint arthroplasty. J Hand Surg 16:61, 1991

Swanson AB, Swanson GG, Leonard JB: Postoperative rehabilitation programs in flexible implant arthroplasty of the digits. In Hunter JM, Mackin EJ, Callahan AD (eds): Rehabilitation of the Hand: Surgery and Therapy. 4th Ed. Mosby, St. Louis, 1995

Swanson AB, Swanson GG, Winfield DC: The pronated index finger deformity in the rheumatoid hand. Bull Hosp J Dis Orthop Inst 44:498, 1989

Utsinger P, Zuaifler N, Ehrlich G: Rheumatoid Arthritis Etiology, Diagnosis, and Management. JB Lippincott, Philadelphia, 1989

Vahuanen V, Viljakka T: Silicone rubber implant arthroplasty of the metacarpophalangeal joint in rheumatoid arthritis: a follow-up study of 32 patients. J Hand Surg 11A:333, 1986

Proximal Interphalangeal and Distal Interphalangeal Joint Arthroplasty

41

Lorie Theisen

Flexible implant arthroplasty may be indicated for the proximal interphalangeal (PIP) or the distal interphalangeal (DIP) joints of the digits. PIP or DIP joint arthroplasty is indicated in the presence of pain, stiffness, deformities, instability about a joint, and loss of cartilage. These findings may be a sequela of osteoarthritis, rheumatoid arthritis, or trauma (Fig. 41-1).

An acceptable alternative procedure to flexible implant arthroplasty of the distal joints is arthrodesis. The advantages and disadvantages of each procedure are weighed carefully by the surgeon. Because hand function is significantly limited by a decrease in range of motion (ROM) at the PIP joints, particularly of the ulnar fingers, arthroplasty of the PIP joint is often preferred over arthrodesis. Hand function is only minimally limited by a decrease in DIP joint ROM; therefore, arthrodesis is often preferred at the DIP joint. Arthroplasty of the DIP joint is indicated where ROM as well as pain relief is necessary.

DEFINITION

A surgical formation or reformation of the PIP or DIP joints.

SURGICAL PURPOSE

The surgical management of acquired or post-traumatic arthritis of the PIP or DIP joints can improve function and joint alignment. Two basic types of arthroplasty can be used: Silastic joint spacers or a soft tissue interpositional joint spacer. Relief of pain and improvement of joint motion is of primary importance in undertaking these operations.

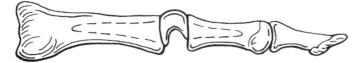

Fig. 41-1. Flexible implant arthroplasty of a PIP joint.

TREATMENT GOALS

The usual postoperative treatment goals regarding wound healing, edema control, and scar management apply. The encapsulated process and associated rehabilitation principles described in postoperative guidelines for metacarpophalangeal (MCP) joint arthroplasty also apply. Specifically, following PIP arthroplasty of the ring and small fingers the goal is pain-free active ROM (AROM) to 70 degrees flexion and neutral extension. For the index and middle fingers, less flexion is acceptable. Following DIP arthroplasty, the goal is 30 degrees flexion and neutral extension. Tendencies toward deformities such as boutonniere or swan neck should be addressed. Finally, the surgeon should be contacted if there is any question regarding joint stability and progression of the mobilization phase of rehabilitation.

POSTOPERATIVE INDICATIONS/ PRECAUTIONS FOR THERAPY

    I. Indications
       A. Rehabilitation is indicated following surgical reformation of a joint and surgical implant of a flexible Silastic spacer.
   II. Precautions
       A. The initiation of the remobilization program depends on the stability of the joint. Consult the physician about the timing of the ROM exercise program.
       B. Additional surgical procedures, such as ligament repair, tendon repositioning or reconstruction, tenolysis, or volar plate release may require adherence to additional rehabilitation principles and precautions.

POSTOPERATIVE THERAPY

    I. PIP arthroplasty
       A. For a preoperative stiff PIP joint requiring joint release procedures.
          1. 3 to 5 days postoperatively begin AROM of the PIP joint, avoiding any lateral deviation.
          2. Continuous static extension splinting (Fig. 41-2), except during exercise, for 6 weeks postoperatively. Alternatively,

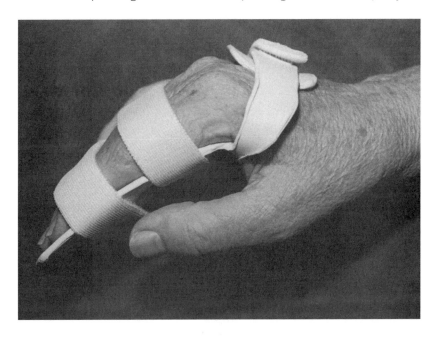

Fig. 41-2. Static PIP extension splint may be used following arthroplasty for a stiff PIP joint.

dynamic PIP extension splinting with intermittent active flexion in the splint may be used. The dynamic splint should be designed to control lateral forces (Fig. 41-3).

3. Dynamic flexion splinting, to gain 70 degrees, may be initiated after the third week postoperatively (Fig. 41-4).

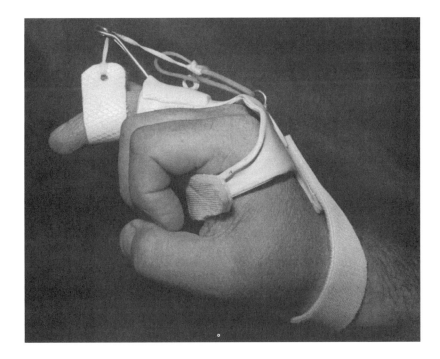

Fig. 41-3. Dynamic PIP extension splint may be used following arthroplasty for a stiff PIP joint.

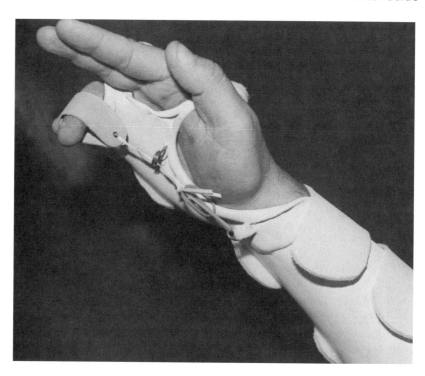

Fig. 41-4. Dynamic flexion splinting may be used to improve PIP flexion.

B. For a boutonniere deformity, the main goal is to maintain PIP extension and DIP flexion.
   1. Maintain static protective splinting with the PIP joint in full extension and continue for 3 to 6 weeks postoperatively. Active DIP flexion exercises with the PIP joint extended are indicated to maintain the oblique retinacular ligament length.
   2. 10 to 14 days postoperatively: active flexion and extension exercises of the PIP joint are initiated with the MCP joint in extension. Static extension splinting continues with intermittent AROM exercises up to 10 weeks postoperatively.
   3. Buddy splinting may be indicated to protect against lateral forces (Fig. 41-5).
C. For a swan-neck deformity, the main goal during the postoperative rehabilitation process is to maintain PIP flexion and DIP extension.
   1. 0 to 10 days postoperatively: continue digital static extension splinting with the PIP in 10 degrees to 20 degrees of flexion and DIP in full extension.
   2. 10 to 14 days postoperatively: initiate AROM. During exercise maintain 10 degrees of flexion at the PIP joint, and avoid extreme flexion at the DIP joint.
   3. 14 days postoperatively: initiate gentle passive exercises in flexion and extension.[1,2]

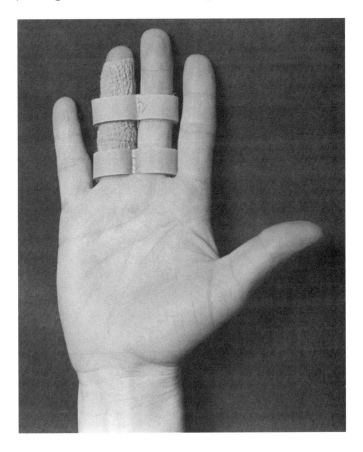

Fig. 41-5. Buddy splint may be used following arthroplasty for a boutonniere deformity.

II. DIP arthroplasty
   A. Without Kirschner wire (K-wire) fixation.
      1. PIP and DIP joints are in extension for 2 weeks.
      2. DIP joint is held in extension for an additional 2 weeks and PIP joint AROM is initiated.
      3. Gentle active flexion is initiated after this immobilization period. Flexion should be performed gradually, progressing to 30 degrees of flexion. Night extension splinting continues for an additional 6 weeks.
   B. With K-wire fixation.
      1. 3 to 4 weeks of fixation followed by an additional 4 weeks of DIP extension splinting (Fig. 41-6).
      2. Gradual AROM to 30 degrees of DIP flexion may be initiated after removal of fixation.
      3. Night DIP extension splinting for another 2 months.
III. Adjunctive treatment
   Consider the use of a continuous passive movement unit as an adjunct to treatment.

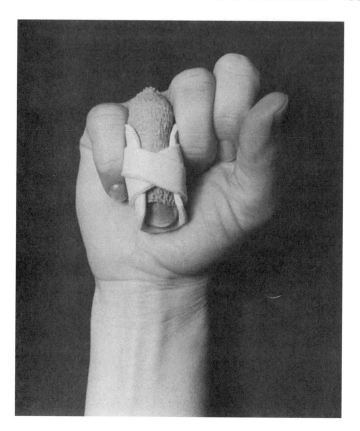

Fig. 41-6. DIP extension splinting follows K-wire immobilization for a DIP arthroplasty.

POSTOPERATIVE COMPLICATIONS

I. PIP arthroplasty
   A. Flexor tendon adherence
   B. Malalignment
   C. Extension lag
   D. Fracture of the prosthesis
   E. Synovitis
II. DIP arthroplasty
   A. Malalignment
   B. Mallet finger
   C. Fracture of the prosthesis
   D. Synovitis

EVALUATION TIMELINE

I. PIP arthroplasty
   A. 3 to 5 days postoperatively: initial AROM measurements.
   B. Re-evaluation every 2 weeks thereafter.
   C. Strength measurements once joint stability is well established. A modified blood pressure cuff may be indicated for strength testing.[3]

II. DIP arthroplasty
    A. 4 weeks postoperatively: initial AROM measurements
    B. Re-evaluation every 2 weeks thereafter
    C. Strength measurements once joint stability is well established. A modified blood pressure cuff for testing may be indicated.

REFERENCES

1. Swanson AB, Swanson-deGroot G, Leonard J: Post-operative rehabilitation programs in flexible implant arthroplasty of the digits. p. 133, 142. In Hunter J (ed): Rehabilitation of the Hand. 2nd Ed. Mosby, St. Louis, 1984
2. Swanson AB, Maupin BK, Gajjar NV: Flexible implant arthroplasty in the proximal interphalangeal joint of the hand. J Hand Surg 10A:796, 1985
3. Melvin JL: Evaluation of muscle strength. p. 291. In Surgical Rehabilitation, Rheumatic Disease Occupational Therapy and Rehabilitation. 2nd Ed. FA Davis, Philadelphia, 1982

SUGGESTED READINGS

Adamson GJ, Gellman H, Brumfield RH et al: Flexible implant resection arthroplasty of the proximal interphalangeal joint in patients with systemic inflammatory arthritis. J Hand Surg 19A:3, 1994

Beckenbaugh RD, Linscheid RL: Arthroplasty in the hand and wrist. p. 167. In Green DP (ed): Operative Hand Surgery. 2nd Ed. Vol. 1. Churchill Livingstone, New York, 1988

Milford L: Reconstruction after injury. p. 283. In: Campbell's Operative Orthopaedics. 7th Ed. Vol. 1. Mosby, St. Louis, 1987

Pellegrini D, Burton R: Osteoarthritis of the proximal interphalangeal joint of the hand: arthroplasty or fusion? J Hand Surg 15A:194, 1990

Smith RJ: Balance of kinetics of the fingers under normal pathological conditions. Clin Orthop 104:92, 1974

Stanly JK, Evans RA: What are the long term follow up results of silastic metacarpophalangeal and proximal interphalangeal joint replacements. Br J Rheumatol 31:839, 1992

Stephens J, Pratt N, Parks B: The reliability and validity of the Tekdyne hand dynamometer: part I. J Hand Therapy 9:10, 1996

Stephens J, Pratt N, Michlovitz S: The reliability and validity of the Tekdyne hand dynamometer: part II. J Hand Therapy 9:18, 1996

Swanson AB, Swanson-deGroot G: Treatment considerations and resource materials for flexible (silicone) implant arthroplasty. Orthopedic Research Dept., Blodgett Memorial Medical Center, Grand Rapids, 1987

Swanson AB, Swanson-deGroot G: Postoperative Care for Patients with Silastic Finger Joint Implants (Swanson Design). 4th Ed. Orthopaedic Reconstructive Surgeons P.C., Grand Rapids, 1985

Swanson AB, Swanson-deGroot G, Leonard JB: Postoperative rehabilitation programs in flexible implant arthroplasty of the digits. p. 1351. In Hunter JM, Macklin EJ, Callahan AD (eds): Rehabilitation of the Hand: Surgery and Therapy. 4th Ed. Mosby, St. Louis, 1995

Zimmerman NB, Shuhey PV, Clark GL, Wilgis EFS: Silicone Interpositional Arthroplasty of the Distal Interphalangeal Joint. J Hand Surg 14A:882, 1989

Thumb Carpometacarpal Joint Arthroplasty

42

Rebecca J. Saunders

Basal joint arthroplasty is indicated when there is significant arthritis of the trapeziometacarpal joint and/or adjacent joints of the thumb, which results in disabling pain and loss of hand function. Surgical intervention may be necessary if the patient fails to respond to a conservative management regimen of splinting, nonsteroidal anti-inflammatory drugs (NSAIDs), and/or steroid injection. Some authors advocate strengthening exercises for the "muscles of the thenar cone, as well as the extrinsic abductor, long extensor, and long flexor."[1] Arthritic changes can be degenerative, traumatic, or caused by systemic disease as in rheumatoid arthritis. Disease of the thumb carpometacarpal (CMC) joint occurs more frequently in women than in men and is thought to be related to activities that require "continuous tone in the thenar musculature during thumb flexion — adduction."[2]

Surgical options in basal joint arthroplasty include silicone implant or soft tissue reconstruction. Implant arthroplasty is usually reserved for the relatively low demand rheumatoid hand because of the potential complications of silicone synovitis and/or subluxation. Many different types of soft tissue reconstructions are performed and the following protocol is based on the Burton–Pellegrini procedure. Range of motion (ROM) after this procedure is approximately the same as it was before surgery. Functionally, a slight decrease in grip and pinch strength is to be expected because of the slight shortening of the first ray, although these functions are now less painful.[3] As with any surgical procedure involving the hand, close communication with the surgeon is necessary to facilitate complete patient care.

DEFINITION

The trapezium is excised and the base of the first metacarpal is resected. A soft tissue spacer is constructed from either the palmaris longus or part of the flexor carpi radialis (FCR) and inserted in the trapezial space; then the joint capsule is closed. Ligamentous stability is often augmented by taking part of the FCR through a drill hole in the first metacarpal and then suturing it back on itself. The abductor pollicis longus tendon is also sometimes imbricated to increase stability (Fig. 42-1).

SURGICAL PURPOSE

Surgical correction of arthritis of the CMC joint of the thumb is designed mainly to relieve pain. Secondary gains are the improved positioning of the thumb with greater active range of motion (AROM) as a result of the decreased pain. This provides better thumb function and appearance. When there is secondary deformity of the metacarpophalangeal (MCP) joint, it may also have to be surgically corrected.

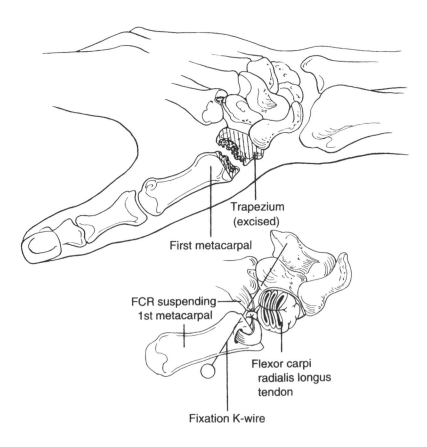

Fig. 42-1. Reconstruction of thumb CMC joint.

TREATMENT GOALS

    I. Edema control.
    II. Pain control.
    III. Increase ROM, strength, and functional use of the hand.
    IV. Promotion of a stable, mobile, and pain-free joint.

POSTOPERATIVE INDICATIONS/ PRECAUTIONS FOR THERAPY

MCP joint hyperextension can be a concurrent problem and this may necessitate additional surgical procedures such as MCP fusion or capsulodesis. Consult the operative note when possible.

POSTOPERATIVE THERAPY

    I. 0 to 2 weeks: The patient is immobilized in a thumb spica cast.
    II. 2 to 4 weeks.
       A. The bulky, postoperative dressing and sutures are removed and the use of elastic stockinette or Coban can be initiated for edema control.
       B. The patient is fitted with a thumb spica cast or splint with the interphalangeal (IP) joint left free for ROM (Fig. 42-2).
       C. The cast or splint is used continuously until the initiation of active ROM (AROM) of the CMC at 4 to 6 weeks postoperatively.

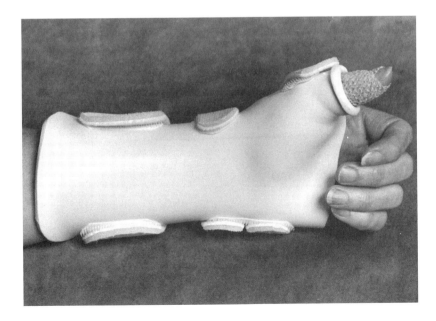

Fig. 42-2. Coban used for edema control may be worn with a thumb spica splint.

III. 4 to 6 weeks.
   A. Active assistive ROM and AROM are initiated to the thumb and wrist.
   B. Exercises should emphasize abduction, extension, and opposition to each fingertip.
   C. Early metacarpal flexion and adduction puts undue stress on the reconstructed ligament and should be minimized at this time.
   D. Complete flexion across the palm to the base of the fifth metacarpal should not be attempted until the thumb can oppose each fingertip with ease, and gradually be worked down to the base of the small finger.[2]
   E. Splinting is continued after exercise and at night primarily for patient comfort.
IV. 7 weeks: Dynamic splinting to increase MCP and IP joint motion can be initiated if the CMC joint is well stabilized.
V. 8 to 10 weeks.
   A. Static splint use can be discontinued if the joint is stable and patient is asymptomatic.
   B. Gentle strengthening including grip and pinch strengthening can be initiated if the joint is stable and relatively pain free.[4]
VI. 10 to 12 weeks: Normal use of the hand may be resumed without restrictions if the joint is stable and the patient is asymptomatic.

POSTOPERATIVE COMPLICATIONS

I. The carpal tunnel is in close proximity to the basal joint, and postoperative edema can exacerbate an underlying median nerve problem or cause an acute carpal tunnel. This responds well to conservative management. If a concurrent carpal tunnel release was performed, the patient may take longer to regain strength.
II. De Quervain's syndrome may become symptomatic during therapy. If recognized, it responds well to conservative treatment, including splinting, NSAIDs, and/or injection.[3]
III. Hypersensitivity of the thenar region and incisional area is not an uncommon complication and when present needs to be treated with desensitization and pain control techniques. The therapist should be on the alert for signs and symptoms of reflex sympathetic dystrophy (RSD), as prompt diagnosis and early intervention are the most effective treatments for this disabling disease.

EVALUATION TIMELINE

I. Preoperative evaluation, when possible, should include:
   A. ROM
   B. Grip and pinch strength
   C. Sensation
II. Postoperative evaluation
   A. 2 weeks: Blocked active and passive MCP and IP ROM.

B. 4 weeks.
  1. MCP and IP ROM.
  2. CMC abduction and extension.
  3. Opposition, active only.
  4. Wrist ROM.
C. 8 weeks.
  1. Thumb ROM (CMC, MCP, IP).
  2. Wrist ROM.
  3. Grip and pinch strength (providing the CMC joint is stable and the patient is asymptomatic).
  4. Sensation.
D. Functional assessment of activities of daily living, vocational, and avocational activities.

REFERENCES

1. Burton R: Basal joint implant arthroplasty in osteoarthritis. Hand Clin 3:473, 1987
2. Burton R: Complications following surgery on the basal joint of the thumb. Hand Clin 2:265, 1986
3. Eaton R: Trapezometacarpal osteoarthritis staging as a rationale for treatment. Hand Clin 3:455, 1987
4. Cannon NM, Eaton R, Glickel S (eds): Soft tissue reconstructions CMC joint. In Diagnosis and Treatment Manual for Physicians and Therapists. 3rd Ed. Hand Rehabilitation Center of Indiana PC, Indianapolis, 1991

SUGGESTED READINGS

Amadio P, Millender L, Smith R: Silicone spacer or tendon spacer for trapezium, resection arthroplasty—comparison of results. J Hand Surg 7:237, 1982

Burton R, Pellegrini V: Surgical management of basal joint arthritis of the thumb. Part II. Ligament reconstruction with tendon interposition arthroplasty. J Hand Surg 11A:324, 1986

Eaton R, Glickel S, Littler W: Tendon interposition arthroplasty for degenerative arthritis of the trapeziometacarpal joint of the thumb. J Hand Surg 10A:645, 1985

Florack TM, Miller RJ, Pellegrini VD et al: The prevalence of carpal tunnel syndrome in patients with basal joint arthritis of the thumb. J Hand Surg. 17A:624, 1992

Froimson A: Tendon interposition arthroplasty of carpometacarpal joint of the thumb. Hand Clin 3:489, 1987

Le Viet DT, Kerboull L, Lantieri L, Collins DE: Stabilized resection arthroplasty by an anterior approach in trapeziometacarpal arthritis: results and surgical technique. J Hand Surg 21A:194, 1996

Pellegrini VD: Osteoarthritis of the trapezio-metacarpal joint: the pathophysiology of articular cartilage degeneration. I. Anatomy and pathology of the aging joint. J Hand Surg 16A:967, 1991

Tomaino MM, Pellegrini VD, Burton RI: Arthroplasty of the basal joint of the thumb: long-term follow-up after ligament reconstruction with tendon interposition. J Bone Joint Surg 77A:346, 1995

Wolock BS, Moore JR, Weiland AJ: Arthritis of the basal joint of the thumb: a critical analysis of treatment options. J Arthroplasty 4:65, 1989

Ulnar Collateral Ligament Injury of the Thumb

43

Arlynne Pack Brown

The function of the thumb metacarpophalangeal (MCP) joint depends on its stability rather than its mobility.[1] Progression through all rehabilitation procedures should be based on continual reassessment of the stability of the ulnar aspect of the joint.

Ulnar collateral joint ligament (UCL) injuries to the thumb MCP joints can be divided into two categories for the purposes of rehabilitation. One category consists of incomplete ligament tears and nondisplaced bony avulsions treated with immobilization. The other category consists of complete tears and displaced bony avulsions treated with surgery and immobilization.

The major distinction between partial and complete ligament tears is the likelihood for complete tears to become Stener lesions.[1a] Stener lesions are formed by avulsed ligaments sliding out from under the adductor aponeurosis and flipping on top of the adductor aponeurosis. These lesions require surgical repair to restore lateral stability. Conversely, if the ligament is partially torn and the joint demonstrates minimal instability, the joint can be immobilized in plaster. The surgeon may position the joint in slight flexion and ulnar deviation to ensure stability (Fig. 43-1).

Rehabilitation for the two categories follows identical progression, with the exception of the amount of time the joint is immobilized. According to the literature, incomplete ligament tears and nondisplaced avulsion fractures are immobilized for 3 to 6 weeks. Surgically repaired injuries are immobilized for 4 to 6 weeks or longer. The precise amount of time of immobilization should be determined by the surgeon given his or her knowledge of the actual repair and subsequent expectations.

During the immobilization period, the primary goal is to maintain range of motion (ROM) of the unaffected joints. Distinct attention should be given to the thumb interphalangeal (IP) joint to prevent tendon adhesions.

369

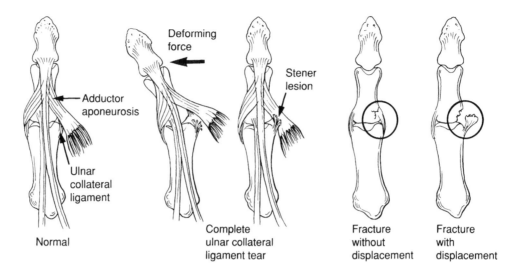

Adductor aponeurosis

Ulnar collateral ligament

Normal

Deforming force

Complete ulnar collateral ligament tear

Stener lesion

Fracture without displacement

Fracture with displacement

Fig. 43-1. Normal anatomy of thumb MCP joint and associated injuries.

Once the splint is removed, active ROM (AROM) is initiated. Following this, passive ROM (PROM) and dynamic splinting begin in 1-week increments.

Gentle, resistive strengthening for partial tears may begin at status post 8 weeks and for repaired complete tears at 10 to 12 weeks. Unrestricted activities for partial tears may begin at 10 to 16 weeks and for repaired complete tears at 12 to 16 weeks.

DEFINITION

   I. Incomplete tears of UCL: partial tears of UCL with minimal lateral instability.
  II. Nondisplaced bony avulsions: injury to bone at attachment of UCL without displacement.
 III. Complete tear of UCL.
    A. Stener lesions: complete UCL tears *with* adductor pollicis tendon interpositioning.
    B. Complete UCL tears *without* adductor pollicis tendon interpositioning.
    C. Displaced avulsion fractures.
 IV. Other names for UCL injuries
    A. Gamekeeper's thumb
    B. Skier's thumb
    C. Stener's lesion
    D. Breakdancer's thumb

TREATMENT AND SURGICAL PURPOSE

The UCL of the thumb MCP joint stabilizes that joint against forces applied in a radial direction to the thumb. If the ligament's integrity is lost, the thumb tends to "run away" from the index finger, and the power of pinch is significantly reduced. The treatment protocol depends on the consideration of how much of this ligament is torn and how unstable the joint may become. Management ranges from simple splinting to operative repair including internal fixation. The goal is to recognize the extent of the injury early and begin appropriate care.

Late reconstruction can seriously compromise the stability and ROM of the thumb MCP joint when compared with normal.

TREATMENT GOALS

I. Maintain full ROM of all uninvolved joints of the upper extremity.
II. Promote ligament healing.
III. Avoid pin tract and/or pullout wire tract infection.
IV. Maximize MCP joint AROM and PROM.
V. Maximize lateral stability of MCP joint during grip and pinch activities.
VI. Return to previous level of function.
VII. Prevent reinjury.

NONOPERATIVE INDICATIONS/ PRECAUTIONS FOR THERAPY

I. Indications
   A. Incomplete UCL tears.
   B. Nondisplaced bony avulsions at site of UCL attachment.
II. Precautions
   A. Avoid torque, which would further tear UCL.
   B. Extreme pain.
   C. Extreme edema.
   D. Associated flexor or extensor tendon ruptures.

NONOPERATIVE THERAPY

Following incomplete UCL tears or nondisplaced avulsion fractures.

I. Weeks 1 through 3 to 6: thumb spica plaster or thermoplastic splint immobilization for amount of time directed by surgeon.[1,2-4] Consult surgeon as to whether immobilization of the IP and wrist joints is indicated (Fig. 43-2).

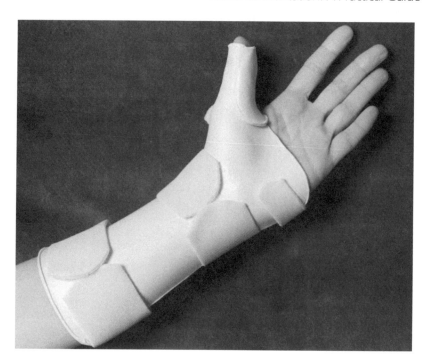

Fig. 43-2. Example of postoperative thumb splint.

Maintain AROM of all joints of the upper extremity while in plaster/splint. Concentrate especially on the IP joint to prevent extensor mechanism adhesions.

II. Week 4: If splint includes the wrist (forearm based), cut it down to exclude the wrist (hand based). Wear splint while sleeping, in crowds, and in other tenuous situations.

Initiate AROM of the MCP joint.

III. Week 5: Begin and progress PROM of the thumb MCP joint.

IV. Week 6: Begin and progress dynamic splinting of the thumb MCP joint as needed.

V. Week 8: Begin and progress strengthening especially of the structures on the ulnar border of the joint, during grip and pinch. Specifically, strengthen the locking of the thumb around a 6 to 8 cm diameter cylinder.[5,6] Strengthening muscles for pinch in lateral, tip, and three jaw positions (Fig. 43-3).

VI. Weeks 10 to 16: Begin unrestricted use. May want to tape protectively during sports activities.[7]

NONOPERATIVE COMPLICATIONS

I. Chronic instability and weakness of pinch.[2,8]

II. Persistent pain and arthritis.[3,8]

III. Decreased ROM of MCP and IP joints.[8]

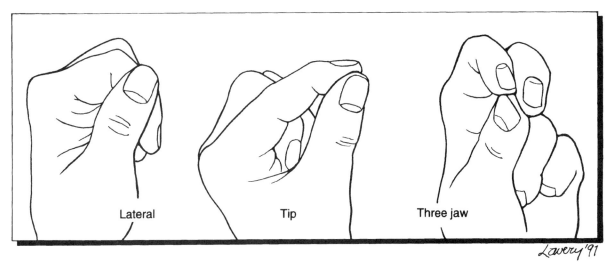

Fig. 43-3. Pinch positions.

POSTOPERATIVE INDICATIONS/ PRECAUTIONS FOR THERAPY

   I. Indications
      A. Complete UCL tears.
      B. Displaced avulsion fractures at site of UCL attachment.
  II. Precautions
      A. Avoid torque to further tear UCL.
      B. Infection
      C. Extreme pain
      D. Extreme edema
      E. Associated flexor or extensor tendon ruptures.

POSTOPERATIVE THERAPY

Following surgical repair and Kirschner wiring (K-wire) pull out wiring

    I. Weeks 1 through 4 to 6: (See Nonoperative Therapy)
   II. Week 4: If surgeon removes cast, K-wire and pull out wire, apply hand-based thumb splint. Continue full-time splinting except for supervised ROM of carpometacarpal and wrist joints.
  III. Week 6: Begin AROM of MCP joint.[4] Protect lateral stability. Splint while sleeping, in crowds, and in other tenuous situations.
  IV. Week 7 to 8: Begin gentle PROM of MCP joint.
   V. Weeks 8 to 10: Begin and progress dynamic splinting of the MCP joint if indicated.

VI. Weeks 10 to 12: Begin and progress strengthening, especially of the structures on the ulnar border during grip and pinch. Specifically, strengthen the locking of the thumb around a 6 to 8 cm diameter cylinder.[5,6] Plus, strengthen the muscles for pinch in lateral, tip, and three jaw positions.

VII. Weeks 12 to 16: Begin unrestricted use.[7] May want to tape protectively during sports activities.[4]

POSTOPERATIVE COMPLICATIONS

I. Chronic instability and weakness of pinch.[2,8]
II. Persistent numbness ulnar aspect of thumb.[8]
III. Persistent pain and arthritis.[3,8]
IV. Decreased ROM of MCP and IP joints.[8]
V. Infection

EVALUATION TIMELINE

I. Incomplete UCL tears.
  A. Week 1: AROM and PROM of all upper extremity joints not included in splint, except thumb and wrist.
  B. Week 4: AROM thumb and wrist joints.
  C. Week 5: PROM thumb and wrist joints.
  D. Week 8: Grip strength and pinch strength, manual muscle testing (MMT) thumb muscles.
II. UCL tears or nondisplaced avulsion fractures.
  A. Weeks 1 to 3: same as incomplete UCL tears.
  B. Week 6: AROM thumb joints.
  C. Week 7: PROM thumb joints.
  D. Week 10: grip strength, pinch strength, MMT thumb muscles.

REFERENCES

1. Miller RJ: Dislocations and fracture dislocations of the metacarpophalangeal joint of the thumb. Hand Clin 4:45, 1988
1a. Stener B: Displacement of the ruptured ulnar collateral ligament of the metacarpophalangeal joint of the thumb. A clinical and anatomical study. J Bone Joint Surg 44B:869, 1962
2. Eaton RG: Injuries of the metacarpophalangeal joint of the thumb. p. 887. In Tubiana R (ed): The Hand. Vol. III. WB Saunders, Philadelphia, 1988
3. Sandzen SC: The Hand and Wrist. Williams & Wilkins, Baltimore, 1985
4. Green DP: Operative Hand Surgery. 2nd Ed. Churchill Livingstone, New York, 1988
5. Kopandji IA: Biomechanics of the thumb. p. 404. In Tubiana R (ed): The Hand. Vol. III. WB Saunders, Philadelphia, 1988
6. Aubriot JH: Injuries of the metacarpophalangeal joint of the thumb. p. 184. In Tubiana R (ed): The Hand. Vol. III. WB Saunders, Philadelphia, 1988
7. Gieck JH, Maxer V: Protective splinting for the hand and wrist. Clin Sports Med 5:795, 1986
8. Helm RH: Hand function after injuries to the collateral ligaments of the metacarpophalangeal joint of the thumb. J Hand Surg 12:252, 1987

SUGGESTED READINGS

Bowers WH: Sprains and joint injuries in the hand. Hand Clin 2:93, 1986

Eaton RG: Joint Injuries of the Hand. Charles C. Thomas, Springfield, 1971

Fess EE, Gettle KS, Strickland JW: Hand splinting principles and methods. Mosby, St. Louis, 1981

Flynn JE: Hand Surgery. 3rd Ed. Williams & Wilkins, Baltimore, 1982

Jupiter JB, Sheppard JE: Tension wire fixation of avulsion fractures of the hand. Clin Orthop 214:113, 1987

Milford L: The Hand. Mosby, St. Louis, 1982

Stener B: Acute injuries to the metacarpophalangeal joint of the thumb. p. 895. In Tubiana R (ed): The Hand. Vol. III. WB Saunders, Philadelphia, 1988

Weeks PM: Management of acute hand injuries. 2nd Ed. Mosby, St. Louis, 1978

Reflex Sympathetic Dystrophy

44

Anne Edmonds

Reflex sympathetic dystrophy (RSD) is a vasomotor dysfunction that can be localized to one area of an extremity, involve an entire extremity, or involve more than one extremity. Pain is commonly the most outstanding complaint, and swelling is most often the outstanding physical feature.

RSD can be divided into three stages: acute, subacute, and chronic. The acute stage begins at onset of injury and continues for approximately 3 months. Pain usually reaches its peak by the end of the first stage or beginning of the second stage. Swelling is apparent at this stage as is redness, hyperhidrosis, and limitation of motion secondary to the pain. Radiographs may reveal demineralization and osteoporosis. The second stage usually extends from about the third to the ninth month with maximum pain and continued limited motion. The swelling is brawny and fixed. Redness begins to diminish during this stage, and hyperhidrosis decreases as well. Stiffness continues with considerable periarticular thickening about the joints of the fingers. Atrophy of the skin and subcutaneous tissue along with palmar thickening of the longitudinal bands are noted in this stage. Osteoporosis is quite pronounced.

The third stage may last from many months to several years. The edema and pain may subside, but considerable joint stiffness continues because of fibrotic changes. Skin color may appear pale and glossy. There is little hope of obtaining good motion at this stage.

Because of the immense pain experienced by RSD patients, it is helpful to enlist various measurements to assess the pain throughout the course of treatment. A regimen devised by Davidoff, as shown by Walsh,[1] to determine the efficacy of treatment of RSD follows:

1. Distal joint pain by palpation (scale of 0 to 4).
2. Volumetric measurements by water displacement of the extremity.
3. Skin temperature measurement.

4. Active range of motion (AROM) of affected limbs.
5. McGill pain questionnaire.
6. Visual analog scale.

Despite a wide range of subjectivity, these tools help quantify pain and determine appropriate treatment.

There are also body diagrams, such as the one described and used by Walsh[1] with qualitative descriptions. The patient can use this to quantify discomfort either verbally or visually.

DEFINITION

A vasomotor dysfunction characterized by very severe pain, swelling, stiffness, and discoloration (Fig. 44-1). It may appear following surgery, trauma, or local and systemic disease. It is variable in duration.

TREATMENT PURPOSE

The cause of RSD is poorly understood. Its effects can be devastating to the patient and the involved part. It may occur after injury or surgery no matter how major or trivial. Its characteristics of pain, tenderness, swelling, and joint stiffness, when recognized or suspected, should be addressed immediately to ensure correction and restoration of maximum

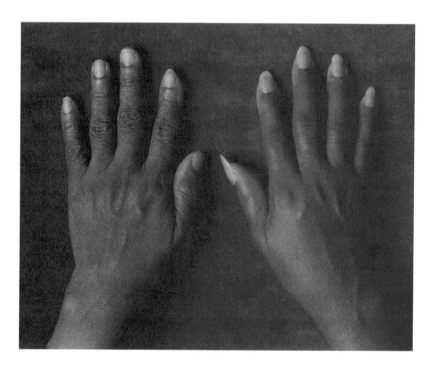

Fig. 44-1. RSD is a vasomotor dysfunction as seen in hand on right.

function. Early recognition of RSD leads to a better outcome of treatment. The diagnosis may sometimes be difficult and other pain-creating conditions must be ruled out to maximize the care of RSD patients.

TREATMENT GOALS

  I. To decrease or eliminate pain and edema.
  II. To restore maximum mobility.
  III. To restore maximum function.

NONOPERATIVE INDICATIONS FOR TREATMENT

  I. Four cardinal signs and symptoms.
     A. Pain
     B. Swelling
     C. Stiffness
     D. Discoloration[2,3]
  II. Secondary signs and symptoms that are most often but not always present.
     A. Osseous demineralization
     B. Sudomotor changes
     C. Temperature changes
     D. Trophic changes
     E. Vasomotor instability
     F. Palmar fibromatosis[3]
     G. Allodynia[1]

NONOPERATIVE THERAPY

  I. Blocks
     A. Stellate: interrupted or continuous (Fig. 44-2).
     B. Bier.
     C. Periodic perineural infusion.
     D. Sympatholytic medication.
     E. Sympathectomy.
     F. Oral steroids.[1]
  II. Therapy
     A. Acute stage
        1. Gentle active exercise and massage without pain: PROM as tolerated by patient.
        2. Elevated hot packs.
        3. Contrast baths.
        4. High voltage galvanic stimulation (Fig. 44-3).
        5. Transcutaneous electrical nerve stimulation (TENS).

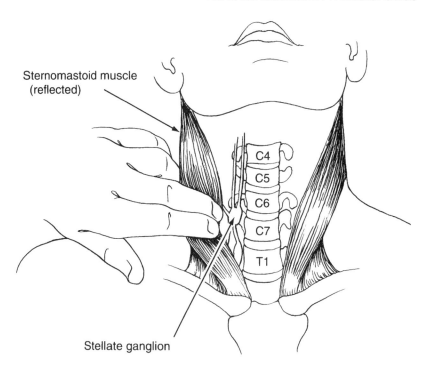

Fig. 44-2. Stellate ganglion block.

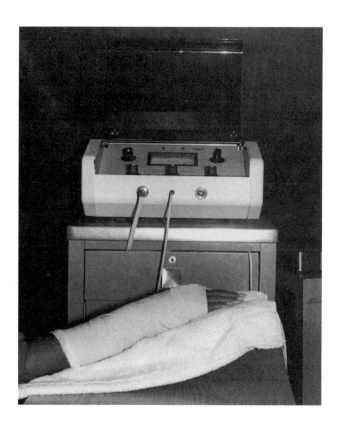

Fig. 44-3. High voltage galvanic stimulation treatment.

6. Desensitization.
7. Phonophoresis.
8. Splinting, protected, as indicated by patient's pain level.
B. Subacute, chronic
   1. All of the above mentioned in the acute stage.
   2. Splinting: progressing to dynamic when tolerated by the patient.
   3. Stress loading (Fig. 44-4).
   4. Functional activities.
   5. Strengthening.

NONOPERATIVE COMPLICATIONS

I. High incidence of traumatic carpal tunnel syndrome.
II. Late diagnosis and treatment can worsen and prolong the already established RSD.

EVALUATION TIMELINE

I. Acute
   A. Initial range of motion (ROM) measurement and every 3 to 4 weeks thereafter.
   B. Initial strength measurement.

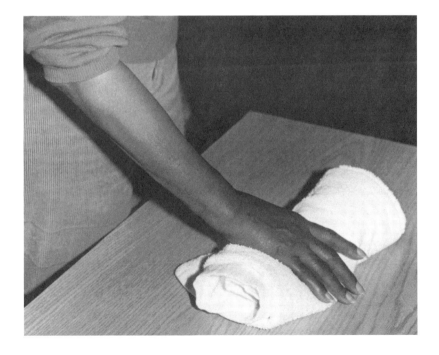

Fig. 44-4. Stress loading.

C. Pain scale — visual or verbal.
D. Initial edema measurement and at each visit — before and after exercise.
E. Sensory screening.
II. Chronic
A. Continued ROM measurements every 3 to 4 weeks.
B. Continued strength assessment every 3 to 4 weeks.
C. Ongoing strength assessment every 3 to 4 weeks.
D. Sensory screening every 3 to 4 weeks.
E. Monitor edema each visit — before and after exercise.

REFERENCES

1. Walsh MT: Therapist's management of reflux sympathetic dystrophy. In Hunter JM, Mackin EJ, Callahan AD (eds): Rehabilitation of the Hand: Surgery and Therapy. Mosby, St. Louis, 1995
2. Lankford LL: Reflex sympathetic dystrophy. In Hunter JM, Mackin EJ, Callahan AD (eds): Rehabilitation of the Hand: Surgery and Therapy. Mosby, St. Louis, 1995
3. Lankford LL: Reflex sympathetic dystrophy. In Green DP (ed): Operative Hand Surgery. Vol. 1. Churchill Livingstone, New York, 1982

SUGGESTED READINGS

Lankford LL: Reflex sympathetic dystrophy. In Hunter JM, Schneider LH, Mackin EJ, Callahan AD (eds): Rehabilitation of the Hand. Mosby, St. Louis, 1990
Ramamurthy S: Anesthesia. p. 23. In Green DP (ed): Operative Hand Surgery. Vol. 1. Churchill Livingstone, New York, 1982
Schutzer SF, Gossling HR: The treatment of reflex sympathetic dystrophy syndrome. Current Concepts Review. J Bone Joint Surg 66A:625, 1984
Schwartzman RJ, McLellan TL: Reflex sympathetic dystrophy. Arch Neurol 44:555, 1987
Waylett-Rendall J: Therapists management of reflex sympathetic dystrophy. In Hunter JM, Schneider LH, Mackin EJ, Callahan AD (eds): Rehabilitation of the Hand. Mosby, St. Louis, 1990

Congenital Hand Differences

45

Mallory S. Anthony

The therapist treating patients with congenital differences will be challenged by the diversity and uniqueness of each one. Each patient and family come to the clinic with his or her own individual set of expectations and goals. Some may opt for function rather than appearance when trying to decide about surgical intervention.

The decision on timing and on whether to intervene with surgery depends on each situation and on each deformity. In some cases, the choice is obvious, and in others, the decision is very difficult. If a patient is able to functionally compensate for his or her deformity, surgery may be unnecessary. In other cases reconstructive surgery can do little to improve function, and families need to be informed and understand these surgical limitations. Some decisions about surgery may be postponed to observe the child and monitor growth and functional adaptation to the deformity. In cases of constriction band syndrome, where vascularity to the digit is compromised, early surgical intervention is necessary. Also, in patients with syndactyly, digits may need to be separated early to allow proper bone growth and prevent flexion contracture of the longer digit.[1] Tendon anomalies should be corrected early to provide better dynamic balance across joints.[1] Other procedures such as pollicization or web widening can usually wait. Because cortical control of placing the upper limb in space and control of strong grasp are well developed by 1 year of age, however, many hand surgeons feel pollicization should be performed by age 2 years.

Recognizing the family's need for proper counseling, support, and guidance is extremely important. Families making decisions for very young patients need to realize the impact their decision will have on the patient when he or she reaches adolescence. The importance of a team approach cannot be overemphasized. The pediatrician, surgeon, therapist, genetic counselor, and possibly psychologist or social worker need to work closely together with the family to help them focus on realistic goals, and help provide them with proper emotional support.

Most children with congenital malformations of the hand are mentally normal, and most anomalous hands have normal sensibility.[1] A great majority of malformations arise either at the moment of conception, or during the second month because the human arm bud appears and fully differentiates between the 25th and 50th day after fertilization. Other systems may also be affected, and many congenital hand anomalies have associated defects frequently involving the cardiac, musculoskeletal, and hematopoietic systems.

The major goal of the hand surgeon is to improve function and appearance of the affected hand. Our goal as therapists is to provide functional assessment of the affected hand, to provide splinting to stretch soft tissues and/or maintain proper positioning, and to provide instruction in stretching and strengthening exercise programs, as well as instruction in retraining and functional activities. While working with these patients and their families, it is imperative to understand the difficulties and frustrations they may be experiencing, and guide them toward the acceptance of realistic goals.

DEFINITION AND CLINICAL MANIFESTATIONS
(Refer to Appendix 45-1 for General Classification)

    I. Radial club hand (radial deficiencies) (Fig. 45-1)
       A. Refers to a spectrum of abnormalities ranging from minor thumb hypoplasia to total absence of the thumb, its metacarpal, scaphoid, trapezium, and entire radius. The most common radial deficiency is partial absence of radius, and absence of radial carpal bones and thumb.[2]

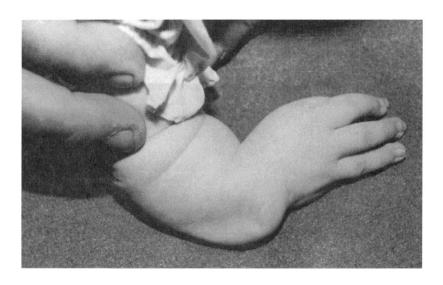

Fig. 45-1. Radial club hand.

B. The ulna is usually curved, shortened, and thickened.[1]

C. Anatomic variations also include deficiencies of the muscular, nervous, and vascular tissues.

D. Classification.
1. Type I: short distal radius.
2. Type II: hypoplastic radius.
3. Type III: partial absence of radius.
4. Type IV: total absence of radius.

E. Common associated abnormalities include blood and cardiac deficiencies.

F. Common clinical picture.[2]
1. Extremity is approximately two-thirds length of the unaffected extremity (bilateral involvement is seen with the same frequency as unilateral).
2. Forearm is bowed to radial side.
3. Hand is deviated radially and amount of deviation depends on degree of absence of radius.
4. Flexion contractures of proximal interphalangeal (PIP) joints of radial digits is common.
5. Thumb may or may not be present and is usually hypoplastic.
6. Metacarpophalangeal (MCP) flexion often restricted and often unstable.
7. Hand is floppy and unsupported because of an unstable wrist.
8. Forearm muscles are less effective in controlling the hand as the amount of radial deviation increases.[3]
9. Elbow usually stable with decreased flexion.
10. Shoulders may be hypoplastic.

II. Brachial plexus birth palsy
A. Refers to brachial plexus injuries resulting from traction on the brachial plexus during delivery.[4] (Since this injury is caused by trauma, it is not a "true" congenital anomaly; however, patients with these injuries are often seen in congenital clinics.)
B. Incidence has decreased over last several years with improved obstetrical management.
C. Generally three types:
1. Lesion of upper roots: Erb's palsy (loss of deltoid, lateral rotators of humerus, elbow flexors, and possibly wrist extensors).
2. Lesion of lower roots: "Klumpke's palsy" (loss of finger flexion/extension, and intrinsic function).
3. Total paralysis (flail upper extremity).

THERAPIST'S EVALUATION

I. Prerequisite to evaluation
A. Knowledge of types of prehension[1] (useful for evaluation of patients older than ten months of age) (Fig. 45-2).

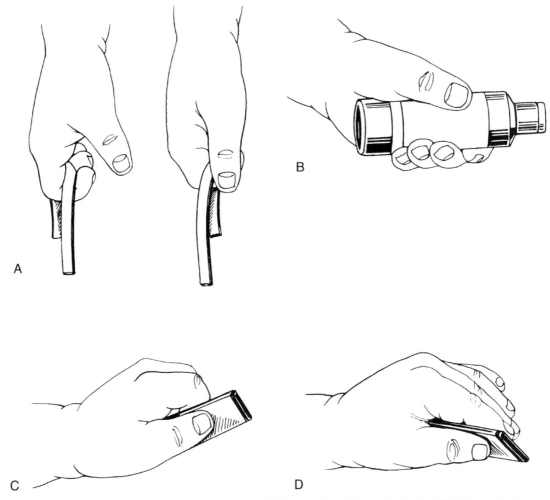

Fig. 45-2. Types of prehension. (**A**) Hook grips. (**B**) Power grip. (**C**) Lateral pinch. (**D**) Palmar pinch.

1. Hook grip.
2. Power grip.
3. Lateral pinch.
4. Precision handling.
   a. Palmer pinch.
   b. Tip pinch.
5. Cylindrical and spherical grips: Descriptive of the object being held rather than of the grip being used.
6. Two most common prehensile movements.
   a. Picking up object.
   b. Holding it for use.
7. Problems which limit manipulation of an object.
   a. Adducted or relaxed position of thumb.
   b. Flat distal transverse arch.
   c. A proximal location of contact (inadequate length of digits).

B. Knowledge of age when normal patterns of prehension develop (useful for evaluation of child younger than 10 months.)
1. Erhardt Developmental Prehension Assessment.[5]
a. Useful tool for assessing development of voluntary grasp (Appendix 45-2).
b. Assesses three areas.
1. Involuntary arm-hand patterns (reflex movements).
2. Voluntary arm-hand movements.
3. Prewriting skills.
c. Components of prehension are grouped into developmental sequence clusters in test booklet.

II. Evaluation[6,7]
A. Evaluation of pinches and grips available to the hand. (Sample evaluation form can be found in Appendix 45-2.)
B. Observe preferred patterns of usage.
C. Measure active and passive range of motion (ROM) of entire upper extremity.
1. Important measurements not to be overlooked.
a. Carpometacarpal (CMC) joint motion of thumb.
b. Finger abduction at MCP joints.
2. For very young patients unable to cooperate for ROM testing, record obvious limitations noted during play.
D. Measure pinch and grip strength.
1. Can rarely be measured accurately in child younger than 5 years old.
E. Size of hand may be relevant to identify inadequate finger and thumb length to span objects in cylindrical grasp.
F. Test sensibility.
1. Note that myelinization is not complete until approximately 2 years of age.
2. Use objective tests for young children (e.g., O'Riain wrinkle test or ninhydrin test).
3. Use standard sensibility tests for older patients (e.g., threshold and functional two-point discrimination testing).
G. Note delays observed in child's developmental sequence, which may be caused by upper extremity anomalies. These may include difficulties in rolling, pushing up on forearms, pushing to sitting, crawling, pulling to standing.
H. Repeated evaluation may be necessary because growth can cause significant changes in congenitally; anomalous hands.

SURGICAL CONSIDERATIONS

Congenital differences of the upper limb in children vary considerably, but each is of serious importance to the parents, child, and family. The deformity should be recognized as the child's "normal" and the limb with which they were born. Surgery will change that "normal" to adapt it for better function, better appearance, or both. This objective must hold up so that when the child reaches maturity there will be no regrets. Careful consideration of each procedure must be thoroughly discussed with the parents, and child if he or she is old enough to be included. There must be a full understanding of the goals to be achieved. Therapists are an integral part of the team considering a surgical decision. It is within the therapist's abilities and skills to document function, know the child's needs, and understand the parent's concerns.

PREOPERATIVE AND POSTOPERATIVE THERAPEUTIC MANAGEMENT

I. Radial club hand
   A. For patients with type I and type II deformities (mild radial deficiencies and stable wrist), serial splinting, and stretching exercises are indicated to help centralize wrist over ulna and to achieve functional elbow flexion.[1] Correction should be maintained with splinting until skeletal maturity[3] (Fig. 45-3).
   B. For some patients with severe type II, as well as types III and IV, surgical correction may be necessary.
      1. Splinting and stretching exercises may be helpful, but not curative preoperatively.
      2. Functional elbow flexion (70 to 90 degrees) should be achieved through stretching exercises and/or splinting.
   C. Pollicization may be indicated in the case of absent thumbs, and a tendon transfer may be necessary in the case of hypoplastic

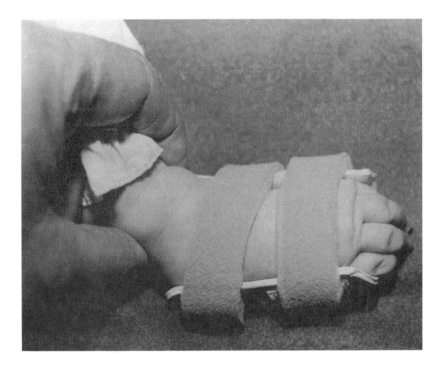

Fig. 45-3. Splinting to assist with correction of radial club hand.

thumb; in either case, postoperative splinting may be required for protective immobilization.

II. Brachial plexus birth palsy

    A. Instruction in ROM and stretching exercises to maintain good passive ROM in all joints in involved upper extremity. Incorporate age-appropriate play activities. (Teach home program to parents. Exercises can be performed at diaper change or bath time.)

    B. Monitor return of muscle function.

    C. A static wrist cock-up splint may be helpful if wrist and finger flexors overpower extensors.

    D. Sensibility testing may be indicated.

    E. Appropriate postoperative management for patients who may undergo nerve grafting, nerve repair, tendon transfers, etc. (Refer to Chs. 6 and 25.)

III. Camptodactyly (flexion deformity of PIP joint, more commonly in little finger)

    A. Nonoperative

       1. Splinting PIP in extension may be indicated in mild to moderate deformities (less than 40 degrees of contracture).[3]

       2. Splinting will not be effective in patients whose cause of contracture is a dynamic muscle imbalance, but may help in cases where lateral bands are malpositioned.[1]

       3. Splints are worn day and night and may need to be continued until skeletal maturity.

    B. Operative

       1. Static splinting is helpful preoperatively to stretch secondary soft tissue contractures, particularly effective with contractures of 40 to 60 degrees (less effective in 60 to 90 degree contractures).[1]

       2. Postoperative splinting in extension is necessary for 3 to 4 weeks, then continued at night for several months.

       3. Patient may require exercises for PIP flexion and extension, postoperatively.

IV. Clinodactyly (curvature of finger in a radioulnar plane, more commonly in little finger).

    A. Conservative management of splinting is not effective in decreasing the progressive angulation of the finger.[1]

    B. Splinting is useful preoperatively to stretch secondary soft tissue deformities on concave side of deviated finger.[3]

    C. Splinting is useful postoperatively to maintain stretched position of soft tissues while corrected bone deformity heals.[3]

V. Clasped thumb (extreme flexion and adduction of thumb into palm).

    A. Splint thumb in abduction and extension in group I patients (those with deficient extension only), who are seen early (before 2 years of age).[1]

    B. Splinting should continue for 3 months. If spontaneous extension is noted at that time, continue for 3 more months to protect the weak extensors from overpowering flexor forces.[2]

    C. Conservative management is effective in two-thirds of these cases if treated early in life before contractures develop.[1]

VI. Miscellaneous surgical procedures: pollicization, tendon transfers, toe-to-thumb, toe phalangeal grafts for short fingers, amputation of extra digits, and web-widening.

    A. Apply appropriate postoperative splint for protection.

    B. Very young patients usually do not require formal therapy postoperatively.

    C. Older children and adults may need exercises and retraining for pollicization, tendon transfers, and toe-to-thumb procedures.

INDICATIONS FOR PEDIATRIC PROSTHETIC USE

Neal B. Zimmerman

Children with transverse deficiencies may be candidates for prosthetic fitting. Longitudinal deficiencies are less suitable for prosthetic usage and are usually better managed by surgical methods.

The most common patient fit for a prosthesis has a transverse terminal deficiency in the proximal to middle third of the forearm. More proximal deficiencies up to the level of shoulder disarticulation can benefit from prosthetic use.

Despite functional gains with prosthetic wear, all patients who have a prosthesis do not choose to make use of it. The prosthesis covers the sensate skin of the residual limb, which some patients view as a deterrent. The longer the residual limb and more retained function, the less likely the child will accept the use of a prosthetic device. For example, the least likely group to accept prosthesis for long-term use is the child with a terminal deficiency at the level of the carpus. A discussion of prosthetic fitting and training is beyond the scope of this book. The reader is referred to several listed works on the subject.

REFERENCES

1. Flatt AE: The Care of Congenital Hand Anomalies. 2nd. Ed. Quality Medical Publishing, St. Louis, 1994
2. Dobyns JH, Wood VE, Bayne LG: Congenital hand deformities. p. 251. In Green DP (ed): Operative Hand Surgery. 3rd. Ed. Churchill Livingstone, New York, 1993
3. Bayne LG: Radial deficiencies. p. 185. In Carter PR (ed): Reconstruction of the Child's Hand. Lea & Febiger, Philadelphia, 1991
4. Carter PR: Brachial plexus birth palsy. p. 49. In Carter PR (ed): Reconstruction of the Child's Hand. Lea & Febiger, Philadelphia, 1991
5. Erhardt RP: Erhardt Developmental Prehension Assessment (EDPA). Therapy Skill Builders, Tucson, 1989
6. Skerik SK, Weiss MW, Flatt AE: Functional evaluation of congenital hand anomalies. Part I. Am J Occup Ther 25:98, 1971
7. Weiss MW, Flatt AE: Functional evaluation of the congenitally anomalous hand. Part II. Am J Occup Ther 25:139, 1971

SUGGESTED READINGS

Byron PM: Splinting of the hand of a child. p. 1443. In Hunter JM, Mackin EJ, Callahan AD (eds): Rehabilitation of the Hand: Surgery and Therapy. 4th. Ed. Mosby, St. Louis, 1995

Cooney WP: Camptodactyly and clinodactyly. p. 209. In Carter PR (ed): Reconstruction of the Child's Hand. Lea & Febiger, Philadelphia, 1991

Dobyns JH: Management of congenital hand anomalies. p. 1425. In Hunter JM, Mackin EJ, Callahan AD (eds): Rehabilitation of the Hand: Surgery and Therapy. 4th. Ed. Mosby, St. Louis, 1995

Gould JS: Syndactyly. p. 128. In Carter PR (ed): Reconstruction of the Child's Hand. Lea & Febiger, Philadelphia, 1991

Jennings JF et al: Reduction osteotomy for triphalangeal thumb: an 11-year review. J Hand Surg 17A:8, 1992

McFarlane RM, Classon DA, Parte AM et al: The anatomy and treatment of camptodactyly of the small finger. J Hand Surg 17A:35, 1992

Radocha RF, Netscher D, Kleinert ME: Toe phalangeal grafts in congenital hand anomalies. J Hand Surg 18A:833, 1993

Scherzer AL, Tscharnuter I: Early Diagnosis and Therapy in Cerebral Palsy. Marcel Dekker, New York, 1982

Slaton DS: Development of Movement in Infancy. Division of P.T., University of North Carolina, Chapel Hill, 1980

Smith RJ: Symposium on congenital deformities of the hand. Hand Clin 1:373, 1985

Sommerkamp TG, Ezaki M, Carter PR, Hentz VR: The pulp plasty: a composite graft for complete syndactyly fingertip separations. J Hand Surg 17A:15, 1992

Swanson AB: A classification for congenital limb malformations. J Hand Surg 1:8, 1976

Watanabe K, Nakamura R, Miura T: Palmar dermatoglyphics in congenital hand anomalies. J Hand Surg 19A:961, 1994

SUGGESTED READINGS FOR PROSTHETIC USE

Bowker JH, Michael JW (eds): Atlas of Limb Prosthetics: Surgical, Prosthetic, and Rehabilitation Principles, 2nd Ed. Mosby, St. Louis, 1992

Wenner SM: Prosthetic management of the upper limb-deficient child. In Hunter JM, Schneider LH, Callahan AD et al (eds): Rehabilitation of the Hand, Surgery, and Therapy. 3rd. Ed. Mosby, St. Louis, 1990

Appendix 45-1

General Classification of Congenital Differences[1]

I. Group I: Failure of formation of parts (arrest of development).
   A. Transverse deficiencies—appear as amputation-type stumps and classified by naming the bony level at which remaining limb terminates.
   B. Longitudinal deficiencies—all failure of formation deficiencies other than the transverse type. Includes failure of formation of radial components (radial club hand), central components (cleft hand deformity), or ulnar components (ulnar club hand). Also includes proximal and distal phocomelias, where proximal and/or distal segments of the arm are missing, and hand may be attached directly to the trunk. (Intercalated defects.)

II. Group II: Failure of differentiation (separation) of parts.
   A. Basic units have developed but the final form is not complete. Syndactyly of the digits, where fingers have failed to separate, is the most common deformity in this category. Also, camptodactyly (flexion contracture of the proximal interphalangeal joint) and clinodactyly (lateral deviation of the digits) are common examples resulting from failure of differentiation of muscles, ligaments, and capsular structures.

III. Group III: Duplication.
   A. Duplication of parts results from insult to the limb bud at early stages of development, so that splitting of the original embryonic part results. Defects range from polydactyly (a common congenital anomaly), to mirror hands (very rarely seen).

IV. Group IV: Overgrowth (gigantism or macrodactyly).
   A. Overgrowth is the pathologic enlargement of skeletal and soft tissues, and may affect the whole limb or parts of the limb, such as the digits.[9] It is very rare.

V. Group V: Undergrowth (hypoplasia).
   A. Hypoplasia results from defective or incomplete development of parts. This can occur in parts of the extremity or the entire extremity. Hypoplasia is most commonly seen in the thumb.[9]

VI. Group VI: Congenital constriction ring syndrome.
   A. These are circumferential constriction bands occurring around the finger, or more proximally. A majority believe they are caused by amniotic bands and that this disorder is nongenetic. Many require early surgery, especially in cases with vascular compromise. Club feet, cleft lip, and cleft palate are common associated anomalies.

VII. Group VII: Generalized skeletal abnormalities.
   A. Defects in the hand may be manifestations of generalized skeletal defects such as Marfan's syndrome, dwarfism, and Madelung's deformity.

Appendix 45-2

Development of Prehension

Developmental Levels		Pattern Components	Grasp of the Dowel (Supine, Prone, or Sitting)

Left	Right			L	R	

10 months — **3-Jawed Chuck Grasp:** Object held with thumb and 2 fingers

9 months — **Wrists** extended

8 months — **Radial-Digital Grasp:** Object held with opposed thumb and fingertips, space visible between

7 months — **Radial-Palmar Grasp:** Object held with fingers and opposed thumb
Wrists straight

5 months — **Palmar Grasp:** Object held with fingers and adducted thumb

4 months — **Primitive Squeeze Grasp:** Contact results in hand pulling object back to squeeze precariously against other hand or body, no thumb involvement

3 months — Sustained voluntary grasp possible if object placed into ulnar side of hand, no thumb involvement
Wrists flexed

— No voluntary grasp, reflexive only

Natal

(From Erhardt,[5] with permission.)

393

Appendix 45-2 (continued)

Sample Evaluation To Record
Grasp Patterns

	Right	Left	Comments
Hook Grip:			
Metacarpophalangeal joints flexed			
Metacarpophalangeal joints extended			
Power Grip:			
Thumb abducted			
Thumb adducted			
Lateral Pinch:			
Standard			
Tip Pinch:			
Standard			
Palmar Pinch:			
Standard			
Cylindrical			
Spherical			
Disc			
Total score			

Scoring:

    0— Patient cannot grasp object

    1— Patient completes grasp in manner of his own adaptation

    2— Patient completes grasp in prescribed manner

General comments:

_____

_____

_____

_____

(From Weiss and Flatt,[7] with permission.)

Conservative Treatment of Arthritis

46

Paige E. Kurtz

Conservative treatment of arthritis can be beneficial for patients in both earlier and more advanced stages to decrease pain and inflammation while increasing range of motion, joint stability, and functional use of the hand and upper extremity. A comprehensive program may include education in disease process and joint protection, use of adaptive equipment and techniques, energy conservation, range of motion (ROM)/exercise program, pain-reducing modalities, and splinting. Conservative management of arthritis may give patients enhanced control over their disease and symptoms, decreasing incidence of deforming and destabilizing forces on joints, and increasing functional use of the hands when incorporated into activities of daily living (ADL).

DEFINITION

Arthritis is characterized by destruction of joint surfaces resulting in pain, stiffness, and inflammation in joints. This may be secondary to either inflammatory processes, as seen in rheumatoid arthritis (RA), or degenerative changes of overuse or trauma, as seen in osteoarthritis (OA).

TREATMENT GOALS

I. Conservative arthritis management program should achieve the following:
   A. Decrease pain and inflammation.
   B. Decrease destabilizing forces on joints.
   C. Increase ROM.
   D. Increase function.

PURPOSE OF CONSERVATIVE ARTHRITIS MANAGEMENT/TREATMENT

Provide a nonsurgical option in treatment to decrease pain and other symptoms while increasing functional use of the involved extremity.

INDICATIONS/PRECAUTIONS FOR THERAPY

 I. Indications
  A. Rheumatoid, osteoarthritis or other forms of arthritis affecting/limiting lifestyle.
  B. Early or later stage arthritis.
  C. Principles of conservative management may also be applied at any point postoperatively to maximize benefits of surgery.
 II. Precautions
  A. Patient compliance and motivation are necessary, with an understanding of rationale for treatment, and the ability to follow through with home program.
  B. Some interventions should be limited if active inflammatory process is present.

CONSERVATIVE MANAGEMENT AND TREATMENT OF ARTHRITIS

 I. Evaluation: a variety of evaluations are available to the therapist. A thorough evaluation should include the following:
  A. History of problem, including onset, history of flares and remissions, medications, and other past treatment interventions.
  B. Joints affected, considering the entire body, with emphasis on the hands, pain levels, and fluctuations.
  C. Range of motion measurements, either detailed or a screening; strength and dexterity.
  D. ADL/functional evaluation: It is important to identify areas where function is limited due to arthritis, as functional improvement is one of the primary goals of conservative management.
   1. Consider common bilateral and daily activities including:
    a. Cooking and eating (e.g., cutting food and serving, stirring, opening jars and cans).
    b. Dressing (e.g., buttoning, tying shoes, managing zippers).
    c. Self-care (e.g., grooming, brushing teeth, hair care, makeup application, toileting, bathing).
    d. Other ADLs (e.g., writing, driving, opening doors, using a key, fastening seatbelt).
    e. Leisure activities (e.g., sewing, reading, gardening).

2. Consider whether the individual is modifying the way in which an activity is performed (awkwardly, or with abnormal motions, or using incorrect postures). It may be helpful to use a functional test to observe the hands in use to note substitution patterns, awkward positions, or other problems.
3. Consider whether an increase in pain accompanies performance of an activity.
4. Consider whether it takes longer than the normal to complete an activity.

II. Splinting

Appropriate splints can help to immobilize and rest a joint to decrease pain and inflammation. Splints protect from destabilizing forces on joints and promote proper positioning and alignment. The therapist should consider the patient's needs with regard to splinting, as well as probable use and wear circumstances. This may affect choice of materials used, and whether a prefabricated or custom-molded splint is more appropriate. Functional use and potential compliance should also be considered, as splints are helpful only if they are used.

A. Rheumatoid arthritis
   1. Antideviation (Fig. 46-1)
   2. Swan-neck (see Fig. 16-3)
   3. Resting (see Fig. 40-3)
B. Osteoarthritis
   1. Carpometacarpal (CMC) support (Fig. 46-2)
   2. Thumb spica (see Fig. 43-2)

III. Patient education

Patients are often more compliant with home programs if education is provided in lay terms about their arthritis, including disease process, effect on joints, and how it progresses. A variety of publications are available for patient education from sources such as the American Occupational Therapy Association and the Arthritis Foundation.

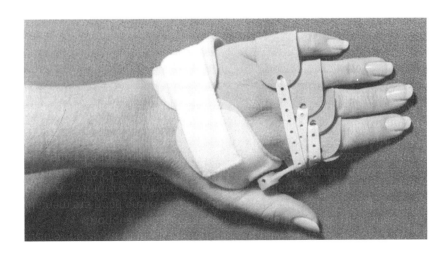

Fig. 46-1. Rolyan hand-based arthritis splint.

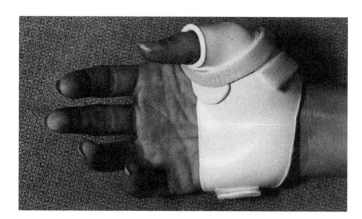

Fig. 46-2. Thumb carpometa-carpal (CMC) splint.

IV. Joint protection

Principles of joint protection should be taught as part of a comprehensive conservative arthritis management program.

A. Respect pain: This is not always noted during an activity; therefore, it is important to develop an awareness of pain with consideration of any activities completed during the previous 12 to 24 hours. Any pain that lingers more than 2 hours after completion of an activity should be considered a warning that the activity should be modified or eliminated.

B. Use larger/strong joints and muscles when able: Protect the more delicate joints of the hands by using larger, more proximal muscles and joints to perform ADLs. For example, using the forearm or shoulder to push open a door protects the fingers. Groceries should be carried in paper bags, with the hip and arm supporting the bag's weight, rather than stressing finger joints by carrying plastic bags with a hook grasp.

C. Avoid tight or prolonged grasp: Build up handles on utensils, tools, and pens. Modify handles with levers. Use adaptive equipment for assistance opening jars, turning knobs, turning keys, and so forth. Change grasp as often as able to avoid static positioning.

D. Avoid positions of deformity: In RA, this often means uses of the hands that push the fingers ulnarly, such as wringing a washcloth or opening jar lids. With OA, stress to the unstable CMC joint is often a problem, and static pinching should be avoided. Good body mechanics should be taught and encouraged.

E. Avoid remaining in one position for a long period of time. This can increase joint pain, strain, and instability. Stop, take a break, and move around as often as possible, preferably every 20 minutes.

F. Balance rest and activity. Plan ahead so rest breaks can be scheduled. Do not start activities that cannot be stopped if needed. Use energy conservation techniques and labor-saving devices. (See sections VII and VIII. Use stress-management and relaxation techniques. Stress, rest, and sleep can have a significant effect on symptoms.

V. Pain management: Modalities should be utilized in the clinical setting and incorporated into a home program.

 A. Heat increases circulation and decreases joint stiffness. It may include application of paraffin, moist heat packs, fluidotherapy, or warm water soaks. Caution: inflammation may be exacerbated by heat if used inappropriately. Make certain clear parameters are explained with regard to appropriate temperatures and application times before adding to a home program. Heat should be used cautiously when significant inflammation or swelling is present.

 B. Cold is best used for reducing pain when there is acute inflammation. For example, during a "flare" or after "overdoing it," particularly if joints feel warm to the touch.

 C. Contrast baths help to "pump" out swelling and pain and are soothing to joints. Techniques and protocols vary, but all alternate between warm and cold water soaks.

VI. ROM and exercise

 Daily use of the hands generally provides more than enough "exercise." The key is to maximize the pain-free arc of active and active-assisted ROM in joints without overstressing them. Appropriate ROM and strengthening exercises should be taught, practiced in the clinical setting, and included in a home program. In addition, low impact exercise benefits the entire body by increasing general health and well-being, as well as strengthening muscles, helping to stabilize joints.

VII. Energy conservation

 Basic principles should be incorporated into patient education. These include sitting when able, planning ahead (gathering needed items together before starting an activity), organizing workspace and storage for accessibility, keeping most commonly used items within easy access, resting during activities as able, and using timesavers such as prepared foods.

VIII. Adaptive equipment and techniques

 These go "hand in hand" with joint protection techniques. Many different catalogs offer equipment, and many stores now carry items such as modified cooking, writing, or cutting utensils. Problem ADLs identified during evaluation should be discussed. Changes in techniques may be suggested and tried out, and use of modified equipment should be practiced in the clinical setting whenever possible. Patients are often resistant to use of adaptive devices, seeing them as a crutch, rather than as an enabler that would increase independence. Sometimes trial use of an item helps an individual see its positive side. Examples of commonly available adaptive equipment include zipper pulls, enlarged handle knives and other utensils, large grip pens, jar openers, and key holder/turner.

SUGGESTED READINGS

Fries J: Arthritis: A Complete Guide to Understanding Your Arthritis. 3rd. Ed. Addison-Wesley, Reading, MA, 1990

Leonard JB: Joint protection for inflammatory disorders. p. 1377. In Hunter JM, Mackin EJ, Callahan AD (eds): Rehabilitation of the Hand: Surgery and Therapy. 4th Ed. Mosby, St. Louis, 1995

Lorig K, Fries J: The Arthritis Helpbook. 3rd. Ed. Addison-Wesley, Reading, MA, 1990

Meenan RF, Mason JH, Anderson JJ et al: AIMS2: the content and properties of the revised and expanded arthritis impact measurement scales health status questionnaire. Arthritis Rheum 35:1, 1992

Melvin JL: Osteoarthritis: Caring for Your Hands. The American Occupational Therapy Association, Bethesda, MD, 1995

Moskowitz R: Osteoarthritis. Arthritis Foundation, Atlanta, 1990

Ouellette EA: The rheumatoid hand: orthotics as preventative. Semin Arthritis Rheum 21:65, 1991

Palmieri TJ, Grand FM, Hay EL et al: Treatment of osteoarthritis in the hand and wrist: nonoperative treatment. Hand Clin 3:371, 1987

Philips CA: Therapist's management of patients with rheumatoid arthritis. p. 1345. In Hunter JM, Mackin EJ, Callahan AD (eds): Rehabilitation of the Hand: Surgery and Therapy. 4th Ed. Mosby, St. Louis, 1995

Pinals R, Zvaifler N: Rheumatoid Arthritis. Arthritis Foundation, Atlanta, 1990

Semble EL: Rheumatoid arthritis: new approaches for its evaluation and management. Arch Phys Med Rehabil 76:190, 1995

Slonaker D, Feinberg J, Holsten D: Taking Care: Protecting Your Joints and Saving Energy. Arthritis Foundation, Atlanta, 1986

Sutej PG, Handler NM: Current principles of rehabilitation for patients with rheumatoid arthritis. Clin Orthop 265:116, 1991

FURTHER INFORMATION

Arthritis Foundation, 1314 Spring Street NW, Atlanta, GA 30309, (800) 283-7800 Offers educational information, programs, and publications. Local chapters may be found in the phone book.

Overuse Injuries of the Upper Extremity in Musicians

47

Jennifer Stephens
Sharon Leilich

Within the last 20 years, information about injuries in performing artists has burgeoned in the literature. The field of performing arts medicine has begun to recognize the unique nature of performance-related injuries in musicians. A survey of more than 2000 symphony orchestra musicians revealed that 76 percent of this population had experienced a problem that affected their performance.[1] The same survey showed that problems differed significantly depending on the instrument (string, brass, woodwind, or percussion), size of the instrument, and gender of the player.[1] This chapter provides the clinician unfamiliar with injuries observed in musicians with a brief overview of common problems, evaluation guidelines, and treatment techniques.

DEFINITION AND GRADES OF INJURIES

When a musician presents with vague complaints of pain that cannot be isolated to a specific tissue or diagnosis, the injury is often categorized as an overuse syndrome. These injuries result when a biological tissue (e.g., muscle, bone, tendon, ligament) is stressed beyond its physiologic limit.[2] Also included under the umbrella of overuse injuries are specific diagnoses such as lateral epicondylitis, De Quervain's syndrome or tenosynovitis, carpal tunnel syndrome, thoracic outlet syndrome (TOS), neuritis, and bursitis.

Various grading scales have been reported in the literature to help classify the irritability of the musician's symptoms. The scale proposed by Fry is broken down into five grades:[3]

Grade I: There is pain in one site while playing. The location and presence of the pain is consistent. Pain ceases when playing stops.

Grade II: Pain is in multiple sites while playing. Other physical findings are vague and transient. Pain does not interfere with
activities of daily living (ADLs).

Grade III: Pain is present in multiple sites while playing. Pain persists
away from the instrument. Pain interferes with other ADLs.
Weakness may be present.

Grade IV: All uses of the hand elicit pain but ADLs may be performed.

Grade V: Loss of hand function secondary to pain and/or weakness.[2]

PREDISPOSING FACTORS FOR OVERUSE INJURIES IN MUSICIANS

I. The following list highlights a few specific factors that may predis-
pose a musician to overuse injuries.

A. Sudden increase in practice time: This often relates to preparation for concerts, recitals, juries, and other performances. Onset
of pain may coincide with attendance at special courses where
a disproportionate amount of playing occurs with respect to the
musician's baseline playing time or with efforts to master technically challenging phrases.[3]

B. Change in instructor: A change in an instructor usually equates
with a change in pedagogy, repertoire, and/or technique. If
such changes are not incorporated gradually, pain may result.

C. Multiple instruments or a change in instrument: Musicians frequently play more than one instrument. Pain that occurs when
playing a primary instrument may actually be the result of playing a secondary instrument or vice versa. Pain syndromes can
also develop when a different instrument is purchased or substituted. Subtle differences in key positions or an increase in the
instrument's weight can change loading demands on muscle
and connective tissue, causing less conditioned tissues to be
overloaded. Injuries may also result from playing on different
instruments, such as pianists encounter when on tour. (It
requires greater force to produce the same musical result on a
piano with stiff keys.)

D. Poorly conditioned muscles: Most athletes know that muscle
strength, flexibility, and endurance play a role in preventing
injuries. Some authors have compared the musician to the athlete as both professions require agility, speed, and neuromuscular coordination.[4] Properly conditioned muscles will be better
able to meet the demand of strenuous rehearsals and performances. Bilateral upper extremity and cervical flexibility and
muscle endurance decrease the chances of static muscle imbalances and minimize the chances of fatigue-related injuries. Digital flexibility will prevent injuries that result from overstretching to reach keys and higher string positions.

E. Poor practice habits: Each practice session should include a
warm-up, rest periods, and a cool down. Soft tissue can be
injured during practice if the warm-up period is inadequate or

absent. At least 5 to 10 minutes of rest every 45 minutes to an hour is suggested. The onset of muscle soreness or pain may be delayed and not appear until 24 to 48 hours after exertion. Therefore, using discomfort, pain, or fatigue as a gauge for incorporating rest periods is not recommended. A cool-down after strenuous playing is advised.

F. Poor technique: To date, most musicians agree that their instrument has no universally accepted proper technique. In fact, developing one's own style and innovative technique may allow virtuoso playing, giving the competitive edge necessary to succeed in today's music world. If these techniques violate proper ergonomic principles and muscle balance, however, they may be detrimental in the long run.

G. Poor posture and muscle imbalances: Repetitive postural deviations such as forward head can result in muscle imbalances. The compression forces of the upper posterior cervical spine increase, and the muscles of the upper posterior cervical spine shorten while the lower posterior muscles and connective tissue lengthen.

H. Previous injury: In a survey of 468 musicians, Dawson[5] found that 51 percent had a traumatic injury which then caused them pain when playing their instruments. Regardless of the origin of the injury, inadequate rehabilitation of a previous injury can result in pain while playing.

I. Aggravating ADLs: The clinician needs to be aware of other activities that the instrumentalist participates in besides those related to music. Job-related activities (filing, typing), sports (golf, tennis), or hobbies (gardening, needlework) may create, exacerbate, or perpetuate pain experienced while playing an instrument.

J. Gender: Data from various studies suggest that there is a higher prevalence of overuse injuries in female musicians as compared to male musicians.[1,6,7]

K. Practice or rehearsal environment: Factors such as insufficient lighting, ambient temperature, and seating within an ensemble can contribute to painful overuse conditions. Poor lighting may cause one to tense his or her muscles while squinting and protracting the head to see the music. Cold or drafty rooms can cause muscles to tighten. The seating arrangement in an ensemble may lead to muscle asymmetries as the musician rotates to see the conductor or to avoid contact with other instrumentalists on crowded stages or in small orchestra pits.

EVALUATION OF THE MUSICIAN

I. Subjective evaluation

The goals of the subjective evaluation should be to obtain an understanding of the musician's practice and playing habits, the location and nature of his or her pain, the irritability of the pain symptoms, previous medical interventions, and his or her general fitness and health. The subjective examination is only as revealing as the clinician's understanding of the significance of the musician's responses to the questions posed. A knowledge of the predisposing factors to injury can assist the clinician in gaining pertinent information.

Typically, musicians are good historians. They often recall the circumstances when they first noted symptoms. A chronologic history of a musician's symptoms may provide clues to the cause of the injury. A self-administered questionnaire can be a time-effective and helpful way to obtain this information (see Appendix 47-1).

II. Physical examination without the instrument

This examination resembles other musculoskeletal examinations. The musician's posture should be observed in sitting and standing, from the front, back, and side, looking at muscle contour for signs of atrophy or hypertrophy. The clinician should observe if there are static muscle imbalances such as forward head, rounded shoulders, reversed curvature of the cervical spine, or an excessive unilateral elevation of the shoulder girdle. Stretch weakness, from poor sitting posture, is often found in scapula adductors with compensatory shortening of the pectoral muscles.[2]

It is also important to look for dynamic muscle imbalances and substitution patterns during movement.[8] Some examples are unequal scapular abduction with shoulder flexion, winging of the scapula with shoulder motion, shoulder girdle motion with neck rotation, and shoulder internal rotation with pronation of the wrist.

Special tests for the cervical spine should be performed to rule out nerve root compression. Tests such as the foraminal compression test, cervical distraction test, vertebral artery test, and cervical quadrant test are all indicated.[9] If peripheral, spinal, or nerve root compression is suspected, sensory testing is indicated.

The examination should include active and passive range of motion (AROM and PROM) of the trunk, cervical spine, and upper extremities. The clinician should look for limitations and/or excessive amounts of joint motion, noting any pain with AROM, PROM, or with over pressure. Joint laxity, or benign hypermobility, may enhance technical performance, but it is more often the reason a musician develops pain in the hand or arm.[10–12]

Manual muscle testing to detect strength deficits in the upper quadrant should be performed. Muscles often overlooked in this examination include muscles of the back, abdomen, cervical spine, shoulder girdle, and the intrinsic muscles of the hand. Special tests to detect shortened muscles, especially for the pectoralis major and minor, latissimus dorsi, scalene muscles, and hand intrinsics, are important to perform.

Musicians may present with specific diagnoses, such as De Quervain's syndrome or tenosynovitis, lateral epicondylitis, medial epicondylitis, TOS, carpal tunnel syndrome, or cubital tunnel syndrome, which are addressed in other chapters of this book. Please refer to the appropriate chapters for evaluation and treatment guidelines for these conditions.

III. Physical examination with the instrument

When evaluating the musician with his or her instrument, the clinician must keep in mind the basic principles of ergonomics and biomechanics. Whether the musician is seated or standing, the clinician should assess the musician's posture to ensure an appropriate base of support and proper vertebral alignment.

It is important to note if joints are in positions which increase pressure on peripheral nerves (i.e., excessive wrist flexion or extension or consistent elbow flexion beyond 90 degrees). The proximal stabilizers (abdominals, paraspinals, rhomboids, latissimus dorsi, serratus anterior, trapezius) should be balanced to allow the arms to move with grace and ease.[13] Additionally, the clinician should observe whether there is excessive tension in muscle groups, for this can lead to premature muscle fatigue.

Musicians who play larger instruments, such as the tuba or string bass, should be evaluated on their technique of transporting the instrument. Heavy cases carried by a handle or a shoulder strap traction the arm, which can aggravate or initiate TOS and other peripheral nerve irritations. Luggage carts or wheeled cases can be used to minimize loading on the upper extremity.

It is important to assess the practice or rehearsal set-up. Playing in an ensemble often requires some spinal rotation to see both the music and the conductor. The clinician should note whether the head position is excessively forward or tilted to one side, as is often the case with the "chin instruments" (violin, viola) and the flute. These postures cause asymmetric loading of the paraspinal and cervical muscles, which can then become painful over time.

The instrument should appear to be an extension of the player; the player should not have to contort himself or herself to fit the instrument.

INSTRUMENT-SPECIFIC PROBLEMS

I. The literature on performing arts medicine reveals that injuries to musicians can be related to the type of instrument played. The prevalence of pain syndromes is significantly higher in string and keyboard players as compared to woodwind, brass, or percussion players.[1,14] It is helpful for the clinician unfamiliar with injuries in instrumentalists to be aware of instrument-specific problems.

A. String instruments

Shoulder problems are common in string players. Three potential injuries are impingement syndrome, subacromial/subdeltoid bursitis, and bicipital tendinitis.[15] Cellists, violinists, violists, and bass players are at risk for developing bicipital tendinitis in their right arm because of the repetitive elbow and shoulder action required for bowing.

Classical guitar players are prone to problems in their right shoulder because of the upper extremity posture needed to clear the edge of the guitar. This posture combined with the picking and strumming action of the fingers can lead to a shoulder injury. Guitar players often position their left wrist in extreme flexion. This position, combined with repetitive digital flexion, makes the left hand susceptible to carpal tunnel syndrome. Repositioning of the instrument to minimize extremes of wrist flexion may help alleviate symptoms. Guitar supports are available that stabilize the guitar on the thigh at an angle that enables proper finger positioning in the left hand with minimal wrist flexion.

Violinists, violists, and cellists may develop cubital tunnel syndrome in either arm. The left arm is more frequently involved because of the sustained position of elbow flexion necessary to reach the fingering board.[15,16] These musicians are also prone to myofascial pain and pain secondary to muscle imbalance. The head and neck are flexed, laterally bent, and rotated with the shoulder elevated to support the instrument. Sustaining this posture (for potentially hours) can lead to muscle pain from active, latent, or chronic trigger points in the shoulder girdle and/or neck musculature.

Harpists usually play with their arms abducted and wrists extended. This position can be taxing to the rotator cuff muscles and increase pressure in the carpal tunnel. Additionally, this instrument requires an enormous amount of tuning. If a small tuning device is used, greater muscle forces are required. Larger, ergonomic tuners can reduce stresses to the hand and should be recommended.

B. Keyboard instruments

Keyboard players are prone to a wide variety of pain syndromes. These include muscle imbalances, myofascial pain, and all the specific diagnoses listed under the umbrella of overuse. For example, De Quervain's syndrome may result from the thumb crossing under the other digits to reach a desired key. Lateral and/or medial epicondylitis may be attributed to techniques using excessive wrist motion. Trigger points are often located in the upper trapezius muscles and levator scapulae from tension and "hunching" the shoulders while playing. Pain from poor body mechanics and/or posture may result from a piano bench that is the improper height or incorrectly positioned. A keyboard player with relatively small hands or limited interdigital web space may experience pain from straining to achieve an octave or more with one hand.

Focal dystonia (often referred to as occupational cramp) is most frequently reported in pianists.[17] It is characterized by impairment or loss of motor control. The condition is often task specific, manifesting as involuntary flexion or extension of the fingers that only occurs while playing the instrument. The etiology and pathology of focal dystonia remains an enigma, and the disorder continues to be frustrating for the clinician and musician. Despite a plethora of proposed treatments, none have been consistently effective.

C. Wind instruments

Flutists are prone to upper quadrant myofascial pain and/or shoulder problems because of the way in which the instrument is designed to be held. One option for positioning the flute is with the head and neck laterally flexed to the right and the right shoulder relaxed, but this positioning can lead to cervical problems. The flutist may elect to keep the head vertical, but this requires static shoulder abduction, which can then lead to tendinitis, impingement syndromes, or pain from chronic trigger points. Flutists are also susceptible to radial digital nerve compression at the base of the left index finger because this area serves as a counterbalance to support the instrument. Piccolo players are subject to cubital tunnel syndrome in either arm because the small size of the instrument requires both elbows to be held in extreme flexion.

Clarinet, oboe, and English horn players may suffer metacarpal joint pain in the right thumb because a large portion of the instrument's weight is supported by the thumb, distal to the interphalangeal joint. Double reed instrumentalists, such as bassoonists and oboists, may develop lateral epicondylitis, sometimes referred to as a *reed-maker's elbow*, from making reeds. Finishing a reed requires holding the reed firmly on a mandrel in one hand, while carefully shaving excess cane from the reed with a knife in the other. The repetitive ulnar deviation and extension of the wrist can lead to tendinitis.

D. Percussion

When percussion instruments are played, rapid deceleration of the forearm muscles occurs on impact with the drumhead, which then causes absorption of vibration forces by muscle and tendon of the forearm. With repetition, inflammation of the connective tissue may result. Percussionists are prone to develop tendinitis of the wrist flexors and extensors, tendinitis of the first dorsal interossei, medial or lateral epicondylitis, and rotator cuff injuries.[18–20] Drummers in rock bands may have pathology of the cervical spine if head thrashing is part of their style.

E. Brass

The majority of problems experienced by brass players relate to the embouchure or the temporomandibular joint.

TREATMENT

I. Goals

Treatment of musicians must be individualized based on the clinical findings of the evaluation. A primary goal of treatment is to identify and reduce unnecessary muscle tension used when playing the instrument. Some examples include pressing more firmly on the keys or strings when playing forte (loud), "tensing up" on difficult, technically challenging passages, and holding the instrument more tightly than necessary. It is also necessary to identify and correct unnecessary tension used in activities of daily living (ADLs), such as carrying objects, driving, and writing.

Musicians will often use coping mechanisms such as refingerings, changes in technique, or changes in repertoire to avoid pain. It is the role of the clinician to identify coping mechanisms used by the musician to avoid pain, to uncover the underlying cause of the pain, and to educate and assist the musician in rectifying the source of the problem.

II. Absolute and relative rest

Most experts agree that rest is the initial treatment of choice.[16,17,21–23] Whether a period of relative rest, meaning a decrease in practice/performance time and elimination of certain aggravating ADLs, or a period of absolute rest is indicated is based on the grade of the injury. Those classified with grade IV and V injuries may initially require absolute rest and immobilization. Musicians advised of relative rest should understand that with the first sign of pain or paresthesia, the aggravating activity should be ceased. It is also important to emphasize that other hand-intensive ADLs, such as gardening, computer work, or needle crafts, should be avoided during the resting phase of treatment. Overuse pain is not something that should be "worked through." The "no pain, no gain" philosophy has no role in the rehabilitation of injured musicians.

III. Exercise programs

Exercise programs should be specific and structured. The clinician must take the time to properly instruct what to feel and expect with stretching and strengthening exercises. Stretching exercises should provide a gentle stretch, not pain. Any discomfort following an exercise program should last no more than 20 to 30 minutes. Pain lasting longer than this is a sign that the exercise was too aggressive. Musicians tend to be very motivated and may be overzealous with exercises. Without appropriate guidelines, an exercise prescription may do more harm than good.

As discussed in Predisposing Factors for Overuse Injuries, the role of proper posture, with and without the instrument, should be addressed. Repositioning of a music stand or seat may be needed to encourage a balanced, neutral posture. If a balanced position cannot be obtained, the musician should be instructed to stretch away from this static posture every 15 minutes while playing and frequently during the day. Some examples of instrument-specific stretches are left lateral bending of the cervical spine for flutists, right lateral bending of the cervical spine for chin instruments, and pectoralis major stretch for cello, oboe, and clarinet players. Muscle imbalances as a result of poor posture can be addressed with range of motion and strengthening exercises.

IV. Role of modalities

As in other cases of acute and chronic tendinitis, bursitis, and nerve compressions, modalities such as ice, heat, phonophoresis, iontophoresis, and electrical stimulation may be indicated for pain reduction.

Biofeedback can be used to help the musician decrease muscle tension with specific tasks and while at rest. When the resting state has improved, the musician should be asked to play, keeping the feedback signal as quiet as possible.

Video analysis can provide visual feedback to the performer. The clinician and musician together can use slow motion videography to look for areas of tension, poor posture, and questionable technique. Sequential videos provide a source of documentation and comparison. In the absence of expensive equipment, mirrors may be an alternative for visual cueing.

Aligning the body properly relieves tension and results in more efficient patterns of movement. The Alexander technique and Feldenkreis are designed to show individuals how their bodies are misused and how to correct detrimental postural and movement patterns. A description of these techniques is beyond the scope of physical and occupational therapy practice; they are best learned from a certified instructor.

V. Patient education

Education of the musician regarding good practice habits and physical fitness can minimize the chance of recurrent injury. A regular warm-up program away from the instrument and on the instrument should be implemented to slowly stretch and warm the muscles before playing. A 5 to 10 minute break should be scheduled every 45 minutes to an hour. This is a must during individual practice time. During ensemble breaks, the musician should put the instrument down, get up, walk around, stretch, and relax. This should be a break from upper extremity use, not time to whittle on a reed or practice a missed passage. If rehearsals do not have scheduled breaks, dangling the arms for a few seconds, resting the instrument in the lap or against the body, and doing gentle finger stretches during measures of rest can help improve circulation to the muscles and alleviate tension.

The musician should be encouraged to have practice time away from the instrument. Individual practice sessions can be taped and reviewed for self-critiquing. Listening to recordings, studying the scores or piano parts, and mentally hearing the way a piece should sound are all methods of enhancing the end performance without touching the instrument. Structured practice sessions with specific goals can maximize the benefits of the session while minimizing the playing time. By preparing well in advance for juries, auditions, rehearsals, and performances, the physical dangers of "cramming" can be avoided.

After an injury, returning to play should be implemented in a scheduled, graduated, progressive manner. The musician should be advised to start with short practice periods and long rest periods. For example, begin with intervals of 5 to 10 minutes of playing and 60 minutes of rest. Keeping a controlled practice schedule will allow both the musician and the clinician to know the irritability and the tolerance level of the involved tissues. The pieces selected should be relatively slow and simple. Warm-up and cool-down exercises must be incorporated. Icing for 15 minutes after practicing can lessen the effects of mild inflammatory responses. With any signs of pain, the duration of play should be lessened.

One of the most important tools for instrumentalists is knowing what to do if their symptoms should return. Most important, they should not ignore pain. The instrumentalist should be instructed to immediately stop playing, try icing the area to control the inflammatory response, rest, and analyze why the problem returned.

VI. Role of splints

Two categories of splints are used in the treatment of injuries in musicians. The first category includes splints to support the instrument and alleviate pain caused by excessive strain on a joint or soft tissue. Some examples include a modified carpometacarpal splint on the right hand of a clarinet, oboe, or English horn player; custom formed chin rests for violin and viola players; and for the flutist, the use of an orthotic device to evenly distribute the pressure on the base of the left index finger. Various commercially available neck straps and posts can be used to support woodwind instruments.

Limitations of these devices include cost, appearance, and acceptance by both the musician and their colleagues. For aesthetic and/or personal reasons, the instrumentalists may be resistant to using these devices during performances; however, even if they are only used for practice, they may be helpful in symptom control.

The second category of splints are those commonly used to treat tendinitis, nerve compression, and other inflammatory conditions. Splints in this category include wrist splints, thumb spica splints, and long arm splints. These splints should be used judiciously, primarily during the acute and, perhaps, the subacute stage of injury. The longer the splints are used, the greater the risk of developing joint stiffness and muscle weakness as a result of disuse. As pain symptoms decrease, splint wear should be gradually weaned with simultaneous incorporation of a progressive strengthening and flexibility program.

VII. Ergonomics of instruments

Instruments were not designed with upper extremity ergonomics in mind. One of the best methods to reduce the risk of overuse injury for a musician is to fit the instrument to their hands and body by modifying the instrument. Instrument manufacturers can be contacted for instrument modification. Examples of ergonomic alterations include extending specific keys on the flute, clarinet, saxophone, or oboe; angling the head joint of a flute 30 degrees, beveling the top right portion of the classical guitar, and reshaping the right edge of the viola or violin. Limitations of these alterations include cost, appearance, and acceptance by both the musician and his or her colleagues.

REFERENCES

1. Middlestadt SE, Fishbein M: The prevalence of severe musculoskeletal problems among male and female symphony orchestra string players. Med Probl Perform Art 41:41, 1989

2. Norris R: The Musician's Survival Manual: A Guide to Preventing and Treating Injuries in Instrumentalists. ed Torch. International Conference of Symphony and Opera Musicians, 1993

3. Newmark J, Lederman RJ: Practice doesn't necessarily make perfect: incidence of overuse syndromes in amateur instrumentalists. Med Probl Perform Art 2:142, 1987

4. Quarrier NF: Performing art medicine: the musical athlete. J. Orthop Sports Phys Ther 17:90, 1993

5. Dawson WJ: Hand and upper extremity injuries in instrumentalists: epidemiology and outcome. Med Probl Perform Art 3:19, 1988

6. Fishbein M, Middlestadt SE, Ottati V et al: Medical problems among ICSOM musicians: overview of a national survey. Med Probl Perform Art 3:1, 1988

7. Roamaryn LM: Upper extremity disorders in performing artists. Maryland Med J 42:255, 1993

8. Kendall FP, McCreary EK: Muscles: Testing and Function. 3rd Ed. Williams & Wilkins, Baltimore, 1983

9. Magee DJ: Cervical spine. p. 21. In Magee DJ: Orthopedic Physical Assessment. W.B. Saunders, Philadelphia, 1987

10. Brandfonbrener AG: Joint laxity in instrumental musicians. Med Probl Perform Art 5:117, 1990

11. Brandfonbrener AG: Joint laxity: help or hinderance? (Editorial). Med Probl Perform Art 9:1, 1994

12. Bird HA, Wright V: Traumatic synovitis in a classical guitarist: a study in joint laxity. Ann Rheum Dis 40:73, 1989

13. Tubiana R, Champagne P, Brockman R: Fundamental positions for instrumental musicians. Med Probl Perform Arts 4:73, 1989

14. Newmark J, Hochberg FH: "Doctor, it hurts when I play": painful disorders among instrumental musicians. Med Probl Perform Arts 2:93, 1987

15. Hoppman RA, Patrone NA: Musculoskeletal problems in instrumental musicians. p. 71. In Sataloff RT, Brandfonbrener AG, Lederman RJ (eds): Textbook of Performing Arts Medicine. Raven Press, New York, 1991

16. Amadio PC, Russotti GM: Evaluation and treatment of hand and wrist disorders in musicians. Hand Clin 6:405, 1990

17. Hoppman RA, Patrone NA: A review of musculoskeletal problems in instrumental musicians. Semin Arthritis Rheum 19:117, 1989

18. Judkins J: The impact of impact: the percussionist's shoulder. Med Probl Perform Art 6:69, 1991

19. Judkins J: A performance application for rehabilitating the rotator cuff in the percussionist. Med Probl Perform Art 7:83, 1992

20. Chong J, Lynden M, Harvey D et al: Occupational health problems of musicians. Can Fam Physician 35:2341, 1989

21. Lederman RJ, Calabrese LH: Overuse syndromes in instrumentalists. Med Probl Perform Art 1:7, 1986

22. Fry JH: The treatment of overuse injury syndrome. Maryland Med J 42:277, 1993

23. Hochberg FH: The upper extremity difficulties of musicians. p. 1197. In Hunter J, Schneider LH, Mackin EJ, Callahan AD (eds): Rehabilitation of the Hand. Mosby, Philadelphia, 1990

Appendix 47-1

Evaluation of Musicians

Name:_____ **Sex:**_____ **Age:**_____

What instrument(s) do you play?

How many years have you been playing each instrument?

How long do you play your instrument daily? (Specify for each instrument)
How many hours are personal practice, rehearsals, and performance?

Have you had a change in your practice, playing, or performance time recently?

Do you have a warm-up routine?

If yes, how long is this routine? Is it with your instrument, without your instrument, or both?

How often do you rest when practicing?

Have you changed teachers recently? Have you changed your playing technique recently?

Have you consulted other musicians concerning your condition or possible technique changes to decrease your symptoms?

In your own words, describe your problem and what you believe to be the cause.

How long has your problem been going on?

When do you have pain? How long can you play pain free?

What do you do to decrease or alleviate your pain?

Do your symptoms increase with arpeggios, scales, trills, or other patterns?

Do you practice technical passages slowly, in small segments, in short time intervals?

Do you tend to practice the same passage over and over until you get it right, no matter how long it takes?

What are you working towards musically at this time?

Do you exercise regularly? (Run, swim, aerobics . . .)

Do you have any other significant health problems?

Do you have a previous history of trauma to your arms, neck, or back?

Have you had any special tests performed? (MRI, EMG, NCV, bone scan, radiographs)

PLEASE CHECK ALL OF THE FOLLOWING THAT APPLY TO YOU:

I have been diagnosed with:

____ Tendinitis ____ Overuse syndrome ____ Fibromyalgia

____ Carpal tunnel syndrome ____ Ulnar nerve compression

____ Thoracic outlet syndrome (TOS)

____ No diagnoses have been made ____ Other

I have had prior therapy including:

____ Non-steroidal anti-inflammatory medications

____ Steroids: oral or injection

____ Splinting ____ TENS ____ Ultrasound

____ Electrical stimulation ____ Acupuncture ____ Chiropractic

____ Moist heat ____ Ice ____ Biofeedback

____ Massage ____ Iontophoresis ____ Phonophoresis

____ Alexander technique ____ Feldenkreis

____ Ergonomic assessment ____ Strengthening/stretching

____ Other ____ NO previous therapy

PLEASE CHECK ANY OF THE FOLLOWING SYMPTOMS THAT YOU EXPERIENCE:

____ Pain ____ Fatigue ____ Swelling

____ Redness ____ Stiffness ____ Pins and needles

____ Weakness ____ Cramping ____ Loss of muscle control

____ Curling of fingers uncontrollably ____ Other: please explain

PLEASE CIRCLE THE SENTENCE THAT MOST ACCURATELY DESCRIBES YOUR PRESENT CONDITION:

1. I have pain in one site while playing. The location and presence of the pain are relatively consistent, but the pain stops very soon after I stop playing.
2. I have pain in multiple sites while playing. The locations of these pains are consistent. The pain stops shortly after I stop playing, and I can perform other activities without pain.
3. I have pain in multiple sites while playing that persists after playing. It now interferes with *some* of my other daily activities.
4. I have pain in multiple sites while playing that persists after playing. It now interferes with *all* of my other daily activities.
5. My hand or arm is now so painful that I cannot use it for anything.

Industrial Rehabilitation Services

48

Donna M. Keegan
Lynne F. Murphy

Hand or upper extremity injuries, including those suffered on the job, can affect that patient's ability to return to work, even at the conclusion of traditional medical treatment and hand rehabilitation. With this in mind, industrial rehabilitation services were developed in the 1970s. During the next decade, focus on these services shifted from dealing with work injuries only from a psychosocial or behavioral model (termed *work adjustment*) to assessment of an injured worker's physical abilities and limitations in the work setting, or what has become known as *industrial rehabilitation*.

Occupational and physical therapists became involved in this field previously addressed primarily by vocational evaluators. These professionals assisted to define functional capacity evaluation and work hardening services. Ideally, these services are best provided by a team of professionals with experience in the vocational, medical, and psychological arenas. By 1989, the Commission on Accreditation of Rehabilitation Facilities (CARF) established specific standards for the practice of work hardening programs.

DEFINITION/TIMELINE

"The Functional Capacity Evaluation Process consists of evaluation procedures, questionnaires, and observations, which document the patient's ability to perform work from a physical, medical, behavioral, and ergonomic perspective... This process will help to determine if that worker can return to work safely."[1] The Functional Capacity Evaluation should take place over at least two client visits to accurately evaluate the client's response to testing and to reduce the cumulative effects of fatigue or pain. Ideally, both sessions should be scheduled so that the evaluation can be completed within 1 week, to more closely simulate work demands. Finally, it should be concluded with a team meeting to formulate appropriate goals and recommendations.

Functional Capacity Evaluation, or a thorough baseline evaluation, is used to determine activities and goal of work hardening. "Work hardening provides a transition between the management of the initial injury and return to work while addressing the issues of productivity, safety, physical tolerances, and work behaviors. Work hardening programs use real or simulated work activities in a relevant work environment in conjunction with physical conditioning tasks. These activities are used to progressively improve the biomechanical, neuromuscular, cardiovascular/metabolic, behavioral, attitudinal, and vocational functioning of the person served."[2] Generally, work hardening is a daily program of either half-day or full-day sessions (up to 8 hours a day) of work simulation, conditioning, and education. The program lasts for an average of 4 weeks, with adjustment as necessary to meet the client's specific goals.

PURPOSE/GOALS

  I. Functional capacity evaluation
     A. Assess the injured worker's abilities and limitations related to work or job demands.
     B. Clarify job demands and vocational status.
     C. Compare current performance of work simulations to required job demands.
     D. Evaluate consistency of effort and pain behaviors as they affect work performance.
     E. Assess work-related behaviors.
     F. Determine whether further services are needed (including work hardening) and provide a thorough baseline for subsequent treatment.
 II. Work hardening
     A. Facilitate gradual, progressive improvement in physical skills and work tolerances.
     B. Physical conditioning and endurance training.
     C. Provide psychosocial preparation for return to work, and identify any related barriers to work performance.
     D. Ensure safety in the workplace, and provide education in topics such as proper body mechanics and injury prevention.

ADMISSION CRITERIA

In general, patients eligible for industrial rehabilitation services should meet the following admission criteria: have physical limitation(s) that may affect job performance or work potential, be medically stable, have a primary diagnosis of musculoskeletal injury, and have written referral or clearance from a physician. To participate in work hardening, the patient should also meet the following criteria: have completed a baseline evaluation or Functional Capacity Evaluation, which documents the probable benefit from a work hardening program, and have a vocational goal or job target. Industrial rehabilitation services are generally initiated when a client has reached maximum benefit from more traditional types of occupational and/or physical therapy. In addition, industrial rehabilitation services are usually covered through worker's compensation insurance carriers, rather than general health insurance companies.

EVALUATION AND TREATMENT GUIDELINES

I. Functional capacity evaluation
  A. Vocational specialist
    1. Interview injured worker/client.
       a. Work history
       b. Educational background
       c. Current employer information
       d. Current source of income
       e. Behavioral and attitudinal status
       f. Cognitive status
       g. Detailed information about job demands and requirements
       h. Social status
    2. Contact client's employer.
       a. Confirm job demands.
       b. Clarify employment status, and/or schedule a job site analysis.
       c. Resolve any return to work issues.
    3. Obtain and review job description with client.
       a. Dictionary of Occupational Titles (DOT)[3]
       b. Client report
       c. Employer's verbal and/or written job descriptions
  B. Exercise physiologist
    1. Assess client's current cardiovascular status.
    2. Determine current fitness level.
    3. Communicate any contraindications for return to work or further participation in Evaluation/Work Hardening program
  C. Occupational/physical therapist
    1. Interview injured worker/client.
       a. History of current injury
       b. Past medical history
       c. Client report of functional abilities/limitations
       d. All current subjective information from client as it relates to injury
    2. Evaluate client's functional abilities/limitations.
       a. Volumetric or circumferential measurement (edema).

      b. Musculoskeletal evaluation, as applicable to client's injury and function.
        1. Range of motion
        2. Manual muscle testing
        3. Sensation
        4. Gross and fine coordination
        5. Grip/pinch strength
        6. Posture, gait, flexibility, balance
      c. Maximum voluntary effort lifting, carrying, pushing and pulling.
      d. Determination of physical demand level and endurance for materials handling.
      e. Consistency of effort using several measures.
      f. Tolerance to working positions.
      g. Work simulations related to specific job demands.
    3. Arrange and facilitate team meeting.
    4. Communicate results and recommendations.
  D. Psychologist
    1. Review client questionnaires related to injury adjustment.
    2. Determine need for psychological services.
    3. Perform initial assessment if warranted.
    4. Refer to social worker if appropriate.
  E. Interdisciplinary team
    1. Attend team meeting to communicate results and develop recommendations.
    2. Contribute to Functional Capacity Evaluation report.
    3. Foster client communication and determine need for treatment.
    4. Develop goals and formulate time frames for intervention.
II. Work hardening
  A. Vocational specialist
    1. Prepare list of job demands specific to job targeted.
    2. May perform job analysis.
    3. May perform transferable skills assessment.
    4. Conduct educational lectures regarding return to work issues.
    5. May assist with resume preparation and job seeking skills.
    6. Act as liaison between employer and team.
  B. Exercise physiologist
    1. Design and implement strengthening/conditioning programs.
    2. Conduct group and/or individual education pertinent to health and fitness.
    3. Supervise clients while performing strengthening/conditioning exercises.
    4. Provide home fitness programs.
  C. Occupational/physical therapist
    1. Act as case manager for work hardening team.
      a. Design individualized treatment plan, including work simulation activities (Fig. 48-1).

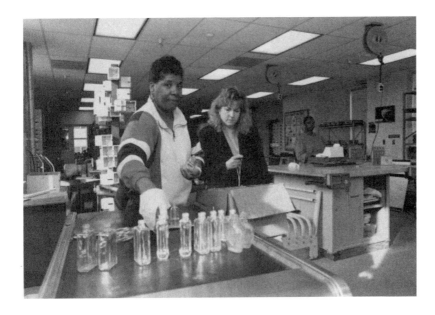

Fig. 48-1. Work simulation.

    b. Orient client to work hardening activities.
    c. Promote client participation in program.
    d. Set short-term and long-term goals.
    e. Consider/implement recommendations of other team members regarding service provision.
    f. Consistently reevaluate client progress.
    g. Complete weekly progress reports.
    h. Communicate with physician, referral source, and all relevant external and internal team members.
    i. Arrange and facilitate team meetings.
    j. Facilitate discharge planning.
    k. Modify treatment plan as needed.
        1. Ensure work simulations are appropriate and progressive during entirety of program.
        2. Ensure conditioning/strengthening activities are appropriate.
  2. Teaches and reinforces proper body mechanics.
  3. Conducts group and/or individual education on pertinent topics.
  4. Makes recommendations for job/tool modifications or any adaptive equipment.
  5. May perform job site analysis or ergonomic consultation.
D. Psychologist
  1. Conduct weekly coping/educational sessions.
  2. Counsel clients individually when necessary.
E. Interdisciplinary team
  1. Participate in weekly client updates, and provide input as needed throughout program to ensure comprehensive client care.

2. Foster client participation in program and client self-advocacy skills.
3. Attend biweekly team meetings with client to assist in discharge planning.
4. Determine appropriate discharge goals and final client disposition/recommendations.
5. Participate in program evaluation and continuous operation improvement activities.

REFERENCES

1. Blankenship K: Industrial Rehabilitation I. American Therapeutics, Inc., Macon, GA, 1990
2. Standards Manual and Interpretive Guidelines for Organizations Serving People with Disabilities. Commission on Accreditation of Rehabilitation Facilities, Tucson, 1994
3. Dictionary of Occupational Titles, 4th Ed. US Department of Labor, Washington, DC, 1991

SUGGESTED READINGS

Bear-Lehman J: Factors affecting return to work after hand injury. Am J Occup Ther 37:189, 1983

Benner C, Schilling A, Klein L: Coordinated teamwork in California industrial rehabilitation. J Hand Surg 12A:936, 1987

Blumenthal S: Vocational rehabilitation with the industrially injured worker. J Hand Surg 12A:926, 1987

Chaffin DB, Andersson GBJ: Occupational Biomechanics. John Wiley & Sons, New York, 1984

Demers L: Work Hardening: A Practical Guide. Andover Medical Publishers, Boston, 1992

Ellexson M: The impact of CARF standards on the practice of work hardening. Work Fall:69, 1990

Good Practice Manual for the Rehabilitation of the Injured Worker. Maryland Rehabilitation Association, Baltimore, 1987

Herbin M: Work capacity evaluation for occupational hand injuries. J Hand Surg 12A:958, 1987

Isernhagen S: Work Injury Management and Prevention. Aspen Publishers, Rockville, MD, 1988

Kuhn M, Kneidel T: Is work hardening effective. Industrial Rehabil Qu 3:1, 1990

Matheson L, Ogden LD, Violette K, Schultz K: Work hardening: occupational therapy in industrial rehabilitation. Am J Occup Ther 39:314, 1985

May V: Work hardening and work capacity evaluation: definition and process. Vocational Evaluation and Work Adjustment Bulletin Summer:61, 1988

Ogden-Niemeyer L, Jacobs K: Work Hardening State of the Art. Slack I, Thorofare, NJ, 1989

Schultz-Johnson K: Assessment of upper extremity-injured persons' return to work potential. J Hand Surg 12A:950, 1987

Social Work Services

49

Ann Leman-Domenici

The clinical skills and services of a social worker have been an integral part of the interdisciplinary treatment offered to hand injured patients.

The social work role in this ambulatory, rehabilitative setting is a consultative one to staff, physicians, patients, and families. The primary focus is to explore the patients' and families' emotional reaction to the hand injury; what the injury means to them in terms of loss and change in their lives, and how they have typically coped with change in the past. It is important to be supportive and challenge the patient and family to use some of those beneficial skills in the present situation. Also, the social worker asks the patient and family to clarify their understanding and expectations of treatment. According to Richard K. Johnson:

> The assessment also might involve exploration of how the injured person is handling grief. The person's sense of grief flows from the experience of loss, a loss of the use of one's hand; if only temporary is significant. The loss triggers not only apprehensions over the future functioning of the hand but also the loss of employment, income and self-image as a productive, contributing person in a company or a family, if only a short while. The stages of grief involving denial, depression and anger are important aspects to be assessed.'[1]

Many psychosocial factors can be triggered as a result of a trauma or injury, including issues of body image, sexuality, and self-identity; physical activity and preinjury recreational/leisure time activities; changes in fulfilling social and familial roles; and responsibilities and employment issues.

The stated message in a psychosocial assessment is that the treatment team wants to learn the best way of treating the whole injured worker so that there will be a successful recovery and rehabilitation. The hand patient requires understanding, empathy, support, and education in establishing realistic goals.

421

The psychosocial support for the hand injured patient should begin as soon as possible following the injury. To accomplish this, in our facility, both Clinical Social Work services and Behavioural Medicine consultations are available to hospitalized hand injured patients. Social Work services are available to patients and families in the outpatient, ambulatory setting during clinic visits, hand therapy, and work hardening programs, both at the hospital and the satellite sites off campus.

It is vitally important for the patient and family to be able to tell their story, the facts of the injury and their feelings associated with those facts to someone on the team.

In the recent past, we used a self-report, screening questionnaire to assist the hand therapists early in treatment to identify patients who could benefit from social work referrals and intervention. This mechanism for identification had dwindled and has become extinct due in part to many other productivity expectations for the hand therapists and myself and the ever changing requirements of managed care payors. Despite such constraints, the hand therapists I work with are knowledgeable and skilled at making early, timely, and appropriate referrals on behalf of their clients.

DEFINITION

Referrals for social work services are typically received from physicians, hand therapists, work rehabilitation therapists, rehabilitation nurses, and family members through direct referrals.

    I. Important indicators for referral include:
       A. Adjustment to injury issues.
       B. Alcohol/drug abuse and/or recovery issues.
       C. Anxiety
       D. Depression
       E. Specific diagnoses
          1. Reflex sympathetic dystrophy (RSD) syndrome.
          2. Traumatic upper extremity amputation.
          3. Chronic pain
          4. Conversion reactions
          5. Factitious disorder
          6. Post-traumatic Stress Disorder (PTSD).
       F. Family problems
       G. Financial issues
       H. High stressors
       I. Lack of social supports.
       J. Marital problems
       K. Previous psychiatric treatment.
       L. Pharmacy assistance/prescriptions.
       M. Transportation to treatment issues.

ASSESSMENT

The social worker will complete a comprehensive written psychosocial assessment, including the following information:

    I. The presenting problem as perceived by the patient.
    II. Insurance coverage (Workers Compensation claim, Medicare, medical assistance, self-pay, commercial insurance), financial and legal status.
    III. Understanding of diagnosis, cause of symptoms, and expectations of treatment.
    IV. Patient's support network, family composition, family/marital status.
    V. Education and/or level of literacy, work history, current job, length of employment, job satisfaction.
    VI. Current affective and cognitive functioning.
    VII. Stressors and emotional state/symptoms of depression.
    VIII. Current medications.
    IX. Alcohol/drug usage.
    X. Activities of daily living (ADL): What is a typical day like?
    XI. Prior mental health treatment.
    XII. Pre-existing/concurrent medical problems.
    XIII. Difficulty with the law.

Once the assessment is complete, the social worker will collaborate with the patient, the hand therapist, the physician, and the rehabilitation specialist to initiate a treatment plan for the patient and to include appropriate plan of action steps and appropriate referrals. This is not a passive process in which the patient is the receiver of the social worker's treatment, but an active process of communication and negotiation to achieve mutual treatment goals.

Additionally, the hand injured patient's spouse or significant other is invited to participate in the sessions. At times a telephone interview is the next best alternative to obtain information and to enlist support toward the recommended plan of treatment. Especially if the recommendation is for a psychiatric evaluation, the spouse or significant other may need assistance also, or couples counseling is recommended.

TREATMENT GOALS

Treatment goals vary depending on the identified and agreed upon problem. Diagnostic indicators for specific problems are presented using the Indicators for Referral list.

    I. Adjustment to injury issues
        A. The treatment goal is to provide information, referral, and emotional support and to advocate on behalf of the patient. Below are a few examples.

1. Basic information on the Workers Compensation system is provided. Patients are redirected back to their representing attorney for specific concerns.
2. Overall orientation to the Hand Center's purpose and philosophy, with clarification of the patient and institution's roles and responsibilities. I encourage patients to take ownership of their care.
3. Information and referral to community resources as appropriate.
   a. Adult literacy and/or GED program to improve skills and to provide a productive, structured activity.
   b. Encourage volunteer employment to reduce boredom, increase activity level, and promote self-esteem.
   c. Referral to the State Division of Rehabilitation Services.
   d. Recommend participation in a senior center for social support and to reduce isolation and symptoms of depression for senior citizens.
   e. Referral to support groups.
   f. Referral to shelters and/or group homes.
   g. Referral to church sponsored programs.

II. Alcohol/drug abuse/addictions (eating, smoking, gambling)

The treatment goal is to identify the problem, educate the patient about the treatment options available, and make a recommendation for treatment to the patient and physician. Also to reinforce and support the program of recovery being used.

A. Documented use (e.g., emergency room) of alcohol/drugs when the injury occurred.
B. Alcohol being used to self-medicate for pain management.
C. Use of prescription narcotics for more than 2 to 3 months after injury and/or surgery.
D. Patient arrives for hand treatment under the influence.
E. Self-identified recovering alcoholic or addict who is working a 12-step program. The stress of the injury and rehabilitation can make the individual high risk for a relapse.
F. Cigarette addiction that is compromising the physical outcome of the hand.
G. Gambling behavior that is interfering with financial resources to engage or follow through with treatment.

III. Anxiety

The treatment goal is to identify the symptoms and provide education and treatment recommendations. Anxiety disorders are treated by a combination of cognitive behavior therapy and medication and usually require a psychiatric evaluation.

A. Phobic disorder: essential feature is the fear of an activity, situation, or object that results in a desire to avoid the same. When the avoidance behavior or fear is a significant source of distress and interferes with social or role functioning, treatment is indicated.
B. Panic disorder: essential feature is sudden onset of intense apprehension, fear, or terror, associated with feelings of impending doom. Symptoms include dyspnea, palpitations, chest pain, dizzi-

ness or unsteady feelings, sweating, faintness, trembling or shaking, hot/cold flashes.

IV. Depression

The treatment goal is to identify the symptoms, educate the patient about available treatment, and make a recommendation for treatment to the patient and physician. Typical treatment involves medication and psychotherapy. Symptoms include:

A. Loss of interest or pleasure in all or almost all usual activities, withdrawal from family and friends.

B. Appetite disturbance, either extreme: increased appetite and weight gain or loss of appetite and weight loss.

C. Sleep disturbance.

D. Concentration difficulties, increased forgetfulness.

E. Suicidal ideation.

V. Specific diagnoses

A. RSD syndrome/chronic pain: treatment goal is to identify symptoms of depression and educate the patient about the benefits of antidepressants in pain management and the symptoms of depression. Also to refer to available RSD support group.

B. Traumatic upper extremity amputation: treatment goal is to identify symptoms of loss, anger, and depression and to provide adjustment to injury counseling. Referrals to the Amputee Association of America is a standard procedure. Psychiatric evaluation is often indicated.

C. PTSD: recognition that the hand patient experienced an event outside the range of usual human experience. The four major characteristics of PTSD:

1. The traumatic event is persistently re-experienced.

2. Recurrent distressing dreams of the event.

3. Sudden acting or feeling as if the traumatic event were recurring (flashback episodes).

4. Persistent avoidance of stimuli associated with the traumatic event.

VI. Conversion reactions

The treatment goal is to identify symptoms and related issues and refer for psychiatric evaluation. The main symptom is a loss or change in physical functioning that suggests a physical disorder but is an expression of a psychological conflict or need. The disturbance is not under the voluntary control of the patient.

VII. Factitious disorder with physical symptoms.

The treatment goal is to identify symptoms and refer for psychiatric evaluation. The essential feature is the presentation of physical symptoms that are not real. An example would be self-inflicted tourniqueting of the upper extremity.

VIII. Family problems

The treatment goal is to identify and educate the patient about available resources.

A. History of physical, sexual, emotional abuse, domestic violence.

B. Bereavement issues when there is a loss of a family member.

C. Child's reaction to a parent's injury.

IX. Financial issues

The treatment goal is to identify the problem and the potential resources and make the necessary referrals.

A. Referral to the Department of Social Services for medical assistance, general public assistance, food stamps, TEMHA (Transitional Emergency Medical Housing Assistance).

B. Referral to the internal mechanisms of the hospital for financial assistance.

X. Stressors are high.

The treatment goal is to identify the stressors and educate the patient in stress management techniques using a cognitive behavioral approach.

A. Progressive muscle relaxation exercises and self-hypnosis.

B. Encourage self-nurturing activities.

C. Affirming positive gains.

XI. Lack of social supports.

The treatment goal is to engage the patient in recognizing the problem and to brainstorm solutions.

A. Encourage and direct the patient to volunteer in some capacity.

B. Encourage the patient to participate in church-related activities.

C. Encourage participation in a support group.

XII. Marital problems

The treatment goal is to identify couples issues as the problem and to refer couples for counseling.

XIII. Previous and/or current psychiatric treatment.

The treatment goal is to obtain the name of the previous or current treating mental health professional and their phone number from the patient. If behavioral changes are observed during the course of hand treatment, contact can be initiated with this resource person.

XIV. Transportation to treatment.

The treatment goal is to facilitate the patient's hand treatment. It may be appropriate to contact the insurance carrier and explain the problem and negotiate a solution.

A. Bus tokens

B. Cab vouchers

SUMMARY

Hand injured patients are just like you or me. We may worry about the past, present, and future; our jobs; our families; the direction and fabric of our lives; and our health and capabilities.

I have experienced the continuum of responses—patients who were initially angry at their physicians for referring them to a social worker and patients who were eternally grateful for the referral. It has always been a privilege for me when another human being willingly or even reluctantly shares thoughts and feelings, fears, frustrations, and sense of loss, in an effort to process individual experience. Social Work services assist the patient and family in this endeavor.

REFERENCE

1. Johnson RK: Psychological evaluation of patients with industrial hand injuries. Occup Injuries 3:567, 1986

SUGGESTED READINGS

Bear-Lehman J: Factors affecting return to work after hand injury. Am J Occup Ther 37:189, 1983

Cone J, Hueston JT: Psychological aspects of hand injury. Med J Aust 1:104, 1974

Grant GH: The hand and the psyche. J Hand Surg 5:417, 1980

Grunert BK, Devine CA, Matloub HS et al: Sexual dysfunction following traumatic hand injury. Ann Plast Surg 1:46, 1988

Grunert BK, Devine CA, McCallum-Burke S et al: On-site work evaluation: desensitizing for avoidance reactions following hand trauma. J Hand Surg 14B:239, 1989

Grunert BK, Matloub HS, Sanger JR, Yousif NJ: Treatment of posttraumatic stress disorder after work related hand trauma. J Hand Surg 15A3:511, 1990

Grunert BK, Smith CJ, Devine CA et al: Early psychological aspects of traumatic hand injury. J Hand Surg (Br) 13B:177, 1988

Hansen F: Psychiatric aspects of the hand patient: their importance in patient assessment. American Physical Therapy Association Hand Section Newsletter I:4, 1983

Lee PWH, Ho ESY, Tsang AKT, Chang JCY: Psychosocial adjustment of victims of occupational hand injuries. Soc Sci Med 20:493, 1985

Louis DS, Lamp M, Greene T: The upper extremity and psychiatric illness. J Hand Surg 10A:687, 1985

Mendelson R, Burech J, Polack EP, Kappel D: The psychological impact of traumatic amputations, a team approach: physicians, therapists and psychologist. Occup Injuries 3:577, 1986

Montague J, Rosner, Stein V: Social work's role in managing chronic pain. Dimens Health Serv 66:23, 1989

Tomlinson WK: Psychiatric complications following severe trauma. J Occup Med 7:454, 1974

Index

Page numbers followed by *t* indicate tables; those followed by *f* indicate figures.